Aging
VOLUME 36

Parkinsonism and Aging

Aging Series

Aging
VOLUME 36

Parkinsonism and Aging

Editors

Donald B. Calne, M.D.

Division of Neurology
University Hospital
Vancouver, B.C., Canada

Donatella Crippa, M.D.

Schering Spa
Segrate
Milan, Italy

Giancarlo Comi, M.D.

Department of Neurology
S. Raffaele Hospital
Milan, Italy

Reinhard Horowski, M.D.

Schering AG
HD Klinische Forschung
Berlin, Federal Republic of Germany

Marco Trabucchi, M.D.

Cattedra di Tossicologia
Universita de Roma
Roma, Italy

Raven Press New York

Raven Press, 1185 Avenue of the Americas, New York, New York 10036

Made in the United States of America

Library of Congress Cataloging-in-Publication Data

Parkinsonism and aging / editors, Donald B. Calne ... [et al.],

        p.   cm. — (Aging : v. 36)
    Proceedings of a symposium held in Milan, Nov. 1987.
    Includes bibliographies and index.
    ISBN 0-88167-502-A
    1. Parkinsonism—Age factors—Congresses. 2. Brain—Aging–
Congresses. I. Calne, Donald B. (Donald Brian) II. Series.
    [DNLM: 1. Aging—congresses. 2. Parkinson Disease—
congresses.
W1 AG342E v. 36 / WL 359 P2472 1987]
RC382.P23 1989
818.8'33—dc19
DNLM/DLC
for Library of Congress   88-36480
                                                 CIP

9 8 7 6 5 4 3 2 1

Preface

Over recent years there has been increasing interest in the argument that Parkinson's disease might result from an early subclinical lesion of the nigrostriatal pathway superimposed on the normal age-related attrition of neurons in the substantia nigra. This volume assembles a range of views both for and against this idea.

The initial two chapters summarized the span between the introduction of levodopa in 1961, and the application of the newest techniques of molecular biology 25 years later. The morphological changes of normal aging and Parkinson's disease were then compared. Neurochemical manifestations of senescence and Parkinson's disease were considered and articles were written on the possible environmental risk factors that might contribute to etiology. In vivo imaging of the brain was reviewed in the elderly and in Parkinson's disease. Other movement disorders of late life were described, and there followed a consideration of therapy for Parkinson's disease, with attention given to both the impact of treatment on symptoms, and the problem of attempting to modify the natural history.

This book is intended for those who have an interest in aging of the nervous system, and in degenerative diseases of the senescent brain. At a time when the large and growing number of the elderly in our society is only just being recognized, it is appropriate to pause and examine the process of normal brain aging, and try to determine the cause of neurodegenerative processes. Athough we need to find better ways of applying our current palliative therapy, of much greater importance is the task of elucidating the causal mechanisms of normal and pathological aging, so that ways might be devised to prevent, or at least slow down the inexorable ravages of time on the central nervous system.

DONALD B. CALNE, M.D.
GIANCARLO COMI, M.D.
DONATELLA CRIPPA, M.D.
REINHARD HOROWSKI, M.D.
MARCO TRABUCCHI, M.D.

Acknowledgment

This volume is based on a symposium held in Milan in November 1987, with the support of Schering A. G.

Contents

Principal Contributors

D. Yves Agid
*INSERM U.289 and Clinique de
Neurologie et Neuropsychologie
Hôpital de la Pitié-Salpêtrière
91, Boulevard de l'Hôpital
F-75634 Paris Cedex 13, France*

Alessandro Agnoli
*I Clinic of Neurology, La Sapienza
University
Viale dell'Università 30
00185 Roma, Italy*

Walther Birkmayer
*LBA Laboratory fuer Bio-Analytic
und MEDINFO Inc.
Schwarzspanierstrasse 15
A-1090 Vienna, Austria*

Donald B. Calne
*Division of Neurology
University Hospital
2211 Wesbrook Mall
Vancouver, B.C., Canada V6T 1W5*

P. J. Delwaide
*University Department of Neurology
Hôpital de la Citadelle
B-4000 Liege, Belgium*

P. C. Emson
*MRC Group
Department of Neuroendocrinology
AFRC Institute of Animal Physiology
and Genetic Research
Cambridge CB2-4AT, England*

Caleb E. Finch
*Andrus Gerontology Center
Department of Biological Sciences
University of Southern California
Los Angeles, California 90089-0191*

Franz Hefti
*Department of Neurology
University of Miami
P.O. Box 016960
Miami, Florida 33101*

Oleh Hornykiewicz
*Institute of Biochemical
Pharmacology
University of Vienna
Borschkegasse 8a
A-1090 Vienna, Austria*

Reinhard Horowski
*Schering AG
HD Klinische Forschung
Postfach 650311 Mullerstrasse 170-
178
D-1000 Berlin 65, F.R.G.*

K. Jellinger
*Ludwig Boltzmann Institute of
Clinical Neurobiology
Lainz-Hospital
1, Wolkersbergenstrasse
A-1130 Vienna, Austria*

Amos D. Korczyn
*Department of Physiology and
Pharmacology
Sackler Faculty of Medicine
Tel-Aviv University
Tel-Aviv 69978, Israel*

J. William Langston
*California Parkinson's Foundation
2444 Moorpark Avenue, Suite 316
San Jose, California 95128*

Klaus L. Leenders
*Paul Scherrer Institute
CH-5234 Villigen, Switzerland*

W. R. Wayne Martin
Division of Neurology
U.B.C. Health Sciences Centre
  Hospital
Vancouver, B.C. Canada V6T 1W5

Reijo J. Marttila
Department of Neurology
University of Turku
SF-20520 Turku, Finland

P. L. McGeer
Kinsmen Laboratory of Neurological
  Research
University of British Columbia
2255 Wesbrook Mall
Vancouver, B.C., Canada V67 1W5

Eldad Melamed
Department of Neurology
Beilinson Medical Center
Petah Tiqva 49 100, Israel

C. W. Olanow
Department of Neurology
University of South Florida
Tampa, Florida 33606

J. M. Rabey
Tel-Aviv Medical Center
Ichilov Hospital
6 Weizman Street
Tel-Aviv 64239, Israel

P. Riederer
Klinische Neurochemie
Universitäts-Nervenklinik
Füchsleinstr. 15
8700 Würzburg, F.R.G.

Urpo K. Rinne
Department of Neurology
University of Turku
SF-20520 Turku, Finland

Robert Schwarcz
Maryland Psychiatric Research
  Center
P.O. Box 21247
Baltimore, Maryland 21228

Peter S. Spencer
Institute of Neurotoxicology
Albert Einstein College of Medicine
1300 Morris Park Avenue
Bronx, New York 10461

Eduardo Tolosa
Department of Neurology
Hospital Clinic I Provincial
University of Barcelona
Villarroel 170, 08036
Barcelona, Spain

Marco Trabucchi
Cattedra di Tossicologia
Università di Roma via O. Raimondo
Torvergata
00173 Roma, Italy

Erik C. Wolters
Belzberg Laboratory of Clinical
  Neuroscience
Department of Medicine
U.B.C. Health Sciences Centre
  Hospital
Vancouver, B.C., Canada V6T 1W5

Dean F. Wong
Division of Nuclear Medicine
Department of Radiology
The Johns Hopkins University School
  of Medicine
Baltimore, Maryland 21205

Parkinsonism and Aging, edited by
Donald B. Calne et al., Raven Press, Ltd.,
New York © 1989.

The L-Dopa Story

Walther Birkmayer and Joerg G. D. Birkmayer

LBA Laboratory fuer Bio-Analytic und MEDINFO Inc., A-1090 Vienna, Austria

The time from the discovery of a biological substance and its action to its clinical application varies considerably. With L-dopa, it took almost 50 years after its detection by Guggenheim in 1913 (1) and its first clinical use in 1961 by Birkmayer (2) for the treatment of patients suffering from Parkinson's disease. Retrospectively, the present therapeutic concept of this neurological movement disorder developed in a five-stage process: stage 1: L-dopa alone; stage 2: L-dopa plus decarboxylase inhibitor; stage 3: L-dopa plus dopamine receptor agonists; stage 4: L-dopa plus monoamine oxidase-B inhibitor; and stage 5: L-dopa plus iron.

STAGE 1: L-DOPA ALONE

The trigger of the clinical application of L-dopa was the observation of Carlsson and co-workers in 1957 (3) that the inhibitory effect of reserpine on the motor activity of rabbits can be antagonized by dopamine. Carlsson realized immediately the possible implication of extrapyramidal diseases (4). This idea gained more relevance when a decreased concentration of dopamine in certain basal ganglia of Parkinson patients was detected (5).

As a logical consequence, L-dopa was applied to Parkinson's patients for the first time by Birkmayer and Hornykiewicz in 1961 (2). The effect was remarkable. A few minutes after intravenous injection of L-dopa, akinetic patients were able to get up and walk around.

The reason for application of L-dopa instead of dopamine is the fact that dopamine cannot pass through the blood–brain barrier, whereas L-dopa can. The latter is rapidly degraded to dopamine by dopa decarboxylase, an almost ubiquitous enzyme. Independent of our very first clinical observations, Barbeau and co-workers reported the positive effect of L-dopa on Parkinson patients (6). They were the first to confirm our discovery.

The fascination with the clinical efficacy of L-dopa was twofold: for the patient, it was the benefit in improving the disability; for the doctor, it was the principle of its action. With a single chemically defined biological sub-

1

stance, it was possible to correct the symptoms of a neurological disease. At that time, this was a unique experience for all neurologists.

STAGE 2: L-DOPA PLUS DECARBOXYLASE INHIBITOR

After a period of enthusiasm, it became clear that the duration of action of L-dopa was very short at 15 to 30 min and thus raised difficulties in its practical therapeutic use. At that time, it was known that the effect of L-dopa is caused by the formation of dopamine by the enzyme dopa decarboxylase. This opinion was derived from the observation that the action of L-dopa can be suppressed by α-methyl-dopa, an inhibitor of dopa decarboxylase. This substance was used quite efficiently in the treatment of chorea syndrome. It can reduce the hyperkinetic movements of these patients. It was in 1965 when Pletscher from Hofmann La Roche (Basel) asked me to test a new substance against anxiety and hypertony. This substance, called benserazide, was claimed to be 100 times more effective as an inhibitor of dopa decarboxylase than α-methyldopa. If this is actually the case, it should be very beneficial to patients with chorea syndrome. When we tested this substance in my hospital in Vienna, it turned out that it worsened the symptoms of chorea. According to my clinical experience, a drug that is beneficial for chorea will harm Parkinson patients and vice versa. I was convinced that benserazide should improve Parkinson symptoms if it harms chorea symptoms. I therefore applied L-dopa together with benserazide to Parkinson patients. The clinical effect was better and longer lasting than that of L-dopa alone (7).

Instead of minutes, the effect lasted half a day. When I reported my clinical observation to the Hofmann La Roche scientists, they accepted it with more than routine skepticism. How could an inhibitor of the decarboxylase, which diminishes dopamine production, improve the Parkinson symptoms, which are caused by a lack of dopamine?

The biochemical explanation for the clinical effect was found by Bartholini and Pletscher (8) in showing that benserazide does not pass the blood–brain barrier. Due to this, it was concluded that only the dopa decarboxylase in the periphery is blocked by benserazide, leading to a higher portion of L-dopa in the brain. On the basis of this higher dopa level, a larger pool of dopamine accumulates, leading to a longer-lasting effect. The combination of L-dopa with benserazide was the beginning of rational therapy for Parkinson's disease. Another decarboxylase inhibitor, carbidopa, showed the same effect as benserazide (9).

STAGE 3: L-DOPA PLUS DOPAMINE RECEPTOR AGONISTS

During these years of dopa research, it became clear that dopamine acts by its transmission via receptors at the postsynaptic membrane, similar to adrenergic receptors, the sensitivity of which changes according to the environment. If only a few transmitter molecules are present in the vicinity of the receptor, its sensitivity becomes very high. The higher the transmitter concentration in the environment of the receptor, the higher its insensitivity. A number of substances have been detected that are able to increase the sensitivity of the dopamine receptors. Bromocryptine, lisuride, and terguride are some of them. It was bromocryptine that was given to Parkinson patients in 1974 by Calne et al. (10). His report looked very promising.

One of the disadvantages of bromocryptine is its induction of hypotension, which is hard for patients to cope with. Fewer side effects have been found with lisuride or terguride, which increased their clinical applicability. On the basis of the present theory, receptors become more sensitive when there is less transmitter present in the vicinity. Due to the dopamine deficit in the brain of Parkinson patients, one would assume hypersensitive postsynaptic dopamine receptors. The question is why should they be stimulated by dopamine agonists. A sensitivity-increasing action would be meaningful only in the case of hyposensitivity. Hyposensitivity may be induced by an overload due to therapy with L-dopa. This implies that a dopamine agonist can act only when L-dopa is given simultaneously. On the other hand, a frequent observation of this combined therapy is hyperkinesia. This argues for a high dose of dopamine administered.

According to our experience, dopamine agonists should be used with some degree of caution. Another drawback of dopamine agonists is stimulation of the presynaptic receptor. The presynaptic, also called autonomous, receptor inhibits the enzyme that forms L-dopa, namely tyrosine hydroxylase. The amount of enzyme is already reduced in the substantia nigra of Parkinson patients. It could be further decreased by dopamine agonists due to their capacity to stimulate the presynaptic receptor. The results of treatment with dopamine agonists turned out to be difficult to predict. In a number of patients they work very well; in others, they appear to be ineffective. Due to the considerable side effects, the therapeutic regimen should be individualized.

STAGE 4: L-DOPA PLUS MAO-B INHIBITORS

The dopamine deficit in Parkinson patients may be corrected by another possibility, namely by inhibition of dopamine degradation. Dopamine is metabolized by monoamine oxidase (MAO). A number of MAO inhibitors have been used for treating depressed patients. They were of little benefit for Parkinson patients. As we know now, they are not selective enough for monoamine oxidase-B (MAO-B), the enzyme that acts on dopamine. In 1974, Knoll et al. (11) reported the development of a substance called L-deprenyl, which was claimed to be a specific MAO-B inhibitor. If this was correct, it should be beneficial for Parkinson patients.

According to a suggestion of my former co-worker Riederer (12), I started to treat patients who developed deterioration after 5 years of L-dopa treatment. The outcome of our clinical studies was the following: One group of patients who suffered from Parkinson's disease for 7 up to 15 years exhibited an average disability of 60% before treatment. They were treated for 2 years with Madopar (L-dopa plus benserazide). An overall improvement of 37% in disability was observed. Seven months after adding L-deprenyl to the treatment, the motor disability decreased further to 23%. The normal motoric disability shows a score of 10.

In summary, L-deprenyl exhibits a remarkable effect on the disability of Parkinson patients, in particular after long-term treatment. When a substance is analyzed for its therapeutic capacity, certain criteria have to be fulfilled: (a) improvement of symptoms, (b) prolongation of life, (c) few side effects, and (d) reduction of fluctuations. L-deprenyl was evaluated according to these criteria.

When the improvement of Parkinson symptoms of patients treated with Madopar was compared with those of patients treated with Madopar and L-deprenyl, the beneficial effect of the latter became obvious. The same holds for the side effects of the combination of Madopar and L-deprenyl. L-Deprenyl acts not only in combination with Madopar but also as a single drug. It improves the symptoms of patients at an early stage of the disease, as reported by Yahr in 1981 (13). On the basis of this observation, a multicenter clinical trial has been started in the United States to prove whether L-deprenyl can prevent the progression of Parkinson's disease (S. Fahn, personal communication).

STAGE 5: L-DOPA PLUS IRON

Until the middle of 1986, the therapeutic concept for treatment of Parkinson's disease was a substitutional one. In other words, the dopamine deficit has been overcome by an exogenous supply of L-dopa and by blocking its degradation in order to achieve a higher dopamine level in the brain. As we know from a number of hormones such as cortisone, exogenous substitution will stop endogenous production. If this feedback control works also in the biosynthetic pathway of L-dopa, it will imply that supplemental therapy with L-dopa will further decrease the already reduced endogenous L-dopa production in Parkinson patients. This seems to be the case in a number of patients for whom L-dopa therapy becomes ineffective even after increasing the dosage.

For these patients, the number of which is increasing due to the prolongation of life expectancy, we have to think of other therapeutic concepts. If substitution does not work, stimulation of endogenous biosynthesis might be another possibility. L-Dopa is synthesized from tyrosine by the enzyme tyrosine hydroxlase. It has been found that the tyrosine hydroxylase activity is considerably reduced in certain brain areas of Parkinson patients (14,15) Obviously, this enzyme plays a central role in Parkinson's disease. Indirect evidence for this fact was obtained in 1969 when we found that administration of α-methyl-P-tyrosine, an inhibitor of tyrosine hydroxylase, leads to a considerable deterioration of the motor activity of Parkinson patients (16).

Tyrosine hydroxylase is an iron-containing enzyme with pteridine as its main cofactor (18). Recently, it has been found that tyrosine hydroxylase can be stimulated *in vitro* up to 20-fold by iron (18). The tyrosine hydroxylase from the brain of Parkinson patients showed the same behavior, although not to that extent. To stimulate endogenous L-dopa biosynthesis in the brain, cofactors have to be added because the protein moiety will not pass through the blood–brain barrier. In the 1970s, we tried to add pteridine as an intravenous infusion to our protocol for treating Parkinson patients. No clinical effect could be observed. The findings of Rausch et al. (18) on the stimulation of tyrosine hydroxylase by iron prompted us to try iron as a medication for Parkinson's disease.

From all of the various pharmaceutically available iron compounds, only one proved to be useful. This was oxyferriscorbone, produced by Theraplix (France). When this substance was given to akinetic Parkinson patients, they became mobile within hours, depending on the route of administration. Intravenous injection improved the disability in less than an hour (19,20). At the beginning of our new therapeutic approach, we started with one ampule of oxyferriscorbone every second day. The dosage was increased gradually to one ampule per day. In severe cases, two ampules were given daily in the form of infusions (20). In patients with improved symptoms, the therapy was discontinued after 4 to 8 weeks. Therapy was restarted when the patient's disability returned. Oxyferriscorbone works with all severities of cases of Parkinson's disease. Slight cases need only one injection every third day; severe cases need two ampules per day. Our present experience with oxyferriscorbone involves more than 200 patients.

We can say that this special iron compound leads to excellent improvement in 20% of the patients and to moderate improvement in 40%. Forty percent do not respond at all to the iron treatment. When the beneficial effect of iron in combination with L-dopa is compared with that of L-dopa alone, retrospectively the following conclusions can be drawn: Iron seems to improve the symptoms more the longer the duration of the disease, whereas the efficacy of L-dopa alone decreases with the duration of the disease.

The biological mechanism of the action of oxyferriscorbone is not yet understood. Oxyferriscorbone itself is a rather peculiar substance. Chemically, it is a complex of ferrous and ferric iron with ascorbic acid. Studies of Riederer et al. (21) indicated that the total iron content of substantia nigra nucleus ruber and some other nuclei in the brainstem of Parkinson patients is comparable to that of normal brain. This would mean that the shortage of tyrosine hydroxylase activity is not caused by the lack of iron. Recent nuclear magnetic resonance investigations, however, revealed that a high percentage of Parkinson patients have a reduced iron content in certain basal ganglia (22). This finding represents a rational explanation for the clinical effect of oxyferriscorbone.

For this iron compound to act directly in the basal ganglia, it has to pass through the blood–brain barrier. Nuclear magnetic resonance studies are in progress to determine whether oxyferriscorbone is able to pass through the blood–brain barrier. The results will provide insights into the biological mechanism of action. The clinical effect, however, has the first priority not only for the patient but also for the doctor treating these patients.

CONCLUSION

According to our experience of more than 25 years, the following conclusions may be drawn: L-dopa is the essential drug for therapy of Parkinson's disease. The other compounds discussed in this review are additives that are more or less effective depending on their route of administration. The goal of an optimized therapy is to use the lowest effective dosage of L-dopa in combination with the various additives. The amount of these different drugs should be carefully selected and adjusted to minimize side effects and to avoid exhaustion of this particular neuronal system. The administration of iron represents a new therapeutic principle that works on the basis of stimulation rather than of supplementation. From the biological point of view, stimulation of synthesis is a better principle than supplementation because the negative feedback regulation caused by the latter, which stops endogenous dopa production, is not induced by stimulation of biosynthesis. Since the first administration of L-dopa in 1961, we have achieved great progress in treating Parkinson patients. Their life expectancy has increased due to new therapeutic aids. We have reached an advanced stage where we have to work with a number of effective additives in order to attain an improvement in the patient's symptoms. Research, however, will continue.

It is the lot of the basic scientist to find additional tools for the activation of the biosynthesis of L-dopa in Parkinson patients. If reduced biosynthesis can be alleviated by certain compounds such as iron, the degenerative process may be prevented. Prevention of a disease is the best and most resonable option. As an optimist, I am convinced that we are on the road to new therapeutic tools for the cure and prevention of this disease.

REFERENCES

1. Guggenheim, M. (1913): *Z. Phys. Chem.*, 228:276–280.
2. Birkmayer, W., and Hornykiewicz, O. (1961): *Klin. Wochenschr.*, 73:787.

3. Carlsson, A., Lindquist, M., and Magnusson, T. (1957): *Nature* (Lond.), 180:1200.
4. Carlsson, A., Lindquist, M., and Magnusson, T. (1958): *Science*, 137:471.
5. Ehringer, H., and Hornykiewicz, O. (1960): *Klin. Wochenschr.*, 72:1236.
6. Barbeau, A., Murphy, C. F., Sourkes, T. L. (1962): In: *Monoamines et systeme nerveux central*, Ajuuriaguerra J, eds. Geneva, Masson, p. 132.
7. Birkmayer, W., and Metasti, M. (1967): *Arch. Psych. Z. Ges. Neurol.*, 210:29.
8. Bartholini, G., Burkhard, W. P., Pletscher, A., et al. (1967): *Nature* (Lond.), 215:852.
9. Cotzias, G. C., VanWoert, M. H., Schiffer, L. M. (1967): *N. Engl. J. Med.*, 276:374.
10. Calne, D. B., Teychenne, P. F., and Leigh, P. M., et al. (1974): *Lancet*, 1355.
11. Knoll, J. (1974): *J. Neural Transm.*, 43:177.
12. Birkmayer, W., and Riederer, P. (1975): *J. Neural Transm.*, 37:95.
13. Yahr, M. D. (1981): In: *Research progress in Parkinson's disease*, F. C. Rose and R. Capildeo. London, Pitman Medical, p. 233.
14. McGeer, P. L., McGeer, E. G., and Wada, J. A. (1971): *J. Neurochem.*, 18:1647.
15. Riederer, P., Birkmayer, W., Rausch, W. D., et al. (1979): In: *CNS and adrenal gland tyrosine hydroxylase and the influence of drug treatment on cAMP-activity in Parkinson's disease—human post mortem studies*. Vienna, LB Institute of Clinical Neurobiology.
16. Birkmayer, W. (1969): *Klin. Wochenschr.*, 81:10.
17. Nagatsu, T., Namaguchi, T., Kato, T., et al. (1981): *Clin. Chim. Acta,* 109:305.
18. Rausch, W. D., Riederer, P., Nagatsu, T., et al. (1987): *J. Neurochem.* (in press).
19. Birkmayer, W., and Birkmayer, J. G. D. (1986): *J. Neural Transm.* 67:287.
20. Birkmayer, J. G. D., and Birkmayer, W. (1987): *Ann. Clin. Lab. Sci.*, 17.
21. Riederer, P., and Jellinger, K. (1985): *Proc. E.N.A.A.*
22. Rutledge, J. N., Hilal, S. K., Silver, A. J., et al. (1987): *AJNR,* 8:397.

Parkinsonism and Aging, edited by
Donald B. Calne et al., Raven Press, Ltd.,
New York © 1989.

Studies on the Chemical Anatomy of the Basal Ganglia in Parkinson's Disease and in Animal Models of Parkinson's Disease

P. C. Emson, S. J. Augood, T. N. Buss, S. Shoham,
*J. Price, †A. R. Crossman, and ‡C. D. Marsden

*MRC Group, Department of Neuroendocrinology, AFRC Institute of Animal
Physiology & Genetics Research, Babraham, Cambridge CB2 4AT; *Laboratory
of Embryogenesis, MRC National Institute of Medical Research, London NW7;
†Experimental Neurology Group, Department of Anatomy, University of
Manchester, Manchester M13 9PT; and ‡Institute of Neurology, National
Hospital, London WC1 3BG, England*

The primary characteristic deficit associated with Parkinson's disease is the loss of the majority of large pigmented neuromelanin-containing neurons of the substantia nigra (1). These large neurons are now known to contain the neurotransmitter dopamine. It is the loss of this dopaminergic input to the caudate nucleus and putamen (striatum) that leads to the characteristic symptoms of Parkinson's disease (hypokinesia/bradykinesia, tremor, and rigidity) (2). Such a depletion of the striatal dopaminergic innervation also leads to a complex series of biochemical changes in this denervated area. In this chapter, we review our recent findings using molecular probes to investigate and compare the neurochemistry of the basal ganglia in normal and "parkinsonian" human brain material, as well as in two established animal models of Parkinson's disease. The animal models were produced by the administration of the neurotoxins, 6-hydroxydopamine (6-OHDA) (3) in the case of the rat and N-methyl-4-phenyl-1,2,3,6-tetrahydropyridine (MPTP) for the primate (4–7).

USE OF MOLECULAR PROBES IN ANATOMICAL STUDIES

The recent development of molecular biological techniques, especially gene cloning, now provides the neurochemist and anatomist with a new selection of analytical tools (complementary deoxyribonucleic acid or complementary ribonucleic acid cDNA/cRNA) with which to investigate the chemistry and organization of the basal ganglia. In our laboratory, we have been concentrating on developing and quantitating techniques of radioactive and nonradioactive *"in situ"* hybridization histochemistry (8,9). Such techniques allow us to visualize the sites of gene expression within the brain. Quantitation of these sites in terms in the amount of hybridized probe signal (either radioactive or color) allows us to follow changes in gene expression (usually neurotransmitter or neuropeptide genes).

In order to localize the cellular sites of expression of a particular messenger ribonucleic acid species (mRNA), we have used either small complementary single-stranded or double-stranded DNA probes, or single-stranded complementary (antisense) RNA probes. Routinely these probes are radiolabeled with ^{35}S to a specific activity of $> 10^8$ dpm/μg DNA or RNA and hybridized to lightly fixed cryostat sections (for details, see ref. 10). Posthybridization, these sections are washed under high stringency conditions (11) and exposed to autoradiography film (Hyperfilm Amersham, or Ultrafilm LKB) together with ^{35}S brain paste standards of known radioactive content. These standards enable a dose–response curve to be plotted so that the degree of darkening of the autoradiography film may be used by an image analyzer to estimate the number of counts present in the relevant sample tissue sections exposed to the same film (Fig. 1). To provide a control for nonspecific binding of labeled DNA/RNA probes to the tissue section, consecutive sections are pretreated with RNase A, which digests all mRNA in the tissue prior to hybridization. The image analyzer can then subtract the nonspecific signal from the total signal to produce an image of the specific binding (Fig. 2). Knowledge of the specific activity of the probe and the section thickness also allows us to calculate the number of copies of mRNA per unit area. However, it should be emphasized that this number can only be a semiquantitative, or relative, figure because there is no way of controlling for the loss of mRNA signal during fixation and section processing prior to autoradiography. The principle advantage of this technique is that it allows visualization of the specific localization of sites of gene expression (as reflected by relative amounts of mRNA) at the cellular level, so that regional or local differences may be detected. Alternative techniques such as Northern blotting (11) provide only a rough estimate (also relative) of the total mRNA content in a tissue homogenate.

APPLICATION OF MOLECULAR PROBES TO STUDIES OF GENE EXPRESSION IN NORMAL AND DENERVATED BASAL GANGLIA

In order to study expression of tyrosine hydroxylase mRNA in the substantia nigra of normal and "parkinsonian" material, we have used a rat tyrosine hydroxylase cRNA probe prepared from a riboprobe vector (pSP65) (12) and a small human cRNA probe synthesized from a DNA sequence

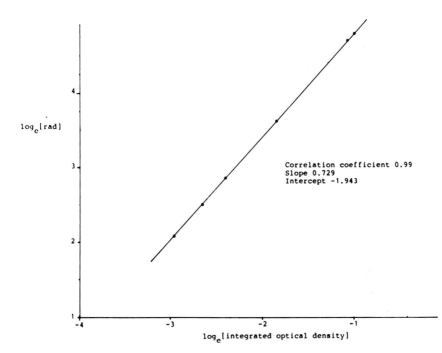

FIG. 1. Standard curve used by the image analyzer to convert degree of film darkening (optical density) into an estimate of counts per unit area. Known amounts of radioactivity (^{35}S) are dissolved in brain paste and sectioned. These standards of known amounts of radioactivity per unit area (determined by scintillation counting) are exposed to autoradiography or X-ray film together with tissue sections.

containing a T7 promoter (HTH-1) (13). Both the rat and human cRNAs demonstrate the presence of tyrosine hydroxylase (the critical enzyme in dopamine synthesis) mRNA within the human substantia nigra pars compacta cells (Fig. 3).

Selective unilateral depletion of the large dopaminergic neurons in the rat substantia nigra may be achieved, as previously mentioned, by a unilateral injection of 6-hydroxydopamine (12 μg free base) into the substantia nigra (Fig. 4) or in the case of the cynomolgus monkey (*Macaca fasicularis*) by a unilateral carotid infusion of MPTP into the brain (6). Such neurotoxin treatment results in an almost complete depletion of the dopamine cells on the injected side, therefore resulting in a corresponding depletion of tyrosine hydroxylase mRNA (Figs. 5 and 6).

Cellular localization of enkephalin gene expression in the primate was investigated using the technique of "*in situ*" hybridization with a ^{35}S-radiolabeled human enkephalin cDNA probe (14). The probe revealed that, as reported by other workers using immunohistochemical techniques (15), the medium-sized spiny enkephalin neurons are grouped together in the matrix

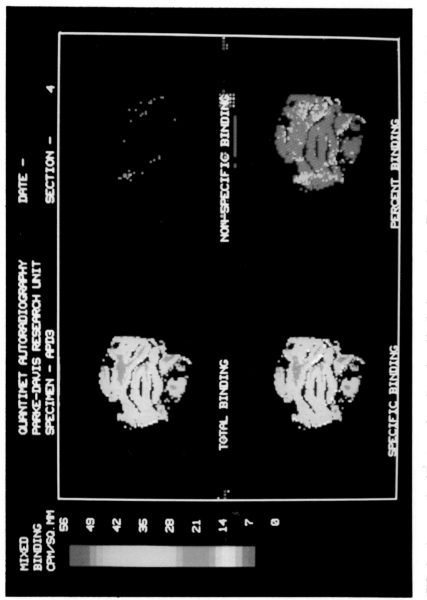

FIG. 2. An example of the type of result produced by the image analyzer. The image analyzer used the standard curve (Fig. 1) to calculate from the autoradiography film the amount of radioactivity localized over a particular part of the film. In this case, a ^{35}S-labeled calcium binding protein cDNA has been hybridized to cerebellum sections. The non-specific binding of the cDNA probe to an adjacent section that has been RNase treated (to digest all cellular mRNA) allows the image analyzer to calculate specific binding. Note the concentration of signal over the molecular layer of the cerebellum.

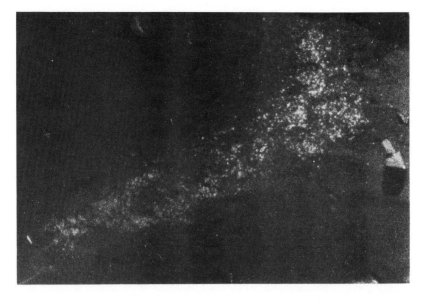

FIG. 3. Localization of tyrosine hydroxylase mRNA in the substantia nigra (pars compacta) of a neurologically normal postmortem human brain. Dark field photograph produced from an X-ray film image ($\times$16.25).

of the striatum. Applying this probe to the denervated primate striatum revealed an increase in enkephalin mRNA content within the neurons, as well as an increase in the number of detectable enkephalin mRNA-positive neurons relative to control tissue (Fig. 7). A similar enkephalin mRNA increase has been reported in the 6-OHDA-treated rat (16), and in this case there is

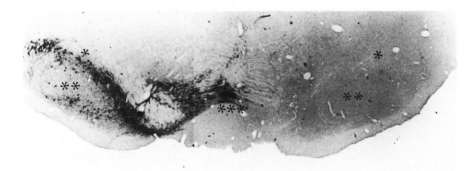

FIG. 4. A montage of the rat substantia nigra to show the effect of a 6-hydroxydopamine injection (12 μg) into the right medial forebrain bundle. Dopamine cells have been visualized using tyrosine hydroxylase antiserum ($\times$32.5). *pars compacta, **pars reticulata, ***ventral tegmental area.

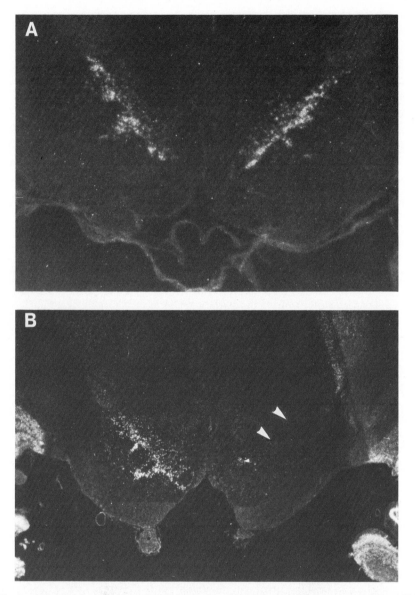

FIG. 5. Effects of a unilateral carotid infusion of MPTP on tyrosine hydroxylase mRNA signal in the monkey substantia nigra. (**A**) Control monkey (no infusion). (**B**) Monkey that received MPTP via the right carotid to produce a unilateral denervation (large arrow heads). Dark field autoradiographs. Note the presence of two or three remaining tyrosine hydroxylase mRNA positive cells (small arrow heads) on the lesioned side (×16.25).

an increase in the amount of enkephalin immunoreactivity in the pallidum (17), suggesting that the additional mRNA is being translated into the neuropeptide product (Fig. 8).

The increase in enkephalin mRNA content within the medium-sized spiny striatal neurons has been quantitated using a Quantimet 720 image analyzer (Cambridge Instruments). The analyzer is initially primed with a standard curve that is calculated from the ^{35}S brain paste standards. The degree of autoradiography film darkening is then quantified in terms of dpm/mm^2. Once programmed, the analyzer constructs a standard curve and then reads off values in terms of dpm/mm^2 for each film image. In order to ensure an accurate value, the mean of triplicate readings was used. The transformed data were then subjected to statistical analysis using the method of analysis of variance followed by the least significance difference test (analysis carried out in conjunction with the MRC Biostatistical Unit, Cambridge). The results calculated are illustrated in Table 1.

From the data it may be seen that the largest increase in enkephalin mRNA content was localized in the putamen. Detailed examination of the exact distribution of this mRNA increase revealed that the ventral part of the putamen appears to exhibit the largest increase.

Further studies aimed at comparing normal human and "parkinsonian" material are underway. Our results so far indicate the feasibility of using *in situ* techniques on human brain tissue, although it is important to obtain material as far as possible matched for sex, age at death, and postmortem delay. Postmortem stability of mRNA is thought to be reasonable, with most mRNA being relatively intact up to 24 h after death (18). Considerations of stability will necessitate the use of internal control probes, i.e., mRNAs not expected to be influenced by degeneration of dopamine cells. Such probes may include actin or neurofilament cDNAs or cRNAs. Internal controls also need to be run on consecutive sections to control for the possibility of general nonspecific loss of mRNA.

THE SEARCH FOR THE MOLECULAR BASIS OF PARKINSON'S DISEASE

The characteristic inclusion in the degenerating dopamine cells in the substantia nigra in idiopathic Parkinson's disease is the Lewy body (19). Lewy bodies are acidophilic, dense-cored spherical inclusions in the cytoplasm of the large pigmented dopamine cells. They also occur in other neurological illnesses (e.g., Alzheimer's disease and supranuclear palsy) and are found in other brain regions including the cerebral cortex and substantia inominata. They are, however, at least as diagnostic of Parkinson's disease as are the senile plaques and neurofibrillary tangles of Alzheimer's disease (20). It is possible that the Lewy body merely represents the "tombstone" of the de-

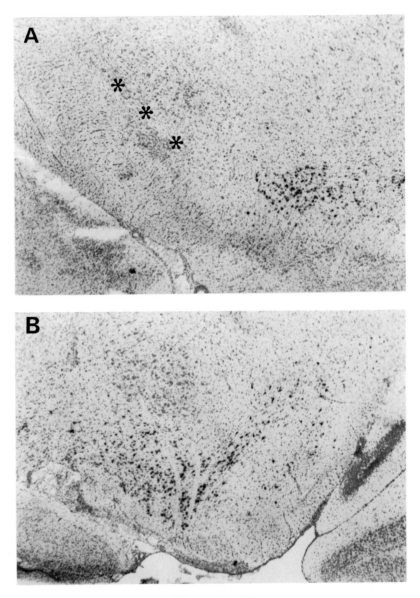

FIG. 6. A and B.

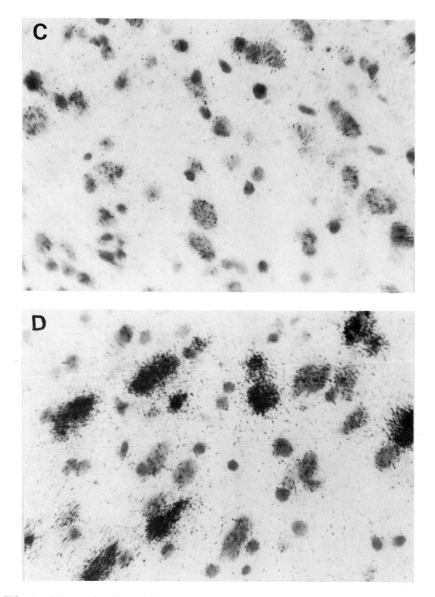

FIG. 6. Effects of unilateral 6-hydroxydopamine injection into the substantia nigra on tyrosine hydroxylase mRNA expression. The normal side (no 6-OHDA injection) contains a number of cells (**B** and **D**) hybridizing strongly with the ^{35}S-labeled tyrosine cRNA probe. On the lesioned side (**A** and **C**), these tyrosine hydroxylase cells are missing (stars) and there is only low nonspecific binding of cRNA probe to nondopamine cells. (**A** and **B** × 32.5; **C** and **D** × 455.)

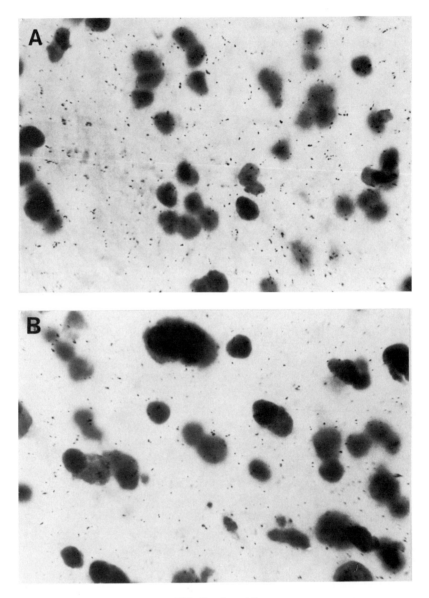

FIG. 7. A and B.

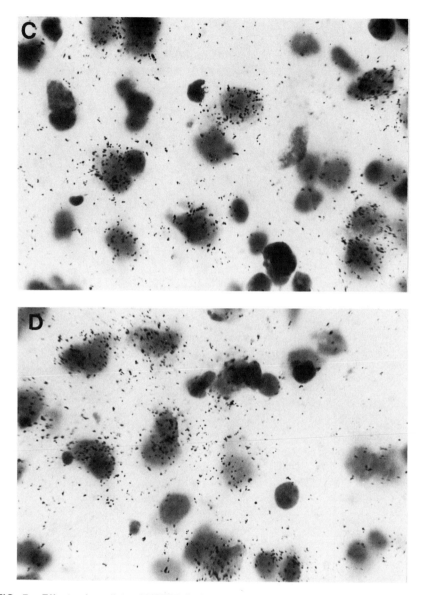

FIG. 7.   Effects of a unilateral MPTP infusion (as in Fig. 5) on enkephalin gene expression in the monkey striatum. (**A**) Caudate control side, (**B**) putamen control side, (**C**) caudate lesioned side, (**D**) putamen lesioned side. Note the substantial increase in enkephalin signal on the MPTP lesioned side. [All sections (× 520).]

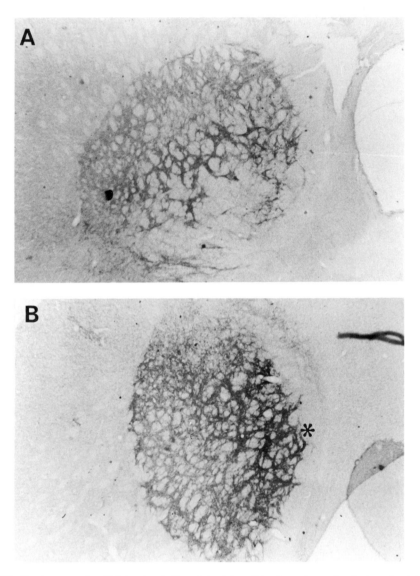

FIG. 8. Increased pallidal enkephalin content in a 6-hydroxydopamine-lesioned rat (as in Fig. 4). The 6-hydroxydopamine lesion results in an increase in enkephalin-like im-munoreactivity in the globus pallidus on the lesioned side (stars), presumably reflecting increased enkephalin synthesis in the denervated striatum ($\times$16.25).

TABLE 1. *Effects of MPTP treatment on enkephalin mRNA expression in the monkey striatum*

		Left side of tissue (dpm/mm^2)	Right side of tissue (dpm/mm^2)
Control—no	Caudate	1.011 ± 0.048	0.985 ± 0.046
treatment	Putamen	0.984 ± 0.052	0.947 ± 0.045
Systemic—MPTP	Caudate	1.167 ± 0.095*	1.144 ± 0.081**
treatment	Putamen	1.181 ± 0.094**	1.183 ± 0.086***

Values are means ± SD. Significantly different from controls. * $p < 0.02$, ** $p < 0.01$, *** $p < 0.001$.
No interarea significant differences were found between the caudate and putamen nuclei for the control animals. Any effect due to intrinsic left–right differences was also considered but no significant differences between sides were observed.

generating nigral cell; however, by analogy with work in Alzheimer's disease, it may perhaps be that the accumulation of protein material in these nigral cells reflects an alteration of gene expression, possibly over expression of a cytoplasmic protein, leading to an accumulation of proteinaceous Lewy body material and eventual death of the cell.

For this reason, it may be feasible to attempt to purify Lewy bodies from substantia nigra or cerebral cortex tissue of patients dying with the diagnosis of idiopathic Parkinson's disease and sequence the proteins present within them. This would represent a major effort; however, work on Alzheimer-related proteins, such as β-amyloid (A4 protein), indicates that this approach would at least be feasible (21–23). Alternatively, it may perhaps be more prudent to wait for the outcome of this current work in Alzheimer's disease before judging the success of this approach. Nevertheless, it is certainly of interest to apply antibodies and cDNA probes specific for β-amyloid protein to "parkinsonian" tissue to see if the antigens or mRNAs are expressed in the cells of the substantia nigra. It remains to be seen whether the Lewy body will provide us with any clues to the etiology of idiopathic Parkinson's disease, or whether the Lewy body merely represents a tombstone unrelated to the cause of cell death.

USE OF RETROVIRUSES OR OTHER VECTORS TO PROVIDE A REPLACEMENT THERAPY IN PARKINSON'S DISEASE

Currently, molecular biological techniques have not yet contributed to the understanding of Parkinson's disease; however, the recent cloning of the human tyrosine hydroxylase gene (24) provides a new opportunity to use this gene in a suitable vector to produce cell lines that could express tyrosine hydroxylase mRNA and protein. A similar approach has already been successfully tried by Ledley and colleagues (25), who used a retrovirus to transfer the related enzyme phenylalanine hydroxylase into two human cell lines. In the case of tyrosine hydroxylase, it would be technically feasible stably to transfer tyrosine hydroxylase activity to human cell lines and use these cells as a possible alternative to the adrenal medulla autografts or fetal neuron grafts currently being used in the treatment of Parkinson's disease. Before such an approach to treatment is tried, it would be necessary to test the cell lines to see if they synthesize or secrete L-dopa (or even dopamine).

In our laboratory, we have demonstrated that it is possible to transfer genetic information into fetal rat striatal neurons before grafting these into the adult rat striatum previously lesioned with ibotenic acid. The retrovirus we have used (βAG) contains the genetic information coding for β-galactosidase activity (from *E. coli*) (26). Rat fetal striatal neurons were dissected out of the rat embryo (day 14) and infected with the βAG virus. These infected neurons were then transplanted back into the striatum of the lesioned adult rat.

Histochemical staining of the striatal grafts after a survival period of 8 months revealed that all the grafts contained β-galactosidase-stained neurons

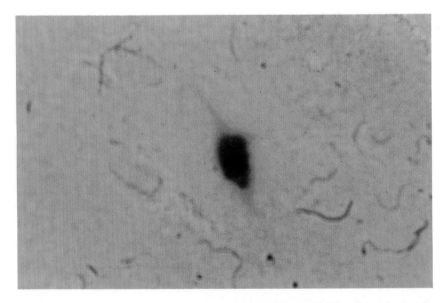

FIG. 9.   A color photograph to show the expression of bacterial (*E. coli*) β-galactosidase by a striatal neuron transplanted into the striatum of an adult rat. The striatal neuron was exposed to a retrovirus containing the *E. coli* β-galactosidase sequence. The neuron has incorporated the retroviral sequence including the information coding for *E. coli* β-galactosidase and is expressing this nonmammalian enzyme. Under the conditions used here, there is no detectable β-galactosidase activity in the host tissues since the cation requirements for mammalian β-galactosidase activity are distinctly different.

(Fig. 9). This enzyme activity was localized in the processes and cell body of the stained neuron. Obviously, in this case, the β-galactosidase enzyme expressed by these infected cells does not repair any existing deficit; however, it does demonstrate the possibilities of this approach. It is important to note that this type of virus cannot produce infectious particles without the help of a packaging cell line. This means that the virus cannot be transferred beyond the "infected" neurons or into the germ line. What is clear, however, is that we will see increasing efforts to diagnose and treat neurological illness with molecular probes.

Acknowledgment: S.J.A. is supported by the U.K. Parkinson's Disease Society. We are grateful to the MRC U.K. for their continued support. Dr. D. Nunez and Dr. A. Davenport developed the use of the image analysis system for quantitation of "*in situ*" signals. We thank Mrs. B. A. Waters for typing the manuscript.

REFERENCES

1. Tretiakoff, C. (1919): Contribution a l'etude de l'anatomia pathologique du locus niger, These, Université Paris.
2. Hornykiewicz, O. (1973): *Fed. Proc.*, 32:183–190.
3. Jonsson, G., Malmfors, T., and Sachs, C. (1975): *Chemical Tools in Catecholamine Research I*, Elsevier, New York.
4. Langston, J., Ballard, P., Tetrud, J., and Irwin, I. (1983): *Science*, 219:979–980.
5. Burns, R. S., Markey, S. P., Phillips, J. M., and Chiveh, C. C. (1984): *Can. J. Neurol. Sci.*, 11:166–168.
6. Mitchell, I. J., Cross, A. J., Sambrook, M. A., and Crossman, A. R. (1985): *Neurosci. Lett.*, 61:195–200.
7. Ballard, P. A., Tetrud, J. W., and Langston, J. W. (1985): *Neurology*, 35:946–949.
8. Nunez, D., Davenport, A., Emson, P. C., and Brown, M. (1988): *Biochem. J.* (in press).
9. Arai, H., Emson, P. C., Christodolou, C., Agrawal, S., and Gait, M. (1988): *Mol. Brain Res.*, 4:63–69.
10. Uhl, G. (1986): *In situ Hybridization*, Plenum Press, New York.
11. Maniatis, T., Fritsch, E. F., and Sambrook, J. (1982): *Molecular Cloning: A Laboratory Manual*, Cold Spring Harbor Laboratory.
12. Lewis, E. J., Tank, A. W., Weiner, N., and Chikaraishi, D. M. (1983): *J. Biol. Chem.*, 258:14632–14637.
13. Emson, P. C., Ichimiya, Y., and Northrop, A. (1988): *Mol. Brain Res.*, 4:255–258.
14. Legon, S., Glover, D. M., Hughes, J., Lowry, P. J., Rigby, P. W. J., and Watson, C. J. (1982): *Nucleic Acid Res.*, 10:7905–7918.
15. Graybiel, A. (1986): Functions of the basal ganglia. *Ciba Found. Symp.* 107:114–143.
16. Normand, E., Popovici, T., Onteniente, B., Fellman, D., Piater-Tonneau, D., Aufray, C., and Bloch, B. (1988): *Brain Res.*, 439:39–46.
17. Voorn, P., Roest, G., and Groenewegen, H. (1987): *Brain Res.*, 412:391–396.
18. Johnson, S. A., Morgan, D. G., and Finch, C. E. (1986): *J. Neurosci. Res.*, 16:267–280.
19. Lewy, F. H. (1923): *Die Letre vom Tonus und der Bewegung*, Springer, Berlin.
20. Forno, L. S. (1986): In: *Advances in Neurology*, Vol. 45, ed by Yahr, M. D. and Bergman, K.-J., pp. 35–43, Raven Press, New York.
21. Masters, C. L., Simms, G., Weinman, N. A., Multhaup, G., McDonald, B., and Beyreuther, K. (1985): *Proc. Natl. Acad. Sci. U.S.A.* 82:4245–4249.
22. Selkoe, D. J., Bell, D. S., Podlisny, M. B., Price, D. L., and Clark, L. C. (1987): *Science*, 235:873–877.
23. Tanzi, R. E., Gusella, J. F., Watkins, P. C., Brown, G. A. P., St. George-Hyslop, P.,

Van Keuren, M. L., Patterson, D., Pagan, S., Kurmit, D. M., and Neve, R. L. (1987): *Science*, 235:881–884.

24. Grima, B., Lamouroux, A., Boni, C., Julei, J-F., Javoy-Agid, F., and Mallet, J. (1987): *Nature* (Lond.), 326:707–711.

25. Ledley, F. D., Grenett, H. E., McGinnis-Shelontt, M., and Woo, S. L. C. (1986): *Proc. Natl. Acad. Sci. U.S.A.*, 83:409–413.

26. Price, J., Turner, D., and Cepko, C. (1987): *Proc. Natl. Acad. Sci. U.S.A.* 84:156–160.

Parkinsonism and Aging, edited by
Donald B. Calne et al., Raven Press, Ltd.,
New York © 1989.

Comparison of Neuronal Loss in Parkinson's Disease and Aging

P. L. McGeer, S. Itagaki, H. Akiyama, and E. G. McGeer

*Kinsmen Laboratory of Neurological Research, Department of Psychiatry,
University of British Columbia, Vancouver, B.C. V6T 1W5, Canada*

A quarter of a century has passed since the loss of substantia nigra (SN) dopaminergic neurons was firmly established as the fundamental lesion of Parkinson's disease. Based on this discovery, drugs have been designed that are capable of affording symptomatic relief, but not of arresting the disease. The most important question—why dopaminergic cells die in idiopathic Parkinson's disease—is still unanswered. Until the answer is found, it is unlikely that any truly effective treatment will emerge. Among causes that have been suggested are abiotrophy (simple degeneration), a pathogenic organism, a toxin, a metabolic abnormality, or an autoimmune phenomenon. Despite much effort, it has so far been impossible to establish or to reject any of these hypotheses. Another, related question that has also remained unanswered is whether there is still active disease at the time of death. The alternative would be a burned-out disease in which an early and heavy loss of dopamine neurons would be followed by the normal mild attrition of aging. This latter mechanism might still lead to the observed onset in later life and progression of symptoms, but would present a much more difficult problem for prevention and therapy. Intervention would need to take place while the disease was still silent.

In this chapter, we present evidence that a burned out disease is not the situation in idiopathic parkinsonism. Not only is there an active disease process at the time of death, but the process itself appears to be occurring at a rate that could not have been sustained for any prolonged period. This conclusion is based on our finding of numerous reactive microglia or macrophages phagocytosing dopaminergic cells in the SN of postmortem parkinsonian brains. Relatively few such microglia are seen in nonparkinsonian SN tissue.

The clear demonstration of phagocytosing reactive microglia has been made possible by the development of an immunohistochemical staining method for HLA-DR, a human glycoprotein of the group II major histocompatibility (MHC) class. HLA-DR is expressed only on the surface of immunocompetent cells. Its major known function is to present antigen to T-helper lymphocytes for the purpose of generating an immune response. It appears on T-lymphocytes, some B lymphocytes, some tissue macrophages, some histiocytes, and, in brain, on reactive microglia. Because HLA-DR is on the cell surface, immunohistochemical staining outlines reactive microglia and other positive cells in a Golgi-like fashion, making their identification much more selective than is possible with the silver methods that have been conventionally used to reveal these cells.

The presence of reactive microglia in the SN in Parkinson's disease has not been previously emphasized in the literature, possibly because of difficulty in detection using conventional methods. However, now that a reliable technique is available, this should become an important part of the pathological description because it indicates the intensity of the disease process. The HLA-DR method highlights phagocytotic activity surrounding dead and dying neurons (1–5) and, as reported here, is a prominent feature in idiopathic Parkinson's disease. Of even greater significance may be the fundamental reason for the presence of the HLA-DR molecule. It could be presenting an antigen or a series of antigens to the immune system, thus stimulating a selective immune response. If this were directed at normal neuronal proteins, an autodestructive process would result.

CELL DEATH IN NORMAL AGING

Regardless of what may cause cell loss in parkinsonism or other disease states, neuronal attrition also occurs as part of the normal aging process. Figure 1 illustrates cell losses in aging from three different subcortical nuclei of the brain: the dopaminergic SN, the noradrenergic locus coeruleus, and the cholinergic nucleus basalis of Meynert. The figure shows the percentage of cells remaining in the nuclei as a function of age. The plots show a remarkably similar decline in the three nuclei. The declines are linear although a different function might be found to apply if a larger series of cases were studied.

The nucleus basalis of Meynert contains 400,000 to 500,000 cholinergic neurons at birth (6) and is the principal source of cholinergic innervation of the neocortex. The SN has a similar complement of dopaminergic neurons (7) that innervate the neostriatum (8) and some structures beyond. The locus coeruleus has fewer than one-tenth as many neurons (9) and provides the principal noradrenergic innervation of the entire forebrain and cerebellum (8). In each nucleus, the neurons project broadly to projection areas that are many, many times larger than the cell body masses themselves. Thus, each neuron may have millions of axonal boutons and should be particularly sensitive to any process that impairs axoplasmic transport.

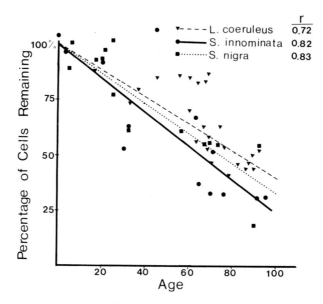

FIG. 1. Percent of neurons remaining vs. age in three areas of human brain. Locus coeruleus data from Vijayashankar and Brody (9), substantia innominata data from McGeer et al. (6), and substantia nigra (SN) data from McGeer et al. (7). The data of Hirai (13) on single sections of the SN give a significant line of correlation, with slope almost identical to that shown above for the SN.

These small nuclei are among the few regions in the brain that have been studied in any detail. Little is known about possible neuronal dropout with age in major areas of the brain. There is computed tomography (CT) and magnetic resonance imaging (MRI) evidence of brain atrophy with age. For example, Takeda and Matsuzawa (10) examined 980 normals ranging in age from 10 to 88 years with no neurological disturbances. They found that the cerebrospinal fluid (CSF) space detected by these imaging modalities increased exponentially with increasing age after the 30s in both men and women. However, substantial changes only began to develop after age 60 years. These data would imply some acceleration of neuronal dropout of a fairly broad degree in people beyond the age of 60 years. So far, however, little can be said about the nature of the process, and simple shrinkage of tissue, rather than neuronal loss, might account for some or all of the effect.

Regardless of the mechanism and cumulative extent of these neuronal losses, the actual rate of loss must be extremely slow. In the case of the three subcortical nuclei (cf. Fig. 1), the slopes would suggest rates of attrition of the order of 0.002% (i.e., 2 per 100,000) of the initial cell complement per day. In the case of the dopaminergic SN, this rate translates to about 8 cells per SN per day on each side. Such a rate of loss would be almost undetectable postmortem by conventional histological techniques. The SN is about 1.2

cm in length and therefore extends over 400 sections of 30 μm or 1,200 sections of 10 μm thickness. The chances of seeing a degenerating profile on any given section would be extremely small. The only evidence that could be readily observed would be cumulative losses determined by counts of remaining cells or reductions in specific metabolic constituents such as tyrosine hydroxylase or dopamine.

CELL DEATH IN PARKINSON'S DISEASE

The cumulative cell losses in Parkinson's disease compared with age-matched controls have been estimated both by counting surviving pigmented cells in the SN and measuring the indices of dopamine metabolism in the striatum. Figure 2 illustrates the results of some typical SN counts. The SN area of a series of cases was cut into 24-μm sections. Every fifth section was mounted and the pigmented cells in every tenth section counted. If

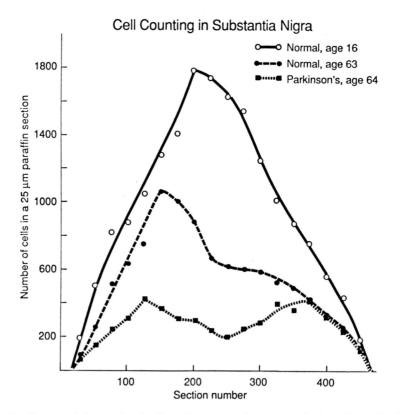

FIG. 2. Representative plots of cell number vs. section number in the substantia nigra for normals, ages 19 and 63 years, and a case of Parkinson's disease, age 64 years.

apparent inconsistencies in the counts of any single section appeared, additional nearby sections were counted so as to develop a reliable profile of cell distribution through the whole of the substantia nigra. Figure 2 is a plot of section number vs. pigmented cell count for a 19-year-old normal, a 63-year-old normal, and a 64-year-old parkinsonian patient. As can be seen from Fig. 2, the number of pigmented cells in the midportion of the SN tends to be considerably higher than the rostral or caudal extremities, although irregularities occur.

We have investigated the nature and extent of immunopathological activity in the SN of parkinsonian patients by staining for HLA-DR, glial fibrillary acidic protein (GFAP), common leukocyte antigen (CLA), and interleukin-2 receptor (IL-2R) by methods that have been previously described (1–5). The results are illustrated in Fig. 3 and are presented in tabular form in Table 1.

All of the cases recorded as having Parkinson's disease had many HLA-DR-positive microglia (Table 1) as recorded by cell counts of five representative high-power fields in single sections of the SN. Traditional pathology in these cases was demonstrated by the presence of Lewy bodies and free melanin, as well as a conspicuous depletion of pigmented dopaminergic cells. By contrast, the cases of deaths from cerebrovascular accidents and nonneurological causes showed relatively few HLA-DR-positive cells in the SN (Table 1).

Figures 3A and 3B illustrate the contrast in HLA-DR activity in the SN of a typical parkinsonian and a typical nonparkinsonian case. Numerous reactive microglia can be seen in close proximity to melanin-containing dopaminergic cells and to free melanin in the tissue of the parkinsonian (Fig. 3A) but not the normal case (Fig. 3B).

Figure 3C illustrates a separate principle with respect to the nature of the cells carrying out the phagocytosis. It is a section doubly immunostained for HLA-DR and GFAP. It illustrates that antibodies to GFAP, which is found in astrocytes, stain a separate cell population from those staining for

TABLE 1. *Mean ages, HLA-DR cell counts in the substantia nigra, and numbers of degenerating dopaminergic neurons (± SD)*

	N	Age (years)	Substantia nigra pathology	
			HLA-DR cells (5 fields)	Deg. DA neurons (one section)
Parkinson's	10	75 ± 10	203 ± 66[a]	9.4 ± 5.8[a]
Controls	8	75 ± 12	16 ± 12	1.6 ± 2.0

[a] Significantly different from controls, $p < 0.001$.

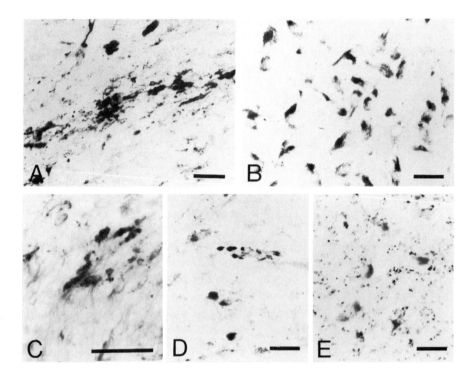

FIG. 3. HLA-DR staining in the substantia nigra. The large dopaminergic neurons can be identified by smooth profiles outlining intracellular melanin pigment. (**A**) Parkinson's disease. There are many HLA-DR-positive reactive microglia in the region of deteriorated cells. (**B**) Comparable stain in the substantia nigra of a suicide case. No HLA-DR-positive reactive microglia are visible. (**C**) Substantia nigra in Parkinson's disease doubly immunostained for HLA-DR and GFAP. The separate populations of reactive microglia (dark stain) and reactive astrocytes (light stain) can readily be distinguished. (**D**) Section of parkinsonian substantia nigra stained for common leukocyte antigen (CLA). Notice the round cells, which are presumed lymphocytes, lining up along the capillary wall. (**E**) Section of parkinsonian substantia nigra stained for interleukin-2 receptor (IL-2R) and counterstained with neutral red. Notice the punctate staining in the tissue matrix, presumably on the surface of specific glial cells. Bars = 50 μm.

HLA-DR, indicating that the phagocytotic cells are not astroglia but microglia.

If HLA-DR is being expressed on the cell surface of the reactive microglia for the purpose of presenting antigen to T cells, then T cells should also be found in the SN of parkinsonian cases. Figure 3D shows the presence of cells positive for common leukocyte antigen (CLA). Round CLA-positive cells were found marginated along the walls of capillaries and, in small numbers, distributed in the matrix itself. Presumably, various leukocytes have the capacity to stick to capillary walls and then penetrate the endothelium to distribute in the tissue matrix.

Activated T cells secrete the lymphokine interleukin-2 (IL-2). This lymphokine is a powerful stimulant for the expression of HLA-DR on the surface of immunocompetent cells. It may also play a role in converting resting microglia to reactive microglia, and/or in stimulating monocytes to enter brain as ameboid cells to become HLA-DR-positive macrophages directly. Figure 3E shows staining of the SN in a parkinsonian case for IL-2R, indicating elaboration of receptors for this lymphokine. These findings demonstrate that, in Parkinson's disease, HLA-DR, an MHC group II glycoprotein specialized for presenting antigen, is vigorously expressed on cells phagocytosing dopaminergic neurons, and that lymphocytes and receptors for a powerful lymphokine, IL-2, are also present in SN tissue. Taken together, they constitute evidence of a chronic inflammatory process possibly generating a cell-mediated immune response in Parkinson's disease.

Table 1 presents quantitative data on the number of neurons being phagocytosed in representative sections of parkinsonian and control SN tissue. The table shows an average of 9.4 cells/30 μm section for the parkinsonians and 1.6 cells for the nonparkinsonians. The table indicates that the number of cells undergoing phagocytosis at the time of death is roughly six times greater in the parkinsonian cases than the normals. We have also estimated numbers of degenerating dopamine neurons for the complete SN in two idiopathic Parkinson's disease cases aged 61 and 64 years by counting the number of SN cells undergoing phagocytosis in every 20th section. The counts for the total SN on one side were 1,540 and 1,380, respectively. Similar counts for a 64-year-old diabetic dying of a myocardial infarct and a 24-year-old suicide were 200 and 0, respectively.

Our previous cell counts in every tenth section across the SN in normal individuals and parkinsonians (7) (Fig. 4) showed a normal cell complement at birth of about 450,000/SN, which declined in an approximately linear fashion to reach a level of about 275,000 by age 60 years. In our study, parkinsonians all had cell counts below 140,000. Three possible routes for reaching the lower cell counts in Parkinson's disease are depicted in Fig. 4: (A) a remote insult caused by an acute disease or environmental toxin at an early age followed by the normal neuronal attrition of aging, (B) accelerated aging, or (C) an active neuropathological process commencing in late life.

If idiopathic Parkinson's disease were merely an aging process superimposed upon some early and burned out disease (route A), then the number of cells being phagocytosed should be the same or less than controls. A lower figure for the parkinsonians might be anticipated because the remaining cells following the initial insult would be only a fraction of the normal complement. Postencephalitic parkinsonism might be one example of such a process. MPTP poisoning might be another (11). Accelerated aging could produce a slightly faster cell loss in idiopathic Parkinson's disease than in normals (route B), but this should not result in more than double the number of SN cells being phagocytosed as compared with controls. Losses sixfold

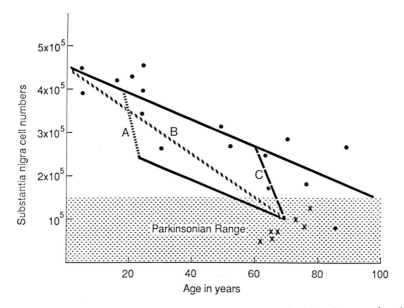

FIG. 4. Dopaminergic cell numbers in some controls (● and ▬) and cases of parkinsonism (x) plotted against age. Possible time sequences for neuronal loss in Parkinsonism are illustrated: **(A)**....▬, remote disease followed by normal aging; **(B)**↘↘, accelerated aging; **(C)**.▬., active disease.

greater than controls, as observed by HLA-DR staining, implies that a much more rapid cell loss is occurring in the disease. This would only be consistent with an active neuropathological process (route C). It is compatible with a previous report of the relative loss of caudate dopamine as a function of time from onset of parkinsonian symptoms (12). Such a process might be the result of chronic infection, an autoimmune phenomenon, or the onset of a relatively severe, age-related degenerative process.

HOW LONG DOES IT TAKE TO PHAGOCYTOSE A NEURON?

While the HLA-DR technique permits estimation of the total number of cells being phagocytosed at the time of death, it cannot give the rate of cell death without knowledge of the time taken to phagocytose a dead nigral neuron. We have approached this problem through model experiments in rats. The results will be reported in detail elsewhere (14). Figure 5A shows a section stained for Ia (the animal equivalent of a Class II glycoprotein) in the SN of a rat 10 days after 6-hydroxydopamine (6-OHDA) administration. Much reactive microglial activity is visible. After 4 weeks, considerable Ia-positive activity still remains (Fig. 5B). A similar time period of appearance

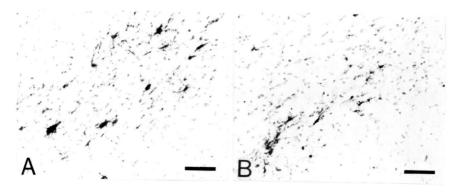

FIG. 5. Staining for Ia in the SN of rats 10 days (**A**) and 4 weeks (**B**) after administration of 6-hydroxydopamine. Note the profusion of Ia-positive microglia at 10 days with somewhat fewer at 4 weeks. Bars = 50 μm.

and decline of Ia-positive reactive microglia has been observed with other model lesions.

These results imply, but do not establish, that most of the cells observed to be undergoing phagocytosis in human material would probably have died in the time range of 4 weeks premortem. Since there are about 400 sections of 30 μm thickness in the SN, the data of Table 1 would suggest cell losses in the range of 1000–3600 neurons in 4 weeks or about 12,000–43,000 per year. Clearly, such losses could not be sustained over many years without total depletion of dopaminergic cells in the SN being the result. By contrast, Fig. 4 indicates a cell loss of only about 3,300 cells per year in normal aging (route A), which would increase to about 5,000–6,000 cells per year if an accelerated aging process were taking place in Parkinson's disease (route B).

Although these results provide no clue as to the reason for cell loss in Parkinson's disease, they do permit rejection of the hypotheses of burned out disease and accelerated aging. They also suggest that appropriate therapeutic intervention early in the disease might drastically reduce the progression of symptoms.

Since one known function of HLA-DR is to present foreign antigen to T-helper lymphocytes, our observation of cells staining positively for leukocyte common antigen and the interleukin-2 receptor in the SN of parkinsonian cases (2,3,5) may be of some importance. The possibility of an autoimmune mechanism contributing to neuronal death should at least be considered. If this were the case, then the process might be slowed and life prolonged by some form of immunosuppression.

Acknowledgment: This research was supported by grants from the Medical Research Council of Canada, the Medical Services Foundation of B.C., the Alzheimer's

Association of B.C., and the Alzheimer's Disease and Related Disorders Association of Chicago. The authors are grateful to Dr. Douglas Walker for supplying the HB104 antibody, to Ms. Joane Sunahara for technical assistance, and to Dr. D. B. Calne and pathologists in the Vancouver area for their help in obtaining specimens.

REFERENCES

1. McGeer, P. L., Itagaki, S., Tago, H., and McGeer, E. G. (1987): Reactive microglia in patients with senile dementia of the Alzheimer type are positive for the histocompatibility glycoprotein HLA-DR. *Neurosci. Lett.*, 79:195–200.
2. McGeer, P. L., McGeer, E. G., Itagaki, S., and Mizukawa, K. (1987): Anatomy and pathology of the basal ganglia. *Can. J. Neurol. Sci.* 14:363–372.
3. Itagaki, S., McGeer, P. L., and McGeer, E. G. (1987): HLA-DR reactive microglia in Parkinson's disease. *J. Neuroimmunol.* 16:81.
4. McGeer, P. L., Itagaki, S., Tago, H., and McGeer, E. G. (1987): Expression of HLA-DR and interleukin-2 receptor on reactive microglia in senile dementia of the Alzheimer's type. *J. Neuroimmunol* 16:122.
5. McGeer, P. L., Itagaki, S., Boyes, B. E., and McGeer, E. G. (1988): Reactive microglia are positive for HLA-DR in the substantia nigra of Parkinson's and Alzheimer's disease brains. *Neurology*, 38:1285–1291.
6. McGeer, P. L., McGeer, E. G., Suzuki, J., Dolman, C. E., and Nagai, T. (1984): Aging, Alzheimer's disease and the cholinergic system of the basal forebrain. *Neurology*, 34:741–745.
7. McGeer, P. L., McGeer, E. G., and Suzuki, J. S. (1977). Aging and extrapyramidal function. *Arch. Neurol*, 34:33–35.
8. Ungerstedt, U. (1971): Stereotaxic mapping of the monoamine pathways in the rat brain. *Acta Physiol. Scand. Suppl.* 367:1–48.
9. Vijayashankar, N., and Brody, H. A. (1979): A quantitative study of the pigmented neurons in the nucleus locus coeruleus and subcoeruleus in man as related to aging. *J. Neuropathol. Exp. Neurol.*, 38:490–498.
10. Takeda, S., and Matsuzawa, T. (1984): Brain atrophy during aging: a quantitative study using computed tomography. *J. Am. Geriatr. Soc.*, 32:520–524.
11. Calne, D. B., Eisen, A., McGeer, E. G., and Spencer, P. (1986): Alzheimer's disease, Parkinson's disease, and motoneurone disease: abiotrophic interaction between ageing and environment? *Lancet*, 2:1067–1070.
12. Riederer, P., and Wuketich, S. T. (1976): Time course of nigrostriatal degeneration in Parkinson's disease. *J. Neural Transm.*, 38:277–301.
13. Hirai, S. (1968): Histochemical study on the regressive degeneration of the senile brain, with special reference to the aging of the substantia nigra. *Adv. Neurol. Sci.*, 12:845–9.
14. Kiyama, H., and McGeer, P. L. (1989): Microglical response to 6-hydroxydopamine induced substantia nigra lesions. *Brain Res.* (in press).

Parkinsonism and Aging, edited by
Donald B. Calne et al., Raven Press, Ltd.,
New York © 1989.

Cytoskeletal Pathology of Parkinsonism and Aging Brain

K. Jellinger

*Ludwig Boltzmann Institute of Clinical Neurobiology, Lainz-Hosptial,
A-1130 Vienna, Austria*

Parkinson's disease (PD) and other neurodegenerative disorders including brain aging are characterized by degeneration of certain vulnerable populations of neurons associated with several types of cytoskeletal pathology often presenting with the formation of abnormal inclusions, e.g., Lewy bodies (LB), Hirano bodies (HB), Marinesco bodies (MB), neurofibrillary tangles (NFT), and other structural changes such as neuritic plaques (NP), grumelous degeneration, dystrophic axons, and deposits of amyloid in the neuronal parenchyma and its vasculature (Table 1). A number of these abnormalities are abundant in certain disorders, e.g., LBs in PD and NFTs in Alzheimer's disease (AD) and senile dementia (SDAT), and therefore are recognized as histopathological hallmarks of these diseases. However, these and other cytoskeletal abnormalities can also be found in normal and aged brain or in various central nervous system (CNS) disorders. Ultrastructural studies have revealed that most of these inclusions are due to either an abnormal accumulation or organization of seemingly normal cytoskeletal components or an accumulation of abnormal filamentous elements. Considerable progress has been made toward the understanding of the structure and chemistry of the three major filamentous structures of the normal cytoskeleton (1–3): (a) microtubules are circular in cross section with 24 nm diameter showing a central 5 nm density within the lucent lumen; they are mainly composed of tubulin with molecular weight (MW) of 54 to 57 kDa; (b) neurofilaments (NF), which are part of a class of 8- to 10-nm intermediate filaments that are most abundant in axons and proximal dendrites and are composed of three proteins with MW of 68, 150–160, and 200 kDA; and (c) microfilaments of 6 to 7 nm in diameter composed mainly of actin with a MW of 42 kDA. The origin and molecular nature of some of these cytoskeletal abnormalities have begun to be understood by modern immunocytochemical and ultrastructural methods using panels of monoclonal and polyclonal antibodies to the major protein subunits of normal and pathological

TABLE 1. *Neuronal cytoskeletal pathology in parkinsonism and aging brain*

Type of lesion (Location)	Ultrastructure	Immunocytochemistry							
		NFP	Tau	MAP	PHF	Ubiquitin	Actin	Tubulin	Thioflavin-S
Lewy body (cytoplasm)	8–10-nm filaments (intermediate type)	++	–	–(+)	++	++	–	+	+
Cortex type	Random arrangement (mainly 10-nm filaments)	+(diff)	–	–(+)	+	++	–	+	+
Brainstem type	Central condensation (core)	+/++	–	–	+	++	–	++	++
	Peripheral radiation (halo)	++	–	–(+)	+	++	–	++	++
Hirano body (juxtanuclear)	6–10-nm filaments (latticework, parallel arrangement)	–	+	+	+	?	++	–	–
Eosinophilic granules (cytoplasm)	Paracrystalline 8.5-nm filaments	–	–	–	–	–	+	+	–
Marinesco body (intranuclear)	10–12-nm (intermediate) filaments, latticework	+	–	?	+	+	–	–	–
Alzheimer neurofibrill. tangles (cytoplasm)	10-nm paired helical filaments twisted at 80-nm intervals + few 15-nm straight filaments	++	+++	+/++	+++	+/+++	–	–	+++
NFTs in PSP (cytoplasm)	15–20-nm straight filaments + few PHF/twisted filaments	++	+/++	+	(+)	+	–	–	++
Granulovacuolar degeneration	Granules and membrane-bound vesicles (hippocamppal neurons)	+	+	?	+	?	–	+	–
Axonal spheroid (presynapt. terminal)	Tubulovesicular, dense bodies, 10-nm filaments, lamellar SER	++	+(–)	?	–	++	–	–	–
Neuritic plaque	Dystrophic neurite terminals, filaments, synapses, glia, amyloid	++	+++	+	+++	+/+++	–	–	+++

NFP = neurofilament protein; MAP = microtubule-associated proteins; PHF = paired helical filament.

cytoskeletal constituents (see refs. 2–4). Because cytoskeletal elements are important in the maintenance of neuronal size and shape, in the intracellular and axonal transport, and in the organization of both cytoplasmic elements and membrane constituents, neurons exhibiting these abnormalities may or may not be able to carry out normal functions. Hence, knowledge of the cytoskeletal pathology of PD and aging brain may provide some insight into the pathogenic role of these lesions. The present overview will outline the current knowledge of cytoskeletal pathology in PD and aging brain with reference to their possible structural and chemical interrelationships and pathogenic relevance.

LEWY BODIES

These intracytoplasmic inclusions were first described by F. H. Lewy (5) in the substantia innominata and dorsal vagal nucleus in a patient with idiopathic PD. He considered these "eosinophilic bodies" as the sequelae of neuronal degeneration. Trétiakoff (6) reported LBs in the substantia nigra and considered them to be the specific anatomical hallmark of PD, although these inclusions were later observed in this and other regions of the nervous system in various disorders and in normal aging (7).

LBs appear in two characteristic forms: (a) The typical or "brainstem" type consists of a single or multiple round or oval eosinophilic structures with a central core surrounded by a less dense peripheral zone and an outermost pale halo that is sharply demarcated from the cytoplasm. (b) The "cortical" type of LBs is not sharply delineated from the cytoplasm and the outline of the central part is rather indistinct. The LBs vary in size from 3 to 20 μm and can be localized in a nerve cell body (classical perikaryal), within nerve cell processes (intraneuronal), and extraneuronal free in the neuropil (7). They are composed of proteins, free fatty acids, sphingomyelin, and polysaccharides; their core contains α-amino acids. Electron probe microanalysis demonstrated a high sulfur content, indicating products of degenerated proteins (8).

Ultrastructurally, LBs are composed of intermediate type filaments, 8 to 10 nm in diameter (with a range from 7 to 20 nm), admixed with vesicular and granular material. In the brainstem type, the central core, showing a chaotic arrangement of filaments, is sharply demarcated from the peripheral portions, consisting of radially arranged filaments (7,9). The cortical type of LBs is rather homogenous, with random arrangement of the filaments without marked dense core and peripheral radiations. Filaments are admixed with membranous and granular material (7,10,11). Similar homogenous, poorly staining intraneuronal hyaline (colloid) inclusions or "pale bodies" composed of randomly arranged collections of 10 nm filaments are found in many neurons in PD (7,12). These pale areas, where the cytoplasm appears

TABLE 2. *Immunocytochemical features of Lewy bodies, neurofibrillary tangles (NFT), and neuritic plaques (NP) with antisera to various cytoskeletal elements*

	Lewy bodies			Neuro-fibrillary tangles	Neuritic plaques
	Typical		Cortical		
Antibodies type	Untreated	PASE			
PHF 3.39 mAb	+ + (CORE) 51%	+ +	+	+ + +	+ + +
PHF 60e pAb	−	−	−	+ + +	+ + +
PHF (phosphoryl. tau)[a]	−		−	+ + +	+ + +
P-NFP (150, 210 kd) SM I-31 mAb	+ (RIM)	−	+	−	−
P-NFP SM I-34 mAb	+ (RIM) 31%	−	+	+	+ + +
P-NFP 200 mAb[a]	−/±		−/±	−/±	−/±
NFP SM I-33 mAb	−	+ (RIM)	+	−	−
MAP 1 (52–68 kd) pAb	−	−	−	−	−
MAP 1 (Goldman) pAb	+[b]				
MAP 2 (200–250 kd) pAb	−	+/−	−	−	−
MAP 2 pAb[a]	+ (RIM)		+ (RIM)	+/+ +	+/+ +
Tau Tau 1 mAb	−	−	−	+/−	+ +
Tau 92 pAb	−	−	−	+	+ +
Tau 55–62 kD pAb[a]	−		−	+ +	+ + +
DF-2 (cross-react ubiquitin) mAb[a]	+ + (RIM)		+ +	+ +	+/+ +
Ubiquitin mAb[a]	+ + (RIM)		+ +	+ +	+/+ +

mAb = monoclonal antibody; pAb = polyclonal antibody; PASE = phosphatase pretreatment.

[a] From ref. 19.

[b] Personal communication (1987), vibratome.

to be devoid of its normal organelles including the Nissl substance and the neuromelanin, are considered to represent the early stage of LB formation (7), from which they may form as a result of concentration of filaments (12).

Immunocytochemical studies (Table 2) demonstrate that LBs react with antisera to NFs (4,13). They show homogenous or peripheral staining with polyclonal antisera that recognize all three of the NF proteins (4,7,13) and with monoclonal antibodies (mABs) to phosphorylated and nonphosphorylated epitopes of NFT (4,14–18). They further react with mABs to tubulin (18), various microtubule polypeptides, occasionally with MAP 1 and MAP 2 (19,20), with some or most of the mAbs to paired helical filaments (PHF) and Alzheimer neurofibrillary tangles (ANFT) (11,18–20), and with ubiquitin (19), a polypeptide required for the ATP-dependent nonlysosomal protein breakdown that recently has been demonstrated to be associated with PHF

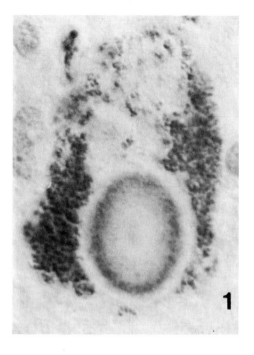

Fig. 1. Lewy body in nigral neuron. Periphery stained with monoclonal anti-phosphorylated NFP (M 1-31) ($\times$ 1,000).

(21,22). LBs do not bind antibodies to actin, high molecular weight microtubule-associated proteins (HMW-MAPs) (4,18), aB to the 200 kDa component of NFs (19), a mAb against isolated PHFs (19), to anti-PHF that preferentially reacts with phosphorylated tau protein (19,23), and the heat-stable microtubule-associated protein tau (4,17–20) that strongly reacts with ANT/PHF (21,24,25).

The *cortical* LBs often display homogeneous staining pattern, particularly with antibodies to NFP and PHF (11,15,17,18,20), whereas MAP 2 stains primarily about the periphery (19). The *classical* LBs show intense staining of the periphery with mAbs to phosphorylated epitopes of NFP (Fig. 1) and MAP 2 (14,17,19,20), while reactivity with MAP 1 appears only on glutaraldehyde-fixed vibratome sections (Goldman, 1987, personal communication). Reactivity with some mAbs to NFP in the periphery of LBs appears only after pretreatment of the sections with phosphatase (Table 2).

Quantitative evaluation revealed that about two-thirds of all subcortical LBs are stained by a monoclonal anti-PHF, but only about one-third with anti-NFP antibodies (20). A mAb to PHF (DF-2) that recognizes ubiquitin (19) and pAbs to ubiquitin have been shown to immunostain virtually all cortical LBs in a diffuse manner and the peripheral rim of the typical LBs (Fig. 2), whereas the cores of the typical LBs and the center of the cortical LBs were less intensely stained or remained unstained. The cores of a large

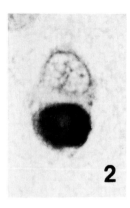

Fig. 2. Lewy body in cerebral cortex diffusely stained with antiubiquitin (× 200).

number of LBs were found to be strongly reactive with a mAb to PHF (Fig. 3) that recognizes determinants of ubiquitin (22).

Immunoelectron microscopy of the LBs confirmed that the strong reactivity with a mAb to isolated PHF was located only in the core of typical LBs, although no PHFs or 15-nm filaments were found in the center of the inclusions (20). This reaction is not due to any common epitope with NFP, since no staining of NF polypeptides on Western blots was observed with this antibody (26). This staining pattern differs considerably from the characteristic reaction of the peripheral ring with anti-NFP (20). Other ultra-

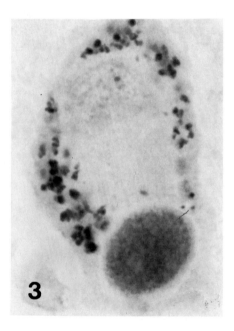

Fig. 3. Lewy body in nigral neuron stained by monoclonal anti-PHF. Intensely stained core surrounded by pale halo (× 1,000).

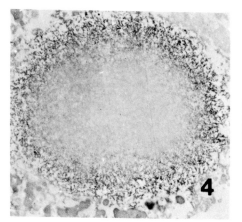

Fig. 4. Typical Lewy body in nigral neuron, showing intense labeling of radiating peripheral filaments with mAb to ubiquitin (courtesy of Dr. S. Kuzuhara) ($\times$ 4,000).

structural studies demonstrated similar anti-NFP reaction in the periphery and less in the core of typical LBs (16), while reaction against DF-2, a mAb to PHF that recognizes ubiquitin, and against pAbs to ubiquitin are located in the filaments exclusively in the periphery, but not in the center (Fig. 4).

The results of recent studies suggest that most of the filamentous material in LBs is related to NFs and contains various antigenic determinants of the NF triplet proteins that, however, undergo biochemical changes within the inclusions during their development. In contrast to ANT, all of the anti-NF antibodies do recognize most of the LBs, particularly their periphery, while the cores of the reactive LBs often remain unstained, although sensitive EM techniques have demonstrated weak anti-NF reactivity in the core (16). The uncovering of NF epitopes by treatment with phosphates indicates that LBs contain epitopes covered with phosphate and that phosphorylation of cytoskeletal elements may play a role in the pathogenesis of LBs. Phosphorylation of cytoskeletal elements is considered to be a posttranslational event rendering neurofilaments more compact and preventing them from proteolytic degradation (19). Under normal circumstances, phosphorylated NF are chiefly found in axons (3). The presence of phosphorylated NFP in perikarya in the form of LBs and other inclusions indicates that in affected neurons phosphorylation processes take place at an abnormal localization, leading to the accumulation of abnormal fibrillary proteins within the nerve cell body (16). This may occur as a cause or consequence of impaired assembling and transport of NF proteins (27,28) that undergo progressive biochemical and structural changes. These changes may represent the molecular correlate of the different appearance and immunoreactivity (IR) of the central core and periphery of LBs, and the different forms of both typical and cortical LBs that probably represent different stages of development. Ballooned neurons in other neurodegenerative dementing disorders, e.g., Pick's disease, corticonigral degeneration, and AD, also contain phosphorylated NF epitopes, but not epitopes unique to ANF and Pick bodies, and have been suggested to result from impaired axoplasmic transport of neurofilaments (28). The fact that proteins with abnormal structure are more readily conjugated to ubiquitin than are most normal proteins (29) could explain the presence of determinants of ubiquitin in both ANT and LBs. The most important function of ubiquitin is in an ATP-dependent proteolytic system responsible for degradation of short-living or abnormal proteins in the cell (29,30). The conjugation of ubiquitin with proteins after covalent binding to degradating enzymes is obligatory for the subsequent protein degradation. Recent data provided evidence for the existence of ubiquitin in both PHF and ANT (19,21,22), which have been shown to contain phosphorylated epitopes of tau protein as a major antigenic component (24,25,31–35). In this respect, the filaments of LBs are distinct from PHF though both are ubiquinated, since they do *not* bind antisera to tau and to PHF containing dominant tau reactivity (19,20). Only the center of LBs strongly reacts with a mAb to PHF that recognizes determinants of ubiquitin while ubiquitin reacts intensely in the periphery of typical and cortical LBs, and reaction products are located only in radiating filaments of the periphery, but not in the densely packed filaments of the center (19).

The frequent coexistence of both LBs and ANT in the same brain of PD patients and in diffuse Lewy body disease (DLBD) (7,10,15,17,19), the occasional presence of both LB and PHF in the same neuronal perikaryon (7,19,36) (Fig. 5), and the sharing of several epitopes have led to the speculation that both types of neuronal inclusions might have a pathogenic relationship. Although LBs and ANFTs are likely to result from alterations of the neuronal cytoskeleton, some of the basic cytoskeletal components involved in these inclusions are different. The function of ubiquitin in LBs is supposedly similar to that in PHF: conjugation to abnormal cytoskeletal proteins, presumably noxious for neurons, that should be removed by deg-

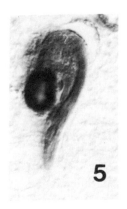

Fig. 5.   Neuron in locus coeruleus in DLBD showing coexisting LB and NFT, both labeled with anti-ubiquitin ($\times$ 200).

radation. However, the ubiquinated proteins in both LBs and PHFs are apparently different, phosphorylated neurofilaments, presumably being the integral component of the LBs and phosphorylated tau proteins being those of PHF. Monoclonal antibodies against LBs have been raised from parkinsonian brain (37), but the molecular basic and principal mechanisms for their development and degradation are still poorly understood. They have been suggested to represent accumulation of phosphorylated NFs undergoing progressive structural breakdown (12) or sequestrated NFs after neuronal regeneration (38) or retrograde degeneration (39). Although ubiquination of abnormal proteins in LBs presumably occurs after filament accumulation and ectopic phosphorylation, it is not known why LBs are resistant to the ATP-dependent proteolysis system despite ubiquination, since no degradation of LBs has ever been observed by light and electron microscopy (7,12,40).

LBs in catecholaminergic neurons show IR with antisera to tyrosine hydroxylase (TH), the rate-limiting enzyme of catecholamine synthesis, suggesting that TH enzyme activity is preserved in neurons involved with LBs or even may play a role in their formation (41). On the other hand, neurons in substantia nigra and locus coeruleus affected by NFTs in PD, progressive supranuclear palsy (PSP), Parkinson–dementia complex (PDC), and AD show positive TH-IR until the perikarya are entirely replaced by NFTs, indicating that these neurons still contain TH enzyme protein, except in the final stages of ghost tangle formation (42). In PD, most of the remaining melanin-pigmented neurons in the substantia nigra and ventral tegmental area and in the noradrenergic locus coeruleus and dorsal vagal nucleus show substantial reduction or less of TH-IR, as do fibers and terminals in the ascending and descending dopaminergic and noradrenergic systems in brain and spinal cord (40,43), indicating severe damage to these catecholaminergic systems. The role of neuromelanin in LB formation has been a matter of speculation (7). Ultrastructurally, melanin granules in nigral and locus coeruleus neurons of PD brains often cannot be distinguished from those in normal individuals (Fig. 6), but there can be a decrease in the very dense component of melanin granules in PD. The substructure of the altered melanin granules including the presence of linear arrays resembles that of lipofuscin (9), but the relationship between these ultrastructural changes and both LB formation and degeneration of melanin-containing cells remains unknown.

LBs occur in 85 to 100% of the brains of patients with idiopathic PD in wide distribution (7,12,40,45) and have been observed in 1 to 25% of the remaining nigral neurons (44). However, they are not found in all cases of PD and some regions showing little loss of pigmented neurons, e.g., the periventricular hypothalamus, are relatively spared from LBs (7). Although the LBs frequently affect aminergic neurons (45), and in the cerebral cortex show a distribution pattern partly corresponding to that of dopaminergic

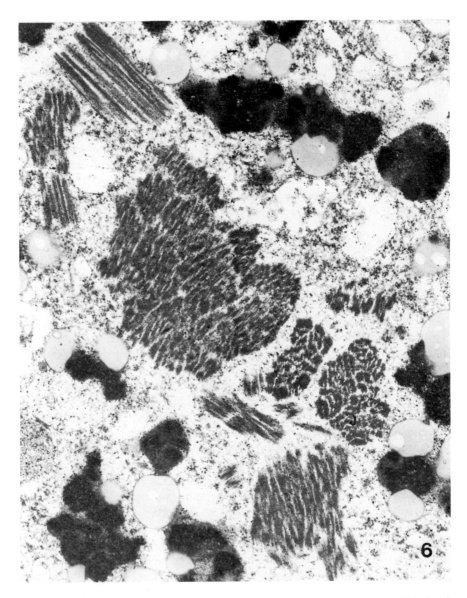

Fig. 6. Intracytoplasmic aggregates of parallel beaded and twisted filaments in nigral neuron ($\times$ 22,950).

axon terminals (46), they appear not to represent a cytoskeletal abnormality specific for any chemically determined neuronal system.

LBs also occur in pigmented brainstem nuclei in 5% of normal controls over the age of 30 years and in 8 to 15% of normal brains over age 65 years (7,12,40), but in 45 to 60% of all cases of AD and SDAT (40,47,48). In addition, LBs in the substantia nigra and brainstem have been found in several cases of PSP (49) and in other CNS disorders, e.g., ataxia–telangiectasia, Hallervorden–Spatz disease, multisystem degenerations, and chronic panencephalitis (7,12,40,49). Hence, LBs are not pathognomonic for PD, but are considered probably to be more characteristic for this disorder than the NFTs, for AD/SDAT (7). Recently, Forno *et al.* (50) reported eosinophilic inclusions in neurons of the substantia nigra, locus coeruleus, and dorsal raphe nucleus in MPTP-treated aged monkeys, suggesting similarity with the pathology of human PD. However, the ultrastructure of these bodies composed of 20-nm filaments appears to differ from human LBs (Forno, 1987, personal communication).

HIRANO BODIES

These rod-shaped eosinophilic intracytoplasmic inclusions, first described in the hippocampus of Guam patients with amyotrophic lateral sclerosis and Parkinson–dementia complex (ALS-PDC) (51), are composed of 6- to 10-nm filaments that are arranged in a regular latticework or as skeins of parallel filaments with adjacent layers that cross obliquely with a periodicity of 20 to 25 nm (2,4). Ultrastructural image analysis indicated that these filaments are helical strands with a pitch of 18.5 nm that appear lattice-like when arranged in parallel (52). At the borders of the bodies, the thin 6-nm filaments may be continuous with the matrix of the inclusion. Immunocytochemically they react with antibodies to actin, tropomyosin, α-actidin, and vinculin (53), but not with NF proteins, and they also share epitopes with the microtubule-associated protein tau (54). Actin appears to be the major cytoskeletal component of HBs that, with high-voltage electron microscopy, shows a purely filamentous nature (53). The presence of these proteins suggests that HBs are derived from an abnormal organization of the neuronal cytoskeleton, their formation presumably being different from that of the LBs and NFTs (53). In humans, HBs are found in the pyramidal cell layer of the hippocampus and subiculum, but also in cerebral cortex and other areas increasing with age. HBs are also seen in PD, AD, Pick's disease, Creutzfeldt–Jakob disease, and motor neuron disease, for example. They also occur in various cell types (neuron, glia, Schwann cells, and muscle) and have been found in other species (2,4,53). In the brindled mouse model, HB formation appears to be consistent with the polymerization of G-actin and/or reorganization of F-actin within dendrites. Its neurochemical basis may be related to the decline in glucose oxidation and acetylcholine synthesis that occurs prior to HB formation (4).

INTRACYTOPLASMIC EOSINOPHILIC GRANULES

The melanin-containing neurons of the substantia nigra and locus coeruleus in normal aged brain, PD, PSP, and various disorders may contain small intracytoplasmic granules composed of aggregates of parallel banded or twisted 8.5 nm filaments (55) (Fig. 6), while others regard them as altered mitochondria (2). Immunocytochemical data are not available so far.

MARINESCO BODIES

These intranuclear eosinophilic inclusions occurring in the pigmental neurons of the substantia nigra and locus coeruleus consist of aggregates of moderately osmiophilic material with a lattice-like meshwork of 10- to 12-nm filaments (56,57). They are often multiple within a single nucleus, and their periphery shows a delicate, sharply demarcated ring of IR with a mAb to PHF (20). These inclusions are found in both PD and normal brains with increasing numbers in advancing age (58). However, their relationship to cytoskeletal abnormalities in aging brain remains to be established.

NEUROFIBRILLARY TANGLES

These flame-shaped or globose intraneuronal inclusions that can be readily identified with silver stains are the most prominent lesions found in AD and aging brain, along with neuritic plaques (NP). NFTs are located in the neuronal perikarya and may enter the axonal hillock or proximal dendrite. They are also found in axon terminals, where they contribute to the neuritic component of NP (59). In AD/SDAT, neuronal dendrites are often packed with PHF and show a complete loss of normal microtubules, which are replaced by PHFs (60). The NFTs appear in two major forms: (a) the Alzheimer NFTs (ANTs) that are mainly composed of PHFs sometimes admixed with 12- to 15-nm straight filaments (22,61,62), which are a major constituent of extracellular tangles (63), and have been observed in continuity with classical PHFs in cerebral cortex (64); occasional filaments display a transition between straight and PHF (65); and (b) the NFTs in PSP that are predominantly made up of 15 nm straight filaments sometimes admixed with typical PHFs (66–68).

Alzheimer Neurofibrillary Tangles

The ANFTs are ultrastructurally composed of close-packed PHFs that are different from normal cytoskeletal filaments. They consist of two helically wrapped 8–12 filaments that cross each other at 65- to 80-nm intervals (69). Each of the 10-nm filaments consists of four protofilaments, each with a diameter of 3 to 5 nm, composed of eight longitudinally connected globules with short sidearms (70). They are composed of bonds of cross-connected proteins sharing antigen determinants with both normal and abnormal brain constituents. Immunocytochemical studies indicate that PHFs react with antibodies against normal cytoskeletal proteins, like NFPs (4,71–74), phosphorylated and hidden NF epitopes (4,75,76), microtubules (31,77), microtubule-associated protein MAP 1 and MAP 2 (32,72), and with the heat-stable microtubule-associated tau protein (23–25,32–35). In addition, ANFTs contain determinants unique to ANFTs (4,23,26,78), and mAbs raised against ANFTs recognize only tangles in cell bodies, neurites in plaques, and numerous fine neuritic processes in areas with many tangles (4), but do not react with any other neuronal or nonneuronal tissue components. The binding sites, detected by immunoelectron microscopy, are located on PHFs (4,65,79). In AD brain, four types of abnormal tau-IR have been recognized (35): NFTs, thickened neurites in plaques, diffuse perikaryal staining in some neurons apparently lacking NFTs, and a dispersed network of randomly oriented thickened neurites not clustered into discrete plaques but found in cerebral cortex rich in NFTs and NFs, indicating widespread abnormality of abnormal tau proteins in AD. Ubiquitin is present in PHFs (19,21,22) that contain phosphorylated epitopes of tau as the major constituent (23–25,31–35). Immunocytochemical staining of ANFTs is identical in AD and SDAT, the most intense IR being found with aBs to PHF and to tau, whereas in nondemented aged controls, neurons react with anti-tau, but none with anti-PHF. Ultrastructural studies using immunogold demonstrated that IR of ANFTs with anti-tau and anti-PHF is associated with PHFs (Fig. 7) that, however, also share epitopes with NFs (4,65,80). Recent studies suggest a stepwise progressive change in the IR pattern of ANT formation, where one can distinguish four stages [with early accumulation of tau (80a)]. The initial stage 0, seen in brains of aged nondemented subjects, shows diffuse IR of neuronal perikarya to anti-tau with completely negative reaction to anti-ubiquitin. This diffuse perikaryal staining seen in neurons apparently lacking NFTs detectable in silver stains appears to indicate a "pretangle" stage (35). Stage I is characterized by small perinuclear cytoplasmic fibrillary inclusions in silver stains that show strong reaction with anti-tau, but only occasional weak reaction with ubiquitin; stage II, the fully developed flame-shaped ANFT, demonstrates strong reactivity to both anti-tau and anti-ubiquitin, indicating progressive loss of tau proteins and increasing ubiquination, whereas in the final stage III, the ghost tangles are almost entirely reactive with ubiquitin but show only little reaction with anti-tau. Transformation of degenerating NFTs into neurofibrillary amyloid substances in AD has been reported (81).

These data indicate that formation of ANFTs is initially characterized by

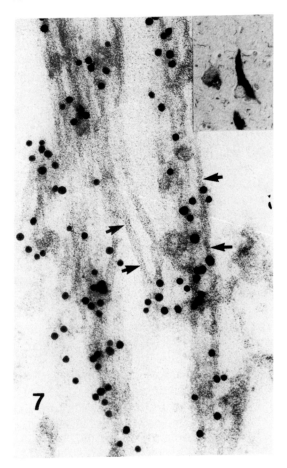

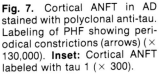

Fig. 7. Cortical ANFT in AD stained with polyclonal anti-tau. Labeling of PHF showing periodical constrictions (arrows) ($\times$ 130,000). **Inset:** Cortical ANFT labeled with tau 1 ($\times$ 300).

the presence of tau protein or phosphorylated epitopes of tau, with progressive loss of IR to tau protein associated with progressive ubiquination in the course of degradation of abnormal neuronal cytoskeletal proteins. While in normal aged brain the majority of neuronal perikarya show persisting anti-tau reactivity without ubiquination during increasing age, in AD, and SDAT, the ANFTs demonstrate progressive loss of IR to tau associated with progressive ubiquination. Abnormal translational phosphorylation of tau (82), resulting in defective assembly of the microtubule system (31), has been suggested as an important mechanism in the formation of ANFTs in which normal microtubules are completely replaced by PHFs (60). An alternative explanation suggests that abnormal phosphorylation of NF high molecular weight polypeptides is an important pathogenic step (76).

ANFTs composed of PHFs are found in increasing density in brains of normal aged subjects and particularly abundant in AD and SDAT, but are also present in PD/AD, postencephalitic parkinsonism (83), Guamanian ALS–PD complex (84), dementia pugilistica (85), and in a variety of other conditions unrelated to AD and PD (86). ANFTs in these various diseases react with anti-NF and anti-ANT/PHF antibodies in a manner similar to that found in AD (4,17,72). Recent studies showed that a substantial number (at least 50%) of cortical NFTs contain cholinesterase activities in both AD and nondemented aged individuals (87). The morphological appearance of NFTs obtained with acetylcholinesterase (AChE) stain was identical to that with silver and thioflavin-S stains. This suggests that some enzyme constituents of NFTs have AChE activities or that such enzymes are passively trapped within the tangle, but the relationship between tangle formation and cholinergic enzyme activities remains poorly understood (87). Whether it contributes to or occurs in response to the tangle remains to be determined. In general, it appears that the formation of ANFTs that involve neurons of varying transmitter specificities, including cholinergic neurons in the basal forebrain and hippocampus (88), is a nonspecific response of the perikaryal cytoskeleton of certain neurons to a variety of noxious factors, the basic mechanisms of which are currently unknown.

Neurofilaments in Progressive Supranuclear Palsy

PSP, a progressive, sporadic, PD-like disorder with ophthalmoplegia, axial dystonia, rigid akinesia, pseudobulbar palsy, and dementia (89), shows widespread NFTs and multisystem neuronal loss, with the hippocampus and neocortex being preserved. The NFTs in PSP differ from the ANFTs in AD/ SDAT, PEP, and Guam PDC in their distribution (90) and ultrastructure. They are made up of 15- to 20-nm straight filaments that are sometimes mixed with PHFs (66–68,79,90,91) and concurrence of straight and paired helical filaments in the same patient or even in the same neuron has been observed (67,68). They are recognized by anti-NF (17,65), anti-ANT, and anti-PHF antibodies (4,17,92), and the antigenetic determinants were considered to be localized to straight filaments (4). Recent studies, however, demonstrate that isolated monoclonal anti-PHF aBs recognize only few PSP tangles mainly due to admixed PHF (79). Immunoelectron microscopy shows that anti-tau reactivity of PSP tangles is associated with straight fibrils, whereas the monoclonal anti-PHF antibody does not stain them (Fig. 8). However, both PHF and straight fibrils were recognized by all antibodies after extraction with an ion detergent (22). These data indicate that the straight PSP filaments contain most, if not all, of the antigens known to be present in PHF, although at least one epitope in PHF seems to be absent on or at least inaccessible in PSP tangles. The coexistence of typical PHF and straight filaments in some cases of AD/SDAT and of PSP, including a continuous morphological transition between PHF and straight filaments,

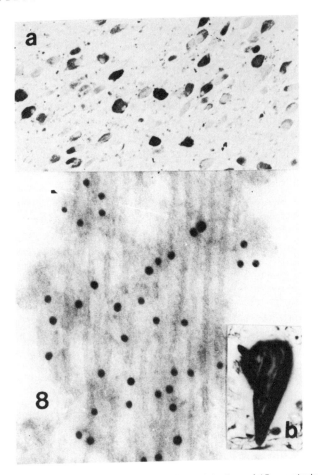

Fig. 8.   NFT of PSP stained with polyclonal anti-tau, labeling of 15-nm straight filaments (× 130,000). **Inset a:** Neurons in locus coeruleus of PSP strongly reactive to tau (arrows) (× 150). **Inset b:** Flame-shaped NFT in magnocellular reticular formation. Bodian (× 700).

may represent different stages of tangle formation, the PSP filaments possibly representing a more immature stage of tangle formation compared to AD/SDAT (79). An alternative explanation might assume that PSP tangles result from alternative pathways of organization of the same components as the PHF, rather than being PHF precursors (22). The pathways for formation of NFTs with different ultrastructural morphology await further elucidation.

GRANULOVACUOLAR DEGENERATION

These cytoplasmic inclusions, found in the pyramidal cells of the hippocampus, and occasionally in the innominata and amygdala, consist of clear vacuoles, 3–5 μm in diameter, with a dense core of 1–2 μm in diameter. At the ultrastructural level, they consist of an outer limiting membrane enclosing a vacuole that contains a granular central core (2). The granules contain tubulin, phosphorylated NFP (38,92a); some show positive (82) and others negative reaction with mAbs to tau (35). These bodies are common in elderly brains, with increasing number with age and much more so in AD/SDAT (2). A strong correlation between the frequency of neurons with GVD, the numbers of ANFTs, and the loss of pyramidal cells in hippocampus has been reported (93). Both the topographic specificity and the origin of these structures are unknown.

GRUMELOUS DEGENERATION AND AXONAL DYSTROPHY

Grumelous degeneration in the reticular zone of the substantia nigra (6) represents spheroid-like or ovoid swellings of axons, considered as a special form of axonal degeneration referred to as axonal dystrophy (94). The spheroids, which include accumulation of organelles, tubulovesicular structures, disarranged 10-nm neurofilaments, dense bodies, abnormal mitochondria, and lamellar profiles derived from the smooth endoplasmic reticulum, involve presynaptic axon terminals. They show positive IR with NF proteins and ubiquitin (Lassmann, personal communication) (Table 2), and have been related to disorders of axonal transport (94). The lesions affect primarily the gracile nucleus and reticulata nigrae in elderly subjects with close relation to age (95), but are also seen in a variety of disorders classified as "neuroaxonal dystrophies" (94). In PD, the incidence of axonal spheroids in the reticulata nigrae is significantly increased after the age of 50 years, and the same relationship to the depletion of melanin-containing neurons in the compacta nigrae with loss of contact to the postsynaptic neurons may be operative (94).

NEURITIC PLAQUES AND AMYLOID

NPs are homogenous or globular spherical densities that occur in the amygdala, hippocampus, neocortex, and in many subcortical areas in aged individuals and, to a much greater extent, in AD, SDAT, and demented cases of PD (38,40,96). Their principal components are dystrophic and degenerating neurites (enlarged axons, nerve terminals, and abnormal dendrites), distended with an excess of straight and PHF resembling components of NFTs, multilamellated lysosomal bodies, abnormals synapses, glia, and extracellular amyloid (38,59,69,96). Three types of NP are distinguished (96): primitive plaques composed of small numbers of amyloid fibers interspersed between degenerating neurites, the "classic" ones of a central amyloid core surrounded by abnormal neurites, and the compact (burnt-out) ones consisting of amyloid only. A further type in which no amyloid or altered neurites are found is considered to represent an initial stage of NP (97). Immunocytochemical studies have uncovered epitopes of NFP, tau, PHF, MAPs, and ubiquitin, most of which are also present in NFTs (Table 2), and a number of neurotransmitter synthesizing enzymes and neuropeptides in proximity to NPs (38,96,97). The transmitter specificities of IR neurites in NPs tend to reflect the distribution of transmitter-associated fibers in normal tissue, suggesting that a variety of transmitter systems are involved in the formation of these neuropil abnormalities (96,98). Formation of NPs has been related to degeneration of neuronal processes, but it is not known whether the abnormal filaments and other cytoskeletal elements are transported from NFT-bearing perikarya or are formed locally within distal axons. In addition, some neurites in NPs may represent regenerating sproutings from unaffected neurons (38,96–98).

The origin of plaque amyloid, composed of extracellular 8- to 10-nm fibrils predominantly made up of β-pleated sheet proteins, and its relation to cerebrovascular amyloid are hitherto unknown (38,96). Some investigators suggest that plaque amyloid may originate from neuronal cytoskeletal elements, e.g., NFTs derived from neurites in NPs (38,81,99), while others believe that blood-derived precursor proteins are an important pathogenic factor (100). Biochemical and immunocytochemical studies of NP and vascular amyloid in AD and aging brain indicate that the amyloid proteins found in these two loci are closely related and share epitopes with certain plasma proteins, but are distinct from intraneuronal PHFs (101–103). These data suggest that the NP and vascular amyloid are made of the same probable blood-derived precursor proteins, although they probably pass through different processing pathways (103). Further studies should help to elucidate the composition and origin of amyloid in the neuropil and cerebral vessels.

CONCLUSIONS

Pathologic changes in both PD and AD/SDAT or aging brain show a preponderance for certain neuronal systems with sparing of other populations. The at-risk neurons may demonstrate several types of cytoskeletal pathology, some of which may serve as diagnostic markers. Based on the morbid anatomy and cytoskeletal pathology, two major types of parkinsonism are distinguished (104): (a) the "Lewy body type," including idiopathic PD that is rather stereotyped and shows good correlation between the clinical picture and the degree of both morphological and biochemical deficits of the dopaminergic striatonigral system (105), and DLBD that encompasses a variety of PD-like disorders with transitions from PD to AD/SDAT (10,11,15,17,40); (b) the "Alzheimer type," morphologically featured by widespread NFTs with or without LBs, which includes a wide variety of disorders ranging from AD with concurrent PD or PD with superimposed AD (AD/PD, PD/

AD), AD extending to the brainstem, PSP, postencephalitic parkinsonism, Guam PD-C, and boxer's dementia (47,106). In addition to classical (pure) anatomical forms of PD and AD, both types of lesion can coexist, suggesting some links between the two disorders (107,108). In autopsy cohorts of PD individuals, the incidence of additional AD/SDAT ranges from 7 to 60% (40,47,107,109,110), whereas among 306 autopsy cases of PD, we observed additional AD pathology in 18.6% of the subjects dying before age 70 years, and in 37% of those dying after age 70 years (47). The severity of cortical lesions, expressed as a total Alzheimer score (four grades of intensity for both NFTs and NPs in the frontal cortex and hippocampus), in PD cases with no or only mild dementia, was similar to age-matched controls, and showed a positive correlation with age, while no such age dependency has been observed in demented PD subjects with additional AD (40,47). This negative relation of AD pathology is well established for AD and younger SDAT subjects, while about 40% of the demented senile PD cases showed associated SDAT (47). On the other hand, additional PD markers have been reported in 27 to 67% of proven cases of AD (47,108). Both clinical and pathological data suggest an increased risk of PD in patients with AD and *vice versa*, although the basis for an association between the two disorders remains to be determined.

The etiology of both PD and AD/SDAT is unknown, and the mechanisms leading to disorganization of the neuronal cytoskeleton with several types of structural changes in these and other aging processes of the CNS are poorly understood. Both the LBs and NFTs, representing the anatomical hallmarks of PD and brain aging, respectively, presumably result from disorganization of the neuronal cytoskeleton, but their overtly different ultrastructural and immunological features suggest that different cytoskeletal components are involved in their formation. The LBs are suggested to originate from an accumulation of phosphorylated neurofilaments, possibly resulting from impaired assembling and/or transport of NF proteins that undergo progressive ubiquination and structural disintegration, but the morphological basis of these changes and their relation with neuromelanin and neuronal loss are obscure. NFTs presumably originate from pathological phosphorylation of microtubule-associated tau protein related to defective assembly of the microtubular system that progressively undergoes ubiquination with loss of tau, progressive structural changes of the affected neuron, and possible transition into amyloid substances. The use of new scientific strategies will hopefully provide new information about biological processes leading to the various types of neuronal cytoskeletal disorders in order to enhance our understanding of some of the causes, mechanisms, and consequences of the cellular and molecular pathology in PD and brain aging.

REFERENCES

1. Bray, D., and Gilbert, D. (1981): *Annu. Rev. Neurosci.*, 4:505–543.
2. Hirano, A. (1985): In: *Textbook of Neuropathology*, edited by R. D. Davis and D. M. Robertson, Baltimore-London-Sidney, Williams & Wilkins, pp. 1–91.

3. Schlaepfer, W. W. (1987): *J. Neuropathol. Exp. Neurol.*, 46:117–129.
4. Yen, S. H., Dickson, D. W., Peterson, C., and Goldman, J. E. (1986): *Prog. Neuropathol.*, 6:63–90.
5. Lewy, F. H. (1912): In: *Handbuch der Neurologie*, edited by M. Lewandowsky, Berlin, Springer, pp. 920–958.
6. Trétiakoff, C. (1919): *Contribution à l'étude de l'anatomie pathologique du locus niger*, Thèse, Université Paris.
7. Forno, L. S. (1986): *Adv. Neurol.*, 45:35–43.
8. Kimula, Y., Utsuyama, M., Yoshimura, M., and Tomonaga, M. (1983): *Acta Neuropathol.*, 59:233–236.
9. Duffy, P. E., and Tennyson, V. M. (1965): *J. Neuropathol. Exp. Neurol.*, 24:398–414.
10. Kosaka, K., Yoshimura, M., Ikeda, K., and Budka, H. (1984): *Clin. Neuropathol.*, 3:185–192.
11. Popovitch, E. R., Wisniewski, H. M., Kaufman, M. A., et al. (1987): *Acta Neuropathol.*, 74:47–104.
12. Gibb, W. R. G. (1986): *Neuropathol. Appl. Neurobiol.*, 12:223–234.
13. Goldman, J. A., Yen, S. H., Chiu, F. C., and Peress, N. S. (1983): *Science*, 221:1082–1084.
14. Forno, L. S., Sternberger, L. A., Sternberger, N. H., et al. (1986): *Neurosci. Lett.*, 64:253–258.
15. Sima, A. A. F., Clark, A. W., Sternberger, N. A., and Sternberger, L. A. (1986): *Can. J. Neurol. Sci.*, 13:490–497.
16. Pappolla, M. A. (1986): *Arch. Pathol. Lab. Med.*, 110:1160–1163.
17. Dickson, D. W., Davies, P., Mayeux, R., et al. (1987): *Acta Neuropathol.*, 75:8–15.
18. Galloway, P., Grundke-Iqbal, I., Autilio-Gambetti, L., et al. (1987): *J. Neuropathol. Exp. Neurol.*, 46:374.
19. Kuzuhara, S., Mori, H., Izumiyama, N., et al. (1987): *Acta Neuropathol.*, 75:345–353.
20. Bancher, C., Lassmann, H., Budka, H., et al. (1988): *J. Neuropathol. Exp. Neurol.*, 48 (in press).
21. Mori, H., Kondo, J., and Ihara, Y. (1987): *Science*, 235:1641–1644.
22. Perry, G., Friedman, R., Shaw, G., and Chau, V. (1987): *Proc. Natl. Acad. Sci. U.S.A.*, 84:3033–3036.
23. Ihara, Y., Nukina, N., Miura, R., and Ogawara, M. (1986): *J. Biochem.*, 99:1807–1810.
24. Delacourte, A., and Defossez, A. (1986): *J. Neurol. Sci.*, 76:173–186.
25. Grundke-Iqbal, I., Iqbal, K., Quinlan, M., et al. (1986): *J. Biol. Chem.*, 261:6084–6089.
26. Grundke-Iqbal, I., Wang, G. P., Iqbal, K., et al. (1985): *Acta Neuropathol.*, 68:279–283.
27. Clark, A. W., Sternberger, N. H., Parhad, I. M., et al. (1986): *J. Neuropathol. Exp. Neurol.*, 45:333.
28. Dickson, D. W., Yen, S. H., Suzuki, K. I., et al. (1986): *Acta Neuropathol.*, 71:216–223.
29. Hershko, A., Athy, E., and Ciechanover, A. (1982): *J. Biol. Chem.*, 257:13964–13970.
30. Ciechanover, A., Finley, D., and Varshavsky, A. (1984): *Cell*, 37:57–66.
31. Iqbal, K., Grundke-Iqbal, I., Zaidi, T., et al. (1986): *Lancet*, 2:421–426.
32. Kosik, K. S., Joachim, C. L., and Selkoe, D. J. (1986): *Proc. Natl. Acad. Sci. U.S.A.*, 83:4044–4048.
33. Wood, J. G., Mirra, S. S., Pollock, N. J., and Binder, L. I. (1986): *Proc. Natl. Acad. Sci. U.S.A.*, 83:4040–4043.
34. Yen, S. H., Dickson, D. W., Crowe, A., et al. (1987): *Am. J. Pathol.*, 126:81–91.
35. Joachim, C. L., Morris, J. H., Selkoe, D. J., and Kosik, K. S. (1987): *J. Neuropathol. Exp. Neurol.*, 46:611–622.
36. Tomonaga, M. (1981): *Acta Neuropathol.*, 53:165–168.
37. Hirsch, E., Ruberg, M., Dardenne, M., et al. (1985): *Brain Res.*, 345:374–378.
38. Price, D. L., Whitehouse, P. J., and Struble, R. G. (1986): *Trends Neurol. Sci.*, 9:29–33.
39. Appel, S. H. (1981): *Ann. Neurol.*, 10:499–505.
40. Jellinger, K. (1987): In: *Movements Disorders*, Vol. 2, edited by C. D. Marsden and S. Fahn, London, Butterworths, pp. 124–165.
41. Nakashima, S., and Ikuta, F. (1984): *Acta Neuropathol.*, 64:273–280.
42. Nakashima, S., and Ikuta, F. (1987): *J. Neurol. Sci.*, 66:91–96.
43. Scatton, B., Dennis, T., Lheureux, R., et al. (1986): *Brain Res.*, 380:181–185.

44. Gibb, W. R. G., and Lee, A. J. (1987): *Acta Neuropathol.*, 73:195–201.
45. Ohama, E., and Ikuta, F. (1976): *Acta Neuropathol.*, 34:311–319.
46. Yoshimura, M. (1983): *J. Neurol.*, 229:17–32.
47. Jellinger, K. (1987): *J. Neural Transm., Suppl*, 24:109–129.
48. Ditter, S. M., and Mirra, S. S. (1987): *Neurology*, 37:754–760.
49. Mori, H., Yoshimura, M., Tomonaga, H., and Yamanouchi, H. (1986): *Acta Neuropathol.*, 71:344–346.
50. Forno, L. S., Langston, J. W., DeLanney, L. E., et al. (1986): *Ann. Neurol.*, 20:449–455.
51. Hirano, A., Dembitzer, H. M., Kurland, L. T., and Zimmerman, H. M. (1968): *J. Neuropathol. Exp. Neurol.*, 27:167–182.
52. Mori, H., Tomonaga, H., Baba, N., and Kanaya, K. (1986): *Acta Neuropathol.*, 71:32–37.
53. Galloway, P. G., Perry, G., and Gambetti, P. (1987): *J. Neuropathol. Exp. Neurol.*, 46:185–199.
54. Galloway, P. G., Perry, G., Kozik, K. S., and Gambetti, P. (1987): *Brain Res.*, 403:337–340.
55. Schochet, S. S., Wyatt, R., and McCormick, W. F. (1970): *Arch. Neurol.*, 22:550–555.
56. Leestma, J. E., and Andrews, J. M. (1969): *Arch. Pathol.* 88:431–436.
57. Janota, I. (1979): *Neuropathol. Appl. Neurobiol.*, 5:311–317.
58. Yuen, P., and Baxter, D. W. (1963): *J. Neurol. Neurosurg. Psychiatry*, 26:178–183.
59. Wisniewski, B. M., and Soifer, D. (1979): *Mechan Ageing Dev.*, 9:119–142.
60. Gray, E. G., Paula-Barbosa, M., and Roher, A. (1987): *Neuropathol. Appl. Neurobiol.*, 13:91–110.
61. Shibayama, H., and Kitch, J. (1978): *Acta Neuropathol.*, 41:229–234.
62. Yagishita, S., Itoh, Y., Wang, N., and Amano, N. (1981): *Acta Neuropathol.*, 54:239–246.
63. Okamoto, K., Hirano, A., Yamaguchi, H., and Hirai, S. (1983): *J. Clin. Electron Microsc.*, 16:77–82.
64. Yoshimura, N. (1984): *Clin. Neuropathol.*, 3:22–27.
65. Perry, G., Manetto, V., Autilio-Gambetti, L., and Gambetti, F. (1987): *J. Neuropathol. Exp. Neurol.*, 46:334.
66. Tellez-Nagel, I., and Wisniewski, B. M. (1973): *Arch. Neurol.*, 29:324–327.
67. Yagishita, S., Itoh, Y., Amano, N., et al. (1979): *Acta Neuropathol.*, 48:27–30.
68. Takauchi, S., Mizuhara, T., and Miyoshi, K. (1983): *Acta Neuropathol.*, 59:225–228.
69. Kidd, M. (1964): *Brain*, 87:307–320.
70. Wisniewski, H. M., and Wen, G. Y. (1985): *Acta Neuropathol.*, 66:173–176.
71. Gambetti, P., Shecket, G., Ghetti, B., et al. (1983): *J. Neuropathol. Exp. Neurol.*, 42:69–79.
72. Perry, G., Rizzuto, N., Autilio-Gambetti, L., and Gambetti, P. (1985): *Proc. Natl. Acad. Sci. U.S.A.*, 82:3916–3920.
73. Cork, L. C., Sternberger, N. H., Sternberger, L. A., et al. (1986): *J. Neuropathol. Exp. Neurol.*, 45:56–64.
74. Miller, C. C. J., Brion, J. P., and Calvert, R. (1986): *EMBO J.*, 5:269–276.
75. Haugh, M. C., Probst, A., Ulrich, J., et al. (1986): *J. Neurol. Neurosurg. Psychiatry*, 49:1213–1220.
76. Sternberger, N. H., Sternberger, L. A., and Ulrich, J. (1985): *Proc. Natl. Acad. Sci. U.S.A.*, 82:4274–4276.
77. Grundke-Iqbal, I., Johnson, A. B., Wisniewski, H. M., et al. (1979): *Lancet*, 1:578–580.
78. Brion, J. P., Couck, A. M., Passareiro, E., and Flament-Durand, J. (1985): *J. Submicrosc. Cytol.*, 17:89–96.
79. Bancher, P., Lassmann, H., Budka, H., et al. (1987): *Acta Neuropathol.*, 74:39–46.
80. Perry, G., Dennis, D. J., Bleck, B. R., et al. (1986): *J. Neuropathol. Exp. Neurol.*, 45:161–168.
80a. Bancher, C., Brunner, C., Lassman, H. (1988): *J. Neuropathol. Exp. Neurol.*, 47:335.
81. Defossez, A., and Delacourte, A. (1987): *J. Neurol. Sci.*, 81:1–10.
82. Grundke-Iqbal, I., Iqbal, K., Tung, Y. C., et al. (1986): *Proc. Natl. Acad. Sci. U.S.A.*, 83:4913–4917.
83. Ishii, T., and Nakamura, Y. (1981): *Acta Neuropathol.*, 55:59–62.

84. Hirano, A., and Llena, J. (1986): *Prog. Neuropathol.*, 6:17–31.
85. Corsellis, J. A. N., Bruton, C. J., and Freeman-Browne, D. (1973): *Psychol. Med.*, 3:270–303.
86. Wisniewski, K., Jervis, G. A., Moretz, R. C. and Wisniewski, H. M. (1979): *Ann. Neurol.*, 5:288–294.
87. Mesulam, M. M., and Moran, M. A. (1987): *Ann. Neurol.*, 22:223–228.
88. Rasool, C. G., Abraham, C., Anderton, B. H., et al. (1984): *Brain Res.*, 310:249–260.
89. Steele, J. C., Richardson, J. C., and Olszewski, J. (1964): *Arch. Neurol.*, 10:333–359.
90. Jellinger, K., Riederer, P., and Tomonaga, M. (1980): *J. Neural Transm., Suppl.*, 16:114–128.
91. Montpetit, V., Clapin, D. F., and Gubermann, A. (1985): *Acta Neuropathol.*, 68:311–318.
92. Gorevic, P. D., Goni, F., Pons-Estel, B., et al. (1986): *J. Neuropathol. Exp. Neurol.*, 45:647–664.
92a. Dickson, D. W., Kszeizak-Reding, H., Davies, P., et al. (1987): *Acta Neuropathol.*, 73:254–258.
93. Ball, M. J., and Lo, P. (1977): *J. Neuropathol. Exp. Neurol.*, 36:474–487.
94. Seitelberger, F. (1986): In: *Handbook of Clinical Neurology*, vol. 5 (49), edited by P. J. Vinken, G. W. Bruyn, and H. L. Klavans, Amsterdam-New York, Elsevier Science Publ, pp. 391–415.
95. Jellinger, K. (1973): *Prog. Neuropathol.*, 2:129–180.
96. Terry, W. (1985): In: *Textbook of Neuropathology*, edited by R. D. Davis and D. M. Robertson, Baltimore-London-Sidney, Williams & Wilkins, pp. 824–841.
97. Probst, A., Brunnschweiler, H., Lautenschlager, C., and Ulrich, J. (1987): *Acta Neuropathol.*, 74:133–141.
98. Struble, R. G., Powers, R. E., Casanova, M. F., et al. (1987): *J. Neuropathol. Exp. Neurol.*, 46:567–584.
99. Kang, J., Lemaire, H. G., Unterbeck, A., et al. (1987): *Nature (Lond.)*, 325:733–736.
100. Glenner, G. G., and Wong, C. W. (1984): *Biochem. Biophys. Res. Commun.*, 120:885–890.
101. Joachim, C. L., Duffy, L. K., and Selkoe, D. J. (1987): *J. Neuropathol. Exp. Neurol.*, 46:396.
102. Selkoe, D. J., Podlisny, M. B., Saperstein, A., and Duffy, L. K. (1987): *Neurology*, 37(suppl. 1):224.
103. Wisniewski, H. M. (1987): *Neurology*, 37(suppl. 1):331.
104. Alvord, E. D., Forno, L., Kusske, J. A., et al. (1974): *Adv. Neurol.*, 5:175–193.
105. Agid, Y., Javoy-Agid, F., and Ruberg, M. (1987): In: *Movement Disorders*, vol. 2. edited by C. D. Marsden and S. T. Fahn, London-Boston, Butterworths, pp. 166–230.
106. Sudhaker, S., Rajput, A. H., Rozdislky, B., and Uitti, R. J. (1987): *Neurology*, 37(suppl. 1):278–279.
107. Boller, F. (1985): In: *Senile Dementia of the Alzheimer Type*, edited by J. T. Hulton and A. D. Kennes, New York, Alan R. Liss, pp. 119–129.
108. Leverenz, J., and Sumi, M. (1986): *Arch. Neurol.*, 43:662–664.
109. Hakim, A. M., and Mathieson, G. (1979): *Neurology*, 20:1209–1214.
110. Perry, R. H., Perry, E. K., Smith, C. J., et al. (1987): *J. Neurol. Transm. Suppl.*, 24:131–136.

Parkinsonism and Aging, edited by
Donald B. Calne et al., Raven Press, Ltd.,
New York © 1989.

Biochemical Changes in Idiopathic Parkinson's Disease, Aging, and MPTP Parkinsonism: Similarities and Differences

Oleh Hornykiewicz, Christian Pifl, *Stephen J. Kish, *Kathleen Shannak, and †Günter Schingnitz

*Institute of Biochemical Pharmacology, University of Vienna, A-1090 Vienna, Austria; *Clarke Institute of Psychiatry, University of Toronto, Toronto, Ontario M5T 1R8, Canada; and †Department of Pharmacology, Boehringer Ingelheim KG, D-6507 Ingelheim, Federal Republic of Germany*

It is now well established that the major neuropathological change in Parkinson's disease is the loss of the melanin and, as we now know, dopamine-containing neurons in the compact zone of the substantia nigra. This nigral cell loss is directly responsible for the most characteristic neurochemical alteration in Parkinson's disease, namely the profound loss of dopamine in the substantia nigra and all basal ganglia regions that are the target areas of the nigrostriatal dopamine pathway, including the putamen, the caudate nucleus, the globus pallidus, and the nucleus accumbens (1).

Although many endogenous and exogenous factors are known to produce damage to the nigral dopamine neurons, the cause of the idiopathic variety of Parkinson's disease is as yet unknown.

The endogenous processes known to be potentially detrimental to the integrity of the nigral dopamine neurons are of special importance: excessive formation from dopamine of free (oxygen) radicals and hydrogen peroxide (either in the course of dopamine auto-oxidation to melanin, or its oxidative deamination by monoamine oxidase); and subnormal functioning, or lack, of biochemical mechanisms, including enzymes, for the removal of destructive oxygen radicals (e.g., catalase, peroxidase, reduced glutathione, glutathione peroxidase and reductase, and superoxide dismutase) (2–5).

Exogenous factors causing damage to the substantia nigra include viral infections (e.g., parkinsonism as a sequela to encephalitis lethargica), environmental toxins (herbicides and pesticides, carbon disulfite, and manganese), as well as the highly selective meperidine analog N-methyl-4-phenyl-1,2,3,6-tetrahydropyridine (MPTP) (6).

In addition to the endogenous and exogenous factors potentially neurotoxic to the substantia nigra, brain aging is known to produce a significant reduction of the dopamine- (and melanin-) containing neurons of the substantia nigra (7,8). The cause of the slow and progressive loss of nigral dopamine neurons with advancing age is unknown, but it has been hypothesized that (accelerated) aging of nigral dopamine neurons, possibly superimposed on a single, or protracted, subclinical nigral insult by a neurotoxic process occurring earlier in life, may be the most important combination of events in the pathoetiology of idiopathic Parkinson's disease (9,10).

Like all hypotheses on the cause, or causes, of idiopathic Parkinson's disease, the nigral dopamine loss due to aging and/or neurotoxic influences presupposes that the basic neurochemical brain dopamine change produced by the proposed mechanisms will be identical with the dopamine changes found in idiopathic Parkinson's disease. This follows from the fact that the striatal dopamine deficiency is the main brain abnormality responsible for the parkinsonian movement disorder (1). Therefore, only a very close replication of the typical dopamine changes will also replicate the clinical picture of this disorder.

In the following discussion, an attempt will be made to compare the striatal dopamine changes found in human subjects during "normal" aging and in MPTP-treated rhesus monkeys with the corresponding changes in patients with morphologically verified idiopathic Parkinson's disease.

STRIATAL DOPAMINE LOSS IN IDIOPATHIC PARKINSON'S DISEASE

A recent detailed study of the interregional and subregional patterns of striatal dopamine loss has permitted a very accurate neurochemical characterization of idiopathic Parkinson's disease (11). In this study, the head of the caudate nucleus and the putamen of eight patients dying with idiopathic Parkinson's disease were subdivided along both the rostrocaudal and dorsoventral extent of the structures, and the resulting interregional and subregional patterns of dopamine loss were compared with the dopamine patterns of ten neurologically and psychiatrically normal control subjects closely matched to the patients with respect to age and postmortem time.

Interregional Dopamine Pattern

Confirming previous observations (12), we found that the dopamine loss in the putamen as a whole was considerably more severe than the dopamine loss in the caudate nucleus. Compared with controls, in the putamen there was an average loss of dopamine by 98%; in contrast, in the caudate head a considerably less severe reduction, by about 81%, was found (Fig. 1). Expressed as a percent of dopamine remaining, in idiopathic Parkinson's

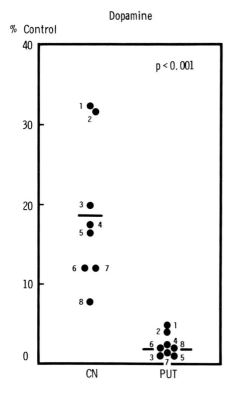

Fig. 1. Interregional pattern of striatal dopamine loss in idiopathic Parkinson's disease. Note the difference between caudate nucleus (CN) and putamen (PUT) with respect to severity of dopamine loss, observed in eight cases with histopathologically verified idiopathic Parkinson's disease. For the purpose of comparison, the individual patients are marked by numbers 1–8. The dopamine changes are expressed in % of the mean values ($n = 10$) of age-matched neurologically normal controls (caudate: 3.29 μg/g; putamen: 4.92 μg/g).

disease the caudate contained about nine times the amount of dopamine found in the putamen. The difference between caudate and putamen was statistically highly significant ($p < 0.001$). Since this dopamine pattern was found without exception in each case with histopathologically confirmed idiopathic Parkinson's disease, it must be concluded that the marked difference between caudate and putamen represents a characteristic feature of idiopathic Parkinson's disease. This conclusion is supported by our data, where, as shown in Table 1, no comparable pattern of striatal dopamine loss was present in any other neurodegenerative brain disease accompanied by striatal dopamine loss and presenting with parkinsonian symptomatology, including postencephalitic parkinsonism (12), progressive supranuclear palsy (13), neuronal intranuclear inclusion body disorder (14), "arteriosclerotic–senile" parkinsonism (12), and dementia–parkinsonism–amyotrophic lateral sclerosis complex (15).

Subregional Dopamine Pattern

Analysis of the subregional dopamine loss revealed that the degree of dopamine changes in the putamen and the caudate nucleus varied in a subre-

TABLE 1. *Striatal dopamine in several neurodegenerative brain disorders with parkinsonian symptomatology—comparison with idiopathic Parkinson's disease*

Brain disorder	Subregion of striatum	Dopamine in % of control[a]		Reference
		Caudate	Putamen	
Postencephalitic parkinsonism	Whole nucleus	1.5	0.6	12
Dementia–parkinsonism– amyotrophic lateral sclerosis complex	Intermediate (between rostral and caudal)	1.4	3.7	15
Neuronal intranuclear inclusion body disorder	Rostral	2.9	0.8	14
Progressive supranuclear palsy	Rostral	20	25	13
"Arteriosclerotic–senile" parkinsonism	Whole nucleus	32	15	12
Idiopathic Parkinson's disease	Whole nucleus	19	2	11

[a] For actual values, see references.

gionally topographic manner. This resulted in a rostrocaudal and dorso-ventral pattern of dopamine loss that was characteristic for each of the two striatal nuclei (11). As summarized in a simplified way in Table 2, in the much more severely affected putamen, all subdivisions were severely depleted of dopamine. The remaining dopamine levels ranged from 4% in the rostral subdivisions of the putamen to nearly total dopamine loss in the caudal part of the nucleus.

In the caudate nucleus, none of the subregions was as severely affected as in the putamen (11). As in the putamen, the subregional dopamine loss

TABLE 2. *Subregional pattern of striatal dopamine loss in idiopathic Parkinson's disease*

Subregional localization[a]	Putamen			Caudate head		
	Controls	Idiopathic PD	% Control	Controls	Idiopathic PD	% Control
Rostral (4/2)	4.60 ± 0.42	0.19 ± 0.08	4.1	2.70 ± 0.26	0.24 ± 0.06	8.9
Intermediate (7/4)	4.64 ± 0.41	0.11 ± 0.02	2.4	3.54 ± 0.42	0.77 ± 0.16	21.8
Caudal (10/10)	5.26 ± 0.48	0.07 ± 0.02	1.3	2.35 ± 0.33	0.72 ± 0.16	30.6

[a] In parentheses are given the analyzed slices, numbered along the rostrocaudal extent of the putamen/caudate; for exact topographic localization of the corresponding slices, see ref. 11, from which the data have been taken. The dopamine levels are means ± SEM, expressed in μg/g wet weight.

in the caudate nucleus was not uniform; however, compared with the putamen, the rostrocaudal dopamine gradient in the caudate was in the opposite
direction. Thus, the rostral caudate head suffered a larger dopamine loss,
by about 91%, than the caudal caudate head, where no more than 69% dopamine was lost (Table 2).

THE NEUROCHEMICAL DEFINITION OF IDIOPATHIC PARKINSON'S DISEASE

It is of great importance to bear in mind that the typical patterns of striatal
dopamine loss described above are a very regular feature of idiopathic Parkinson's disease. A critical evaluation of the data published in the literature
(see ref. 1) reveals that of all the studied neurotransmitter changes, the interregional pattern of striatal dopamine loss is the only change found, without
any exception, in each case with neuropathologically verified idiopathic Parkinson's disease. In contrast to the nondopamine changes, the reduced dopamine levels in putamen as well as in caudate nucleus are, as shown in Fig.
2, in each case well outside the range of the normal control values.

Taken together with the direct relationship that has been established between the degree of striatal dopamine loss and the severity of the parkinsonian movement disorder (12), the characteristic striatal dopamine pattern
can be considered as the most consistent and specific neurochemical marker
of idiopathic Parkinson's disease. The highly specific striatal dopamine
changes are undoubtedly the result of the underlying specific (nigral) pathology. Therefore, they can be taken as being a reliable index of the processes involved in the pathoetiology of idiopathic Parkinson's disease, thus
representing a dependable criterion by which the validity of any etiologic
hypothesis of this disorder can be judged.

Therefore, if the aging/neurotoxin hypothesis of idiopathic Parkinson's
disease is to be valid, at least one of the etiological factors, aging or a MPTP-
like neurotoxin, should mimic the specific dopamine patterns found in the
striatum of patients with idiopathic Parkinson's disease.

AGE-RELATED STRIATAL DOPAMINE CHANGES IN NEUROLOGICALLY NORMAL SUBJECTS

There is sufficient evidence to show that the human nigrostriatal dopamine
neurons are especially sensitive to the aging process (7,8). The age-related
decay of the nigral dopamine results in an average loss of striatal dopamine
levels of approximately 6 to 8% per decade of life. Thus, by the end of the
sixth decade, a 40 to 50% reduction of striatal dopamine can be expected
to occur as a consequence of this, due to the nigral dopamine neurons' "normal" aging process. By itself, this "physiological" loss of striatal dopamine

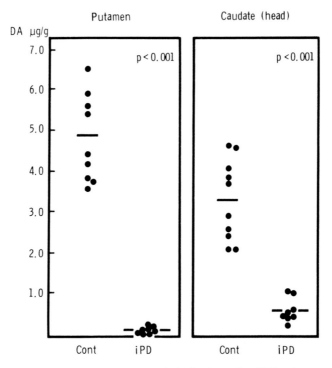

Fig. 2. Comparison between the ranges of single dopamine (DA) values, expressed in μg/g wet weight, in the putamen and caudate (head) of control cases (Cont) and of cases with histologically confirmed idiopathic Parkinson's disease (iPD). Note that in no single instance of idiopathic Parkinson's disease is there any overlap with control values.

is not sufficient to produce overt symptoms of Parkinson's disease. From studies in patients with Parkinson's disease (12) as well as monkeys with experimental nigral lesions (16), it can be concluded that symptoms do not become manifest unless 80% or more striatal dopamine has been lost. Deficits due to lower degrees of dopamine depletion can be offset by increased activity in the remaining dopamine neurons, which possess an exceptionally high capacity for functional compensation (1).

Recently, we measured the concentration of dopamine in the caudate and putamen in a group of five senescent neurologically normal controls (mean age of 79 years) and compared the results with dopamine values found in a younger group of five neurologically normal controls (mean age of 30 years). As shown in Fig. 3, the results of this preliminary study indicate that the dopamine level in the caudate nucleus of the senescent subjects was only 39% of the dopamine level found in the caudate nucleus of the younger subjects. In the putamen, the corresponding dopamine level in the senescent group was 50% of the dopamine level measured in the younger subjects. This observation is, in principle, in accord with an earlier report (17) and

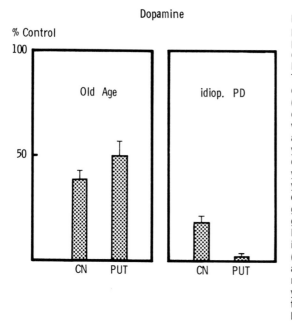

Fig. 3. Interregional (caudate/putamen) pattern of striatal dopamine loss due to old age—comparison with idiopathic Parkinson's disease (idiop. PD). The dopamine changes in caudate nucleus (CN) and putamen (PUT) are expressed in % of the corresponding mean of control values. Controls for the "old age" group (mean age of 79 years, $n = 5$) served a group of five neurologically normal younger cases (mean age of 30 years). The actual dopamine levels in the younger reference group were for caudate: 6.66 μg/g and for putamen: 8.85 μg/g. For the group of patients with idiopathic Parkinson's disease (mean age of 71 years, $n = 8$), age-matched neurologically normal controls (mean age of 75 years, $n = 10$) were used (for actual dopamine means, see the legend to Fig. 1).

shows that, although the age-related decay of the nigrostriatal dopamine is real, the resulting interregional pattern of striatal dopamine loss is opposite to the dopamine pattern typical of idiopathic Parkinson's disease (Fig. 3).

As regards the subregional dopamine patterns in the caudate nucleus and the putamen, we have some tentative data suggesting that in the senescent brain these patterns resemble, although not on the quantitative level, the dopamine patterns found in idiopathic Parkinson's disease. Despite this possible similarity, the main conclusion that can be drawn from our observations is that aging could only play a role in the pathoetiology of idiopathic Parkinson's disease if it combined with another factor that would produce a very region-selective neurotoxic damage to those neurons of the substantia nigra that provide the putamen with its dopamine innervation.

Does perhaps MPTP represent such a region-specific neurotoxin, selective for the putamen dopamine?

MPTP-INDUCED STRIATAL DOPAMINE CHANGES IN THE RHESUS MONKEY

Since so far it has not been possible to obtain data on striatal dopamine in patients with MPTP-induced parkinsonism, we recently studied the interregional and subregional patterns of striatal dopamine loss in rhesus monkeys with permanent MPTP parkinsonism (18).

TABLE 3. *Dopamine in the caudate nucleus and putamen in rhesus monkeys with MPTP-induced permanent parkinsonism*

	Dopamine (μg/g)		
	Controls[a]	MPTP[a]	% of control
Caudate	8.54 ± 0.64	0.037 ± 0.018	0.43
Putamen	10.48 ± 1.34	0.054 ± 0.008	0.52

[a] Number of monkeys = 4. Data taken from Ref. 18.

In four adult rhesus monkeys, permanent symptoms of typical Parkinson's disease (bradykinesia, akinesia, freezing episodes, flexed posture, and postural tremor) were produced by repeated intramuscular injections of small doses of MPTP (single doses between 0.15 and 0.4 mg/kg; total doses between 2.1 and 6.45 mg/kg). After a survival time of 1.5 to 7 months, the striatal nuclei were dissected and analyzed for dopamine, and the results compared with dopamine values obtained in four untreated monkeys.

Compared with the mean values obtained in control animals, the striatal dopamine concentrations in the MPTP-treated monkeys were severely reduced to less than 1% of control values (Table 3). This confirms published observations (19–28) and establishes MPTP as a very efficient parkinsonism-inducing agent in the primate.

However, our results demonstrate that doses of MPTP that induce permanent parkinsonism deplete the striatum completely unselectively of its dopamine. In these MPTP monkeys, there were no apparent interregional or subregional differences typical for idiopathic Parkinson's disease. Thus, in sharp contrast to idiopathic Parkinson's disease, in our monkeys with persistent parkinsonism, the dopamine loss in the caudate nucleus (− 99.6%) was at least as severe as in the putamen (− 99.5%) (Table 3). There was also in these MPTP animals no unequivocal indication of a significant rostrocaudal dopamine gradient; both the rostral and the caudal subdivisions of the caudate nucleus and the putamen seemed about equally affected by (maximal) dopamine loss. Thus, in our rhesus monkeys, MPTP mimicked more closely the diffuse and profound striatal dopamine loss found in postencephalitic parkinsonism (12) (see Table 1) rather than the discrete dopamine pattern typical of idiopathic Parkinson's disease.

In a preliminary study, repeated daily administration of subclinical doses of MPTP (0.1 mg/kg for 32 days) resulted in a less complete striatal dopamine depletion (with approximately 5 to 20% dopamine still detectable) and a subregional dopamine loss qualitatively (but not quantitatively) somewhat similar to the rostrocaudal dopamine loss typical of idiopathic Parkinson's disease. However, despite this rough similarity, in this animal the interregional pattern of dopamine loss was just the reverse of the dopamine pattern characteristic of idiopathic Parkinson's disease, with the caudate nucelus being more affected by dopamine loss than the putamen.

If one assumes that in humans the MPTP-induced striatal dopamine changes are qualitatively identical with the dopamine changes we have observed in our rhesus monkeys, the apparent inability of MPTP to replicate the interregional pattern of striatal dopamine loss typical of idiopathic Parkinson's disease makes the notion unlikely that a neurotoxic factor with a MPTP-like mechanism of action may be involved in the etiology of idiopathic Parkinson's disease.

CONCLUSIONS

We have compared the characteristic behavior of striatal dopamine in three conditions that are accompanied by significant loss of this basal ganglia neurotransmitter, i.e., in idiopathic Parkinson's disease, in senescent neurologically normal human subjects, and in MPTP-treated rhesus monkeys.

From our study, which is still in progress, we conclude that there are substantial qualitative differences between these three conditions as regards the observed patterns of striatal dopamine loss. This suggests that with respect to the etiological factors that may underly the pathological processes responsible for the respective changes in striatal dopamine, these three conditions appear to represent three separate entities, each with a specific etiology of its own.

The most distinctive neurochemical feature of idiopathic Parkinson's disease that is not mimicked by any of the other examined conditions is the marked degree and pattern of dopamine loss in the putamen as compared with the caudate nucleus. This suggests that one of the central aspects of the pathoetiology of idiopathic Parkinson's disease must involve a mechanism that is preferentially operative in those nigral dopamine neurons that control the functioning of the putamen.

In this respect, Hassler's observations may be relevant that those nigra (compacta) cell groups that have the highest neuronal density are precisely the sites that, in idiopathic Parkinson's disease, are most markedly affected by neuronal degeneration (29).

REFERENCES

1. Hornykiewicz, O., and Kish, S. J. (1986): Biochemical pathophysiology of Parkinson's disease. In: *Advances in Neurology*, Vol. 45, edited by M. D. Yahr and K. J. Bergmann, pp. 19–34. Raven Press, New York.
2. Cohen, G. (1983): The pathobiology of Parkinson's disease: biochemical aspects of dopamine neuron senescence. *J. Neural Transm.*, 19(suppl):89–103.
3. Cohen, G. (1984): Oxy-radical toxicity in catecholamine neurons. *Neurotoxicology*, 5:77–82.

4. Halliwell, B. (1987): Oxidants and human disease: some new concepts. *FASEB J.*, 1:358–364.
5. Southorn, P. A., and Powis, G. (1988): Free radicals in medicine. I. Chemical nature and biological reactions. *Mayo Clin. Proc.*, 63:381–389.
6. Langston, J. W., Irwin, I., and Ricaurte, G. A. (1987): Neurotoxins, parkinsonism and Parkinson's disease. *Pharmacol. Ther.*, 32:19–49.
7. Hornykiewicz, O. (1987): Neurotransmitter changes in human brain during aging. In: *Modification of Cell to Cell Signals During Normal and Pathological Aging*, NATO ASI Series, Vol. H9, edited by S. Govoni and F. Battaini, pp. 169–182. Springer-Verlag, Berlin-Heidelberg.
8. Hornykiewicz, O. (1985): Brain dopamine and aging. *Interdiscipl. Topics Gerontol.*, 19:143–155.
9. Calne, D. B., McGeer, E., Eisen, A., and Spencer, P. (1986): Alzheimer's disease, Parkinson's disease, and motoneurone disease: abiotropic interaction between aging and environment? *Lancet*, 2:1067–1070.
10. Langston, J. W. (1985): MPTP and Parkinson's disease. *Trends Neurosci.* 8:79–83.
11. Kish, S. J., Shannak, K., and Hornykiewicz, O. (1988): Uneven pattern of dopamine loss in the striatum of patients with idiopathic Parkinson's disease. *N. Engl. J. Med.*, 318:876–880.
12. Bernheimer, H., Birkmayer, W., Hornykiewicz, O., Jellinger, K., and Seitelberger, F. (1973): Brain dopamine and the syndromes of Parkinson and Huntington. *J. Neurol. Sci.*, 20:415–455.
13. Kish, S. J., Chang, L. J., Mirchandani, L., Shannak, K., and Hornykiewicz, O. (1985): Progressive supranuclear palsy: relationship between extrapyramidal disturbances, dementia, and brain neurotransmitter markers. *Ann. Neurol.*, 18:530–536.
14. Kish, S. J., Gilbert, J. J., Chang, L. J., Mirchandani, L., Shannak, K., and Hornykiewicz, O. (1985): Brain neurotransmitter abnormalities in neuronal intranuclear inclusion body disorder. *Ann. Neurol.*, 17:405–407.
15. Gilbert, J. J., Kish, S. J., Chang, L-J., Morito, C., Shannak, K., and Hornykiewicz, O. (1988): Dementia, parkinsonism, and motor neuron disease: neurochemical and neuropathological correlates. *Ann. Neurol.*, 24:688–691.
16. Poirier, L. J., Sourkes, T. L., Bouvier, G., Boucher, R., and Carabin, S. (1966): Striatal amines, experimental tremor and the effect of harmaline in the monkey. *Brain*, 89:37–52.
17. Carlsson, A. (1981): Aging and brain neurotransmitters. In: *Strategies for the Development of an Effective Treatment for Senile Dementia*, edited by T. Crook and S. Gershon, pp. 93–104. M. Powley Associates, New Canaan, CT.
18. Pifl, Ch., Schingnitz, G., and Hornykiewicz, O. (1988): The neurotoxin MPTP does not reproduce in the rhesus monkey the interregional pattern of striatal dopamine loss typical of human idiopathic Parkinson's disease. *Neurosci. Lett.*, 92:228–233.
19. Bédard, P. J., DiPaolo, T., Falardeau, P., and Boucher, R. (1986): Chronic treatment with L-DOPA, but not bromocriptine induces dyskinesia in MPTP-parkinsonian monkeys. Correlation with [^{3}H] spiperone binding. *Brain Res.*, 379:294–299.
20. Cohen, G., Paski, P., Cohen, B., Leist, A., Mytilineou, C., and Yahr, M. D. (1984): Pargyline and deprenyl prevent the neurotoxicity of 1-methyl-4-phenyl-1,2,3,6-tetrahydropyridine (MPTP) in monkeys. *Eur. J. Pharmacol.*, 106:209–210.
21. Deutch, A. Y., Elsworth, J. D., Goldstein, M., et al. (1986): Preferential vulnerability of A8 dopamine neurons in the primate to the neurotoxin 1-methyl-4-phenyl-1,2,3,6-tetrahydropyridine. *Neurosci. Lett.*, 68:51–56.
22. DiPaolo, T., Bédard, P., Daigle, M., and Boucher, R. (1986): Long-term effects of MPTP on central and peripheral catecholamine and indoleamine concentrations in monkeys. *Brain Res.*, 379:286–293.
23. Eidelberg, E., Brooks, B. A., Morgan, W. W., Walden, J. G., and Kokemoor, R. H. (1986): Variability and functional recovery in the N-methyl-4-phenyl-1,2,3,6-tetrahydropyridine model of parkinsonism in monkeys. *Neuroscience*, 18:817–822.
24. Elsworth, J. D., Deutch, A. Y., Redmond, D. E., Sladek, J. R., and Roth, R. H. (1987): Effects of 1-methyl-4-phenyl-1,2,3,6-tetrahydropyridine (MPTP) on catecholamines and metabolites in primate brain and CSF. *Brain Res.*, 415:293–299.
25. Elsworth, J. D., Deutch, A. Y., Redmond, D. E., Sladek, J. R., and Roth, R. H. (1987):

Differential responsiveness to 1-methyl-4-phenyl-1,2,3,6-tetrahydropyridine toxicity in sub-regions of primate substantia nigra and striatum. *Life Sci.*, 40:193–202.

26. Jenner, P., Rupniak, N. M. J., Rose, S., et al. (1984): 1-Methyl-4-phenyl-1,2,3,6-tetrahydropyridine-induced parkinsonism in the common marmoset. *Neurosci. Lett.*, 50:85–90.
27. Mitchell, I. J., Cross, A. J., Sambrook, M. A., and Crossman, A. R. (1985): Sites of the neurotoxic action of 1-methyl-4-phenyl-1,2,3,6-tetrahydropyridine in the Macaque monkey include the ventral tegmental area and the locus coeruleus. *Neurosci. Lett.*, 16:195–200.
28. Schultz, W., Studer, A., Jonsson, G., Sundström, E., and Mefford, I. (1985): Deficits in behavioral initiation and execution processes in monkeys with 1-methyl-4-phenyl-1,2,3,6-tetrahydropyridine-induced parkinsonism. *Neurosci. Lett.*, 59:225–232.
29. Hassler, R. (1938): Zur Pathologie der Paralysis agitans und des postenzephalitischen Parkinsonismus. *J. Psychol. Neurol. (Leipz.)*, 48:387–476.

Parkinsonism and Aging, edited by
Donald B. Calne et al., Raven Press, Ltd.,
New York © 1989.

Tyrosine Hydroxylase, Dopamine, and Energy Metabolism: Role in Parkinson's Disease and Aging

P. Riederer, E. Sofic, *W. D. Rausch, and G. †Hebenstreit

*Klinische Neurochemie, Universitäts-Nervenklinik, 8700 Würzburg, F.R.G.;
*Institut für Medizinische Chemie, Vet. Med. Universität, 1030 Wien, Austria;
and †Landeskrankenhaus, 3362 Amstetten/Mauer, Austria*

Selective degeneration of dopaminergic neurons within the substantia nigra and damage of noradrenergic cell bodies within the locus coeruleus with resultant reductions of dopamine (DA) and noradrenaline (NA) in the striatum and other projection areas seems to be a causative pathogenic process leading to Parkinson's disease (PD). It is not clearly understood, however, how these lesions are triggered and why they undergo a time-dependent progress. Neurotoxins, such as 1-methyl-4-phenyl-1,2,3,6-tetrahydropyridine (MPTP), do not cause progressive parkinsonism in acute trials (1,2) and this holds true for other toxins like acute carbon monoxide (3) or manganese (4) intoxication. Only severe cases of manganese intoxication might become progressively worse at a relative slow rate for long periods of time (5). Therefore, only a chronic exogenous or endogenous toxic noxa is able to reduce cell somata down to a denervation-induced threshold number at which compensation is not any more effective. Then, a self-driving, irreversible, and still unknown pathogenic process of endogenous origin seems to cause this deleterious progression. With the exception of a chronic intake of neurotoxins by foodstuffs (6–8) at work (3–5) or accidentally (9), it might be endogenous substances accumulating due to enzymopathies including aging processes that trigger a malignant or benign time course of PD.

Endogenous radicals, generated by hydrogen peroxide (10), toxic α,β-unsaturated aldehydes that could react with glutathione (11,12), or metabolic compounds of the catecholamine metabolism, such as 5-S-cysteinyldopamine (13), are potent candidates to trigger PD (Table 1).

Tyrosine hydroxylase (TH), the rate-limiting enzyme in catecholamine synthesis, shows highly reduced activity in PD. Therefore, it is this apparent vulnerability of this enzyme that is worth looking at in more detail. The

TABLE 1. *Experimental intoxications associated with lesions of the striatum possibly due to disturbances of energy metabolism*

MPTP
Kainic acid
Excitotoxic transmitters
Sodium azide
Hydrogen peroxide, $\cdot OH$, O_2^-, etc. (increase of malondialdehyde; catalase potentiates TH)
Tetrahydroisoquinolines
α, β-unsaturated aldehydes
Quinones of autoxidative processes
5-S-cysteinyl dopamine?
6-Hydroxydopamine

intention of this work is to find a link between such pathologic processes and the apparent vulnerability of this enzyme.

POSSIBLE MECHANISMS TRIGGERING THE LOSS OF TYROSINE HYDROXYLASE

Tetrahydrobiopterin System

TH is long known to be significantly decreased in the nigrostriatal DA regions of PD (14–17). There are several lines of thinking to explain this finding (Table 2). Active TH reacts with oxygen and tyrosine in the presence of (6*R*)-L-erythrotetrahydropteridine (BH_4) and iron (II) to form 3,4-dihydroxyphenylalanine, water, quinonoid–dihydrobiopterin (qBH_2), and iron (III) (27,18). Inactive TH is formed, and by some unknown process it may be this inactive TH that accumulates and cannot be transferred back to the active type by physiological processes. In fact, Mogi et al. (19) have found the inactive (or less active) type of TH in human postmortem control brain

TABLE 2. *Tyrosine hydroxylase in Parkinson's disease*

Severely decreased activity
Loss of TH protein
Supersensitivity of residual TH
Reduced tetrahydropteridine
Accumulation of inactive TH?
qBH_2 formed and recycled?
Sufficient amount of NADH + H$^+$ available?
Derangement of the kinase system
Increase of protein-bound iron
Iron (II) stimulatory properties maintained

TABLE 3. *MPTP-induced changes of tyrosine hydroxylase*

MPP^+:
   Inhibits TH activity
   Inhibits dihydropteridine reductase
   Leads to depletion of ATP production
   Blocks $NADH + H^+$ reoxidation

---

tissue. However, whether it accumulates in PD has to be proved in future studies. Although the concentration of BH_4 is reduced in the nigrostriatal system in PD, this figure is significantly less pronounced compared to the loss of TH activity (20). Therefore, it seems that the concentration of BH_4 in PD is sufficient to stimulate the conversion of tyrosine to DOPA. There is, however, no experimental evidence to show that qBH_2 is formed and thereafter recycled to BH_4 via a process requiring $NADH + H^+$ and it is questionable whether $NADH + H^+$ is available in sufficient quantity for process promotion.

Parkinsonism induced by the neurotoxin MPTP resembles PD in humans (1,2) (Table 3). Although not perfect (21), the MPTP model mimics the disease to a high degree. It has been shown by Nagatsu (22) that MPTP's presumed neurotoxic metabolite MPP^+ inhibits TH activity by blocking BH_4 production at the level of "dyspropterin" reductase and sepiapterin reductase. Moreover, dihydropteridine reductase, converting $NADH + H^+$ to NAD^+, is inhibited by MPP^+ (23). It is therefore worth mentioning that NADH ubiquinone oxidoreductase—forming NAD^+ and $CoQH_2$ from $NADH + H^+$ and CoQ—located at the inner mitochondrial membrane is blocked by MPP^+ only after conversion of MPTP by monoamine oxidase-B (MAO-B), which is located at the outer mitochondrial membrane. Thus, especially MAO-B synthesizes the radical MPP^+, which crosses the membrane and exerts there a deleterious effect on the $NADH + H^+/NAD^+$ system. In the glia, therefore, MPP^+ accumulation might lead to depletion of mitochondrial ATP production and NADH reoxidation (1), whereas MPP^+ is taken up by the nigrostriatal neurons via the dopamine uptake system. Once in the DA cell bodies and nerve terminals, the neurotoxic effect is widespread, as described above, and meets both the intrasynaptosomal TH system and mitochondrial processes (24).

Tyrosine Hydroxylase Protein

In a recent study by Mogi et al. (25), it has been shown that the loss of TH in the substantia nigra and striatum is due to loss of TH protein. Furthermore, calculation of TH activity based on TH protein concentration indicates a significant increase of this so-called "homospecific activity" in PD compared to control tissue. This finding is evidence for supersensitive TH due to degeneration of the nigrostriatal DA system. Whether or not the mechanisms mentioned in the previous section contribute to the loss of TH protein is not clear at present. It seems, however, that this supersensitive TH compensates for DA synthesis in PD (25). Up to a certain threshold, this induction of TH activity is sufficient to overcome the loss of DA. Increased DA production and enhanced DA utilization as indicated by an increase of the HVA/DA ratio seem to be the most potent compensatory mechanisms counteracting the progressive denervation.

Stimulation of TH under phosphorylating conditions has shown to be effective with protein kinase in postmortem samples of caudate nucleus of PD only while other phosphorylating agents, e.g., cAMP plus ATP and Ca^{2+}–calmodulin, did not show any stimulatory properties (26). These results may indicate derangement of the kinase systems in samples of PD.

Stimulatory Properties of Iron on TH Activity

TH of bovine adrenal medulla is an iron-dependent enzyme. The pure enzyme contains the (rather underestimated) amount of 0.5–0.75 mol of iron per mole of enzyme (27). Iron dependence has recently been shown also for human brain TH (26). Iron (II) participates in the hydroxylation reaction, and it has been suggested that it is its well-known catalytic activity to decompose hydrogen peroxide (H_2O_2) (28). *In vitro* H_2O_2 reduces TH activity in the gerbil caudate nucleus only at high concentrations (26). In the gerbil caudate nucleus, these stimulatory properties of iron (II) are reduced by H_2O_2 only slightly at 1 mM of both substances while there is a complete loss of stimulation in the pig caudate nucleus (26). That H_2O_2 may be of relevance in inhibiting the enzyme is shown by the TH stimulatory properties of catalase, which decomposes H_2O_2 to oxygen (27). H_2O_2 or H_2O_2-derived radicals (O_2^- and $\cdot OH$) and iron seem to accumulate during aging (29). Furthermore, total iron has been shown to be increased in the substantia nigra of PD (30). We have extended this finding by showing that it is iron (III) that accumulates probably as ferritin (31,32). Furthermore, the increase of total iron seems to be related positively to the grade of degeneration (32).

Therefore, loss of TH activity in PD may be related in part to accumulation of inactive protein-bound iron and in addition to the increase of endogenous H_2O_2. *In vitro* TH activity of both control and PD caudate nucleus can be stimulated up to 1,317 and 1,100%, respectively (26). This finding shows that iron (II) stimulatory properties of TH are maintained in PD although TH protein is lost. There are also *in vivo* and *ex vivo* data supporting this view. Ten years ago, we showed that TH is reduced in postmortem adrenal medulla of PD (33). Recently, Birkmayer and Birkmayer (34) described antiparkinsonian properties of a complexed iron salt, oxyferriscorbone. This iron salt contains both iron (II) and iron (III) bound to alloxanic acid and 2,3-diketogulonic acid, respectively. The peripheral effects of this compound are shown in the substantial increase of homovanillic acid in the urine of patients with PD (Birkmayer, personal communication). This finding clearly shows improved stimulatory properties of otherwise reduced TH activity in the adrenal medulla of PD due to infusions of this special iron salt. It is noteworthy, however, that the peripheral iron status in PD is not abnormal, as determined by measurements of total iron, transferrin, ferritin, hemoglobin, hematocrit, erythrocytes, reticulocytes, and ceruloplasmin (31). It may be speculated that stimulation of TH in PD by iron (II) is inhibited to some extent by as yet unknown compounds that may include endogenous radicals of various origin (O_2^-, $\cdot OH$, aldehydes, organic peroxides, quinolins, etc.). Both increased lipid peroxidation. as shown by the increase of malondialdehyde in SN of PD (35), and the substantial increase of tetrahydroisoquinoline and 2-methyltetrahydroquinoline in parkinsonian brain (36) seem to be in line with this hypothesis. Radicals derived from H_2O_2 (26,27), tetrahydroisoquinoline (37), and very high doses of DOPA (38) inhibit TH activity. However, it is unknown whether the underlying mechanisms involved in this reduction influence iron stimulation.

ENERGY METABOLISM AND PARKINSON'S DISEASE

It is well known that iron plays an important role in the respiratory chain. The various cytochromes, having redox potentials between $+0.22$ and 0.29 V, use iron (II) and iron (III) for electron transfer. Any changes in the redox equilibrium between iron (II) and iron (III) may therefore change the functional activity of the respiratory chain, thus possibly uncoupling the reaction of O^{2-} and $2H^+$. Evidence for a shift in the iron (II)–iron (III) equilibrium in favor of iron (III) has been found in the substantia nigra of PD (39). It may well be that this shift is triggered by an oxidizing compound (for example, H_2O_2) (Table 4). There is experimental evidence that antioxidants partially prevent the neurotoxic effects of MPTP in mice (40,41) while diethyldithiocarbamate, an inhibitor of superoxide dismutase, potentiates it (42). Transition metals like iron (II) potentiate the formation of MPP^+ from MPTP (43,44). On the contrary, metal chelators decrease the toxic effects of MPTP (43). Blockade of mitochondrial NADH oxidation by MPP^+ depletes ATP production and prevents NADH reoxidation. By this, cell death may occur (43). In agreement with this assumption, blockade of NADH–coenzyme Q reductase by rotenone results in the decrease of dopamine (45). In this context, it seems to be of interest to note that, in humans, conditions

TABLE 4. *Evidences for a dissociated energy metabolism in Parkinson's disease?*

A shift of iron (II) to iron (III) may change the redox equilibrium
Formation of H_2O_2 potentiates MPP^+ blockade of NADH reoxidation
Iron (II) potentiates the formation of MPP^+ from MPTP
Metal chelators decrease MPTP's neurotoxicity
Antioxidants partially prevent MPTP's neurotoxicity
Superoxide dismutase inhibitors potentiate MPTP neurotoxicity

leading to severe disturbances of energy metabolism are associated with exogenous bilateral striatal necrosis (3). Such conditions include vascular lesions, hypoxic–hypotensive states, and intoxication with carbon monoxide, cyanide, sodium azide, manganese, and others (Table 5).

CONCLUSION

Evidence is presented to suggest that, during aging and in particular in Parkinson's disease, toxins of endogenous and/or exogenous origin accumulate. Candidates for endogenous neurotoxins are primarily hydrogen peroxide and radicals derived from it, aldehydes and quinones, whereas exogenous intoxications are known to exist for MPTP, carbon monoxide, manganese, and others. Single or combined toxic events may lead to disturbances in energy metabolism including the respiratory chain. The resultant derangements include lipid peroxidation of neuronal membranes and functional disturbances for oxygen and iron (II) requiring enzymes like tyrosine hydroxylase. Neuropathological examinations of human postmortem brain tissue after intoxications with carbon monoxide, manganese, methyl alcohol, or hypoxic–hypotensive states clearly show bilateral lesions of the striatum. Further evidence for the "superoxide theory of oxygen toxicity" is given by the MPTP model, which shows a significant relation to disturbances of energy metabolism induced by MPP^+. Therefore, strategies have to be de-

TABLE 5. *Intoxications associated with lesions*
of human striatum possibly due to
disturbances of energy metabolism

Carbon monoxide
Manganese
Cyanide
Methyl alcohol
Vascular lesions
Hypoxic–hypotensive states

veloped both to improve the antioxidant potential of cells and to reduce the intake of exogenous toxins.

REFERENCES

1. Kinemuchi, H., Fowler, C. J., and Tipton, K. F. (1987): The neurotoxicity of 1-methyl-4-phenyl-1,2,3,6-tetrahydropyridine (MPTP) and its relevance to Parkinson's disease. *Neurochem. Int.*, 11:359–373.
2. Langston, J. W. (1985): MPTP and Parkinson's disease. *Trends Neurol. Sci.*, 8:79–83.
3. Jellinger, K. (1986): Exogenous striatal necrosis. In: *Handbook of Clinical Neurology, Vol. 5, Extrapyramidal Disorders*, edited by P. J. Vinken, G. W. Bruyn, and H. L. Klawans, pp. 499–518. Elsevier Science Publishers, Amsterdam.
4. Barbeau, A. (1984): Manganese and extrapyramidal disorders. *Neurotoxicology*, 5:13–36.
5. Cotzias, G. C. (1958): Manganese in health and disease. *Physiol. Rev.*, 38:503–532.
6. Hirano, A., Kurland, L. T., Krooth, R. S., and Lesell, S. (1961): Parkinsonism–dementia complex, and endemic disease on the Island of Guam. I. Clinical features. *Brain*, 84:642–661.
7. Yase, Y., Matsumoto, F., Yoshi, F., and Masu, Y. (1986): Motor neuron disease in the Kii Peninsula of Japan. *Proc. Aust. Assoc. Neurol.*, 5:335–339.
8. Rajput, A. J., Stern, W., Christ, A., and Laverty, W. (1984): Etiology of Parkinson's disease: environmental factor(s). *Neurology*, 34(suppl 1):207.
9. Markey, S. P., Castagnoli, N., Trevor, A. J., and Kopin, I. J. (1986): *MPTP: A Neurotoxin Producing a Parkinsonian Syndrome*. Academic Press, Orlando.
10. Cohen, G. The pathobiology of Parkinson's disease: biochemical aspects of dopamine neuron senescence. *J. Neural Transm.* 19(suppl):89–103.
11. Riederer, P., Strolin Benedetti, M., Dostert, P., Sofic, E., Heuschneider, G., and Guffroy, C. (1987): Do glutathione and ascorbic acid play a role in the neurotoxicity of 1-methyl-4-phenyl-1,2,3,6-tetrahydropyridine. *Pharmacol. Toxicol.* 60(suppl 1):39.
12. Strolin Benedetti, M., Dostert, P., and Guffroy, C. (1986): The possible reaction of glutathione and MPTP to Parkinson's disease. In: *MPTP: A Neurotoxin Producing a Parkinsonian Syndrome*, edited by S. P. Markey, N. Castagnoli, A. J. Trevor, and J. J. Kopin, pp. 455–460. Academic Press, Orlando.
13. Rosengren, E., Linder-Eliasson, E., and Carlsson, A. (1985): Detection of 5-S-cysteinyl-dopamine in human brain. *J. Neural Transm.*, 63:247–253.
14. Lloyd, K. G., Davidson, L., and Hornykiewicz, O. (1975): The neurochemistry of Parkinson's disease: effect of L-DOPA therapy. *J. Pharmacol. Exp. Ther.*, 195:453–464.
15. McGeer, P. L., and McGeer, E. G. (1976): Enzymes associated with the metabolism of catecholamines, acetylcholine and GABA in human controls and patients with Parkinson's disease and Huntington's chorea. *J. Neurochem.*, 26:65–76.
16. Nagatsu, T., Kato, T., Numata, Y., et al. (1977): Phenylethanolamine-N-methyltransferase and other enzymes of catecholamine metabolism in human brain. *Clin. Chim. Acta*, 75:221.
17. Riederer P., Rausch, W. D., Birkmayer, W., Jellinger, K., and Seemann, D. (1978): CNS-modulation of adrenal tyrosine hydroxylase in Parkinson's disease and metabolic encephalopathies. *J. Neural Transm.* 14(suppl):121.
18. Carlsson, A. (1974): The in vivo estimation of rates of tryptophan and tyrosine hydroxylation: effects of alterations in enzyme environment and neuronal activity. In: *Aromatic Amino Acids in the Brain*, edited by G. E. W. Wolstenholme, and D. W. Fitzsimons, pp. 117–134. Elsevier, Amsterdam.
19. Mogi, M., Kojima, K., and Nagatsu, T. (1984): Detection of inactive or less active form of tyrosine hydroxylase in human adrenals by a sandwich enzyme immunoassay. *Anal. Biochem.*, 138:125–132.
20. Nagatsu, T., Yamaguchi, T., Kato, T., et al. (1981): Biopterin in the brain of controls and patients with Parkinson's disease and related striatal degenerative diseases: application of new biopterin radioimmunoassay. In: *Transmitter Biochemistry of Human Brain Tissue*, edited by P. Riederer and E. Usdin, pp. 281–289. Macmillan Publishers Ltd., London, Basingstoke.

21. Riederer, P., and Youdim, M. B. H. (1987): MPTP induced dopaminergic neurotoxicity—
    a useful model in the study of Parkinson's disease? *Neurochem. Int.*, 11:379–381.
22. Nagatsu, T. (1987): MPTP and its relevance to Parkinson's disease. *Neurochem. Int.*,
    11:375–377.
23. Abell, C. W., Shen, R., Gessner, W., and Brossi, A. (1984): Inhibition of dihydropteridine
    reductase by novel 1-methyl-4-phenyl-1,2,3,6-tetrahydropteridine analogs. *Science*,
    224:405–407.
24. Takamidoh, H., Naoi, M., and Nagatsu, T. (1987): Inhibition of type A monoamine oxidase
    by 1-methyl-4-phenyl-pyridine. *Neurosci. Lett.*, 73:293–297.
25. Mogi, M., Harada, M., Kiuchi, K., et al. (1988): Homospecific activity (activity per en-
    zyme protein) of tyrosine hydroxylase increases in Parkinsonian brain. *J. Neural Transm.*,
    72:77–81.
26. Rausch, W. D., Hirata, Y., Nagatsu, T., Riederer, P., and Jellinger, K. (1988): Tyrosine
    hydroxylase activity in caudate nucleus from Parkinson's disease: effects of iron and phos-
    phorylating agents. *J. Neurochem.*, 50:202–208.
27. Kaufman, S. (1977): Mixed function oxygenases—general considerations. In: *Structure
    and Function of Monoamine Enzymes*, edited by E. Usdin, N. Weiner, and M. B. H.
    Youdim, Vol. 10, pp. 3–22, Marcel Dekker, Inc., New York, Basel.
28. Shiman, R., Akino, M., and Kaufman, S. (1971): Solubilization and partial purification of
    tyrosine hydroxylase from bovine adrenal medulla. *J. Biol. Chem.*, 246:1330–1340.
29. Hallgren, B., and Sourander, P. (1958): The effect of age on the non-heme iron in human
    brain. *J. Neurochem.*, 3:41–51.
30. Dexter, D. T., Wells, F. R., Agid, F., et al. (1987): Increased nigral iron content in post-
    mortem parkinsonian brain. *Lancet*, 2:1219–1220.
31. Riederer, P., Rausch, W. D., Schmidt, B., et al. (1988): Biochemical fundamentals of
    Parkinson's disease. *Mount Sinai J. Med.* 55:21–28.
32. Riederer, P., Sofic, E., Rausch, W. D., Schmidt, B., and Youdim, M. B. H. (1989): *J.
    Neurochem.* (in press).
33. Riederer, P., Rausch, W. D., Birkmayer, W., Jellinger, K., and Danielczyk, W. (1978):
    Dopamine-sensitive adenylate cyclase activity in the caudate nucleus and adrenal medulla
    in Parkinson's disease and in liver cirrhosis. *J. Neural Transm.*, 14(suppl):153.
34. Birkmayer, W., and Birkmayer, J. G. D. (1986): Iron, a new aid in the treatment of Par-
    kinson patients. *J. Neural Transm.*, 67:287–292.
35. Dexter, D., Carter, C., Agid, F., et al. (1986): Lipid peroxidation as cause of nigral cell
    death in Parkinson's disease. *Lancet*, 2:639–640.
36. Niwa, T., Takeda, N., Kaneda, N., Hashizume, Y., and Nagatsu, T. (1987): Presence of
    tetrahydroisoquinoline and 2-methyl-tetrahydroquinoline in parkinsonian and normal
    human brains. *Biochem. Biophys. Res. Commun.*, 144:1084–1089.
37. Nagatsu, T., and Hirata, H. (1987): Inhibition of the tyrosine hydroxylase system by
    MPTP, 1-methyl-4-phenylpyridinium ion (MPP^+) and the structurally related compound
    in vitro and in vivo. *Eur. Neurol.*, 26(suppl 1):11–15.
38. Dairman, W., and Udenfriend, S. (1972): Decrease in adrenal tyrosine hydroxylase and
    increase in norepinephrine synthesis in rats given L-DOPA. *Sciences*, 171:1022.
39. Sofic, E., Riederer, P., Heinsen, H., Beckmann, H., Reynolds, G. P., and Hebenstreit,
    G. (1988): Increased iron (III) and total iron content in post mortem substantia nigra of
    Parkinsonian brain. *J. Neural Transm.*, 74:199–205.
40. Perry, T. L., Young, V. W., Clavier, R. M., et al. Partial protection from the dopaminergic
    neurotoxin N-methyl-4-phenyl-1,2,3,6-tetrahydropyridine by four different antioxidants in
    the mouse. *Neurosci. Lett.*, 60:109–114.
41. Wagner, G. C., Jarvis, M. F., and Carelli, R. M. (1985): Ascorbic acid reduces the do-
    pamine depletion induced by MPTP. *Neuropharmacology*, 24:1261–1262.
42. Corsini, G. U., Pintus, S., Chiueh, C. C., Weis, J. F., and Kopin, I. J. (1985): 1-Methyl-
    4-phenyl-1,2,3,6-tetrahydropyridine (MPTP) neurotoxicity in mice is enhanced by pre-
    treatment with diethyldithiocarbamate. *Eur. J. Pharmacol.*, 119:127–128.
43. Poirier, J., Donaldson, J., and Barbeau, A. (1985): The specific vulnerability of the sub-
    stantia nigra to MPTP is related to the presence of transition metals. *Biochem. Biophys.
    Res. Commun.*, 128:25–33.
44. Barbeau, A., Poirier, J., Dallaire, L., Rucinska, E., Buu, N. T., and Donaldson, J. (1986):

Studies on MPTP, MPP$^+$ and paraquat in frogs and in vitro. In: *MPTP: A Neurotoxin Producing a Parkinsonian syndrome*, edited by S. P. Markey, N. Castagnoli, A. J. Trevor and I. J. Kopin, pp. 85–103. Academic Press, New York.

45. Heikkila, R. E., Nicklas, W. J., Vjas, I., and Duvoisin, R. C. (1985): Dopaminergic toxicity of rotenone and the 1-methyl-4-phenylpyridinium ion after their stereotactic administration to rats: implications for the mechanism of 1-methyl-4-phenyl-1,2,3,6-tetrahydropyridine toxicity. *Neurosci. Lett.*, 62:389–394.

Parkinsonism and Aging, edited by
Donald B. Calne et al., Raven Press, Ltd.,
New York © 1989.

Nerve Growth Factor and Neurotrophic Factors in Parkinson's Disease and Aging

Franz Hefti

Department of Neurology, University of Miami, Miami, Florida 33101

Neurobiological research carried out in recent years revealed that development, maintenance of function, and regeneration of neurons are influenced by proteins called "neurotrophic factors" (1,2). The neurotrophic factors are proteins acting on receptors located on the neuronal surface. These receptors then stimulate mechanisms necessary for survival, neurite growth, and functions related to transmitter production and release. Nerve growth factor (NGF) is the first and best characterized neurotrophic factor and serves as a paradigm for more recently discovered molecules. "Nerve growth factor" is a historical term erroneously implying that this protein affects a majority of neurons. Indeed, the spectrum of neurons influenced by NGF is quite narrow. It has long been known that NGF is a neurotrophic factor for peripheral sympathetic and sensory neurons. More recent findings show that NGF also affects cholinergic neurons in the brain. Other neurotrophic factors characterized so far influence survival and function of parasympathetic neurons, spinal cord neurons, cholinergic motoneurons, retinal cells, and various subpopulations of sensory neurons. These findings have been taken to suggest that there is a multitude of neurotrophic factors with different specificities. Research has not progressed sufficiently far to conclude whether every group of neurons requires a specific neurotrophic factor or whether the various factors have partly overlapping specificities.

The results obtained in basic science studies have obvious implications for neurodegenerative diseases. Based on the new concepts, Appel (3) formulated a general hypothesis stating that the lack of neurotrophic factors is responsible for the degeneration of selective neuronal populations as it occurs in Parkinson's disease, amyotrophic lateral sclerosis, and Alzheimer's disease, and that application of the corresponding neurotrophic factor might prevent the neuronal degeneration. In the first part of this chapter, the present knowledge about NGF is briefly summarized. Special emphasis is given to its role in the function of forebrain cholinergic neurons, which are involved in memory function and are affected in Alzheimer's disease. The

79

trophic control of cholinergic neurons by NGF is well characterized and can serve as a paradigmatic example in the search for other neurotrophic factors acting on central neurons. The second part of the chapter briefly describes the neurotrophic factors that have been characterized so far. The third part summarizes the present knowledge about the trophic control of dopaminergic neurons that are selectively affected in Parkinson's disease. In the fourth part, the possibility is discussed that NGF might improve survival of adrenal medullary cells transplanted into basal ganglia.

NGF AND ITS ACTIONS ON CHOLINERGIC NEURONS OF THE FOREBRAIN

NGF is a protein of known amino acid sequence and structure. Its gene has recently been sequenced and cloned. NGF has been extensively characterized in its role as neurotrophic factor for peripheral sympathetic neurons (1,2). It is essential for the development and maintenance of function of these cells. NGF is synthesized by target tissues of sympathetic neurons and acts on specific receptors located on the sympathetic neurons. These receptors mediate local actions of NGF and its internalization, which initiates retrograde transport to the cell bodies of sympathetic neurons. In the cell body, NGF stimulates the synthesis of proteins essential for survival and expression of transmitter-specific properties by sympathetic neurons. Administration of NGF to rodents produces a hypertrophic reaction of sympathetic ganglia and results in selective stimulation of the synthesis of key enzymes for the production of norepinephrine, the transmitter used by sympathetic neurons. Administration of antibodies to these animals results in atrophy of the sympathetic ganglia. The crucial role played by NGF in the development of sympathetic neurons is best demonstrated in experiments with cell cultures. Sympathetic neurons isolated and placed in culture dishes require NGF for survival, fiber growth, and for the expression of transmitter-specific enzymes. In adult animals, sympathetic neurons remain responsive to NGF. Very recent studies show that transection of sympathetic axons results in local synthesis of NGF by nonneuronal cells, suggesting that NGF-related mechanisms participate in the regenerative growth of sympathetic axons (4).

For many years, neuroscientists have been looking for a function of NGF in the brain. Because, in the peripheral nervous system, NGF affects sympathetic neurons that use catecholamines as their transmitter, the efforts focused on central dopaminergic and noradrenergic neurons. Many studies, however, showed clearly that these neurons do not respond to NGF (5). Around 1980, indirect evidence appeared suggesting that NGF acts as a neurotrophic factor for cholinergic neurons of the forebrain (6). These findings were surprising and were initially met with skepticism. Nevertheless, there is now a substantial body of evidence that conclusively demonstrates this unexpected role of NGF.

The evidence indicating that NGF acts as a neurotrophic factor for cholinergic neurons of the forebrain includes the following points: First, NGF as well as the mRNA coding for NGF are present in the brain. The levels of both protein and its mRNA correlate with the anatomical distribution of cholinergic neurons (7,8). Second, forebrain cholinergic neurons contain receptors for NGF. Recently, these NGF receptors on forebrain cholinergic neurons have been directly demonstrated using autoradiographic immunohistochemical visualization methods (9,10). In the adult brain, cholinergic neurons are the only cells containing such receptors. A third and rapidly growing group of findings provides evidence that the stimulation of NGF receptors on cholinergic neurons mediates trophic influences on these cells. In studies on living animals and on cell cultures, NGF has been found to elevate the activity of choline acetyltransferase, the key enzyme in the synthesis of acetylcholine (6,11,12), and to promote survival and fiber elongation of cholinergic neurons (13,14). These findings show that NGF trophically affects cholinergic neurons of the basal forebrain by acting on specific receptors located on these cells.

Most of the findings reviewed above that indicate that NGF is a neurotrophic factor for cholinergic neurons of the basal forebrain were obtained on newborn animals, healthy young adult rodents, or on cultures prepared with tissue from fetal animals. While clearly indicating that NGF plays an important role in the development and function of cholinergic neurons, these findings are not necessarily relevant for the situation in neurodegenerative diseases that typically are associated with aging. Effects of NGF were therefore studied on adult animals with experimentally induced lesions of cholinergic pathways. These lesions mimic the loss of cholinergic neurons as it occurs in Alzheimer's disease. NGF was given to such animals and its effect on function of the cholinergic neurons and on the behavior of the animals was studied. Since NGF is not able to cross the blood–brain barrier, it had to be administered directly to the brain. Animals were implanted with cannulas reaching into the ventricles, and NGF was applied through them. The experimentally induced lesions reduced the number of cholinergic neurons in the septum and the density of cholinergic fibers in the area of innervation. Intraventricular applications of NGF for several weeks largely prevented this lesion-induced degeneration of cholinergic neurons (13). Lesions of the cholinergic septohippocampal projection reduced the ability of the rats to perform a behavioral task. The animals with lesions exhibited a reduction in their ability to learn a radial maze task, in which they had to pick up food pellets from the various arms of a radial maze without re-entering an arm previously visited. NGF treatment counteracted this lesion-induced deficit. Rats subjected to intraventricular applications of NGF learned the maze problem more rapidly than untreated rats with the same lesions (15). These findings suggest the possibility that the behavioral improvements observed in NGF-treated animals reflect its promotion of survival of cholinergic neurons in the septum. More recently, we have found that chronic long-term administration of NGF to lesioned animals promotes the regrowth of cholinergic axons into the denervated hippocampus (unpublished results). Other investigators showed that NGF administration to aged animals ameliorates the age-related atrophy of cholinergic neurons in rats and to improve the performance of behaviorally impaired aged rats (16). In summary, the findings indicate that NGF is able to promote survival and regeneration of cholinergic neurons in an animal model mimicking some aspects of Alzheimer's disease and to improve the behavioral performance of lesioned and aged animals.

CHARACTERIZED NEUROTROPHIC FACTORS

The number of characterized neurotrophic factors is still very small. These molecules occur in minimal quantities, making their isolation a cumbersome and time-consuming effort. The search for neurotrophic factors normally starts with the characterization of a source (e.g., tissue extract) and an assay system (typically a cell culture system). The active principle is then isolated and purified from the source using a sequence of various protein purification methods. With this approach, ciliary neurotrophic factor (CNTF) was purified from chick eye extracts and rat sciatic neurons. This protein promotes the survival of parasympathetic neurons (17). Brain-derived neurotrophic factor (BNTF) is a protein purified from pig brain that supports that survival of chick sensory neurons and rat retinal ganglion cells (18). Retina-derived growth factor (RDGF) was isolated from bovine retinas and shown to induce neurite growth in a neuroblastoma cell line (19). Glia-derived neurite promoting factor (GdNPF) produced by glial cells and inducing neurite growth of neuroblastoma cells was purified and found to be an inhibitor of cell-derived proteases (20). This finding is in line with other findings suggesting that protease inhibitors are involved in neurite growth and might play a role in regeneration. Very recently, a protein called "neuroleukin" was purified from salivary glands. This factor supports survival of a subpopulation of spinal cord and sensory neurons (21). Several laboratories have reported the initial characterization of neurotrophic factors for spinal cord motoneurons (22). However, no complete purification has been achieved so far.

Besides these neurotrophic factors found by purification, there is a number of earlier characterized growth factors or growth hormones that were found to affect neurons and therefore are considered "neurotrophic factors." Among these are epidermal growth factor (EGF) and basic fibroblast growth factor (bFGF), which stimulate the proliferation of nonneuronal cells but also promote survival of rat brain neurons *in vitro* (23,24). Insulin as well as insulin receptors occur in the brain and this hormone as well as insulin-like growth factor II promote survival of cultured sympathetic and sensory neurons (25). S-100β, a calcium-binding protein, was found to promote the extension of neurites from cultured chick brain neurons (26). Besides the neurotrophic factors described so far, which are saliva proteins, there are membrane-bound molecules promoting adhesion and neurite extension of neurons. Characterized molecules are laminin and fibronectin, both constituents of the extracellular matrix. When applied to the surface of cell culture dishes, laminin and fibronectin promote survival of neuronal cells (27).

As is evident from this brief summary, the field of neurotrophic factors is still in its infancy. Several major questions remain to be answered. First, most of the neurotrophic factors' actions were characterized in cell culture experiments. It remains to be shown that these *in vitro* observations reflect physiological processes. Second, the degree of specificity of neurotrophic factors is not clear. Can we expect to find a selective neurotrophic factor for every major population of brain neurons? The specific effect of NGF on forebrain cholinergic neurons suggests the existence of other factors with a similar degree of specificity for other populations of neurons. However, EGF and bFGF apparently have a much lower degree of specificity and affect a larger number of neuronal populations. It is possible that the number of neurotrophic factors is relatively small and that the very limited specificity of NGF turns out to be exceptional. Third, growth factors characterized so far were shown to play a role in developmental processes. In contrast, much less is known about their function in the adult nervous system. Central cholinergic and peripheral sympathetic neurons remain responsive to nerve growth factor during the entire life span. In contrast, sensory neurons, which respond to NGF during development, lose the receptors for NGF and become independent from the supply of this neurotrophic factor. There seems to be no doubt that more growth factors will be found in the future and that these and the known factors will be more extensively characterized. The future results have to be awaited before general conclusions are drawn regarding the function of neurotrophic factors.

SEARCH FOR NEUROTROPHIC FACTORS FOR DOPAMINERGIC NEURONS

As outlined, NGF was expected to affect central dopaminergic neurons, since catecholaminergic neurons of the peripheral nervous system respond to this factor. However, NGF failed to promote differentiation of dopaminergic neurons (5). Furthermore, these neurons do not express receptors for NGF (9). These findings did not exclude the possibility that injured dopaminergic neurons become responsive to NGF and that application of ex-

TABLE 1. *Effect of intracerebral injections of NGF on survival of cholinergic and dopaminergic neurons after experimental injury in the rat brain*

	% Surviving neurons
Cholinergic neurons in septum[a]	
Controls	42.8 ± 4.2%
NGF	88.9 ± 2.6%*
Dopaminergic neurons in substantia nigra[b]	
Controls	36.7 ± 7.6%
NGF	35.5 ± 7.2%
Insulin	43.7 ± 6.6%

Values given indicate means ± SEM of 5–15 animals per group. * Significantly different from controls, $p < 0.01$.

[a] In adult rats, the cholinergic septohippocampal pathway was destroyed unilaterally by a partial fimbrial transection. Animals were implanted with a cannula through which NGF or a control protein was injected twice weekly during 4 weeks. Cholinergic neurons in the medial septal nucleus and the vertical limb of the diagonal band were visualized using choline acetyltransferase immunohistochemistry. The number of positively stained cell bodies was counted on the lesioned side and expressed as a percentage of the neurons found on control sides (for further experimental details, see ref. 26).

[b] The nigrostriatal dopaminergic pathway was destroyed unilaterally in rats by a hemitransection of the medial forebrain bundle. A 4.5-mm-wide blade was lowered into the brain at an angle of 65° and a starting position 1.0 mm anterior to the bregma and 0.5 mm lateral to the midline. The blade was then lowered to a level 9.2 mm below the dura. The animals were then chronically implanted with a guiding cannula and were injected at the site of the lesion with NGF (5 µg twice weekly), insulin (5 µg daily), or a control protein. After 2 weeks, the dopaminergic neurons in the substantia nigra were visualized using tyrosine hydroxylase immunohistochemistry. The number of stained cells on the lesioned side was expressed as a percentage of the number of neurons on control sides.

ogenous NGF to injured neurons might promote their survival and regeneration. To test for this possibility, we injected NGF intracerebrally into rats with experimental lesions of the dopaminergic pathway. The medial forebrain bundle, which carries the nigrostriatal dopaminergic neurons, was transected in adult rats. This lesion resulted in loss of dopaminergic cell bodies in the zona compacta of the substantia nigra. Chronic intraventricular injections of NGF or injections at the lesion side failed to prevent the loss of dopaminergic neurons (Table 1). These findings are in clear contrast to the positive findings obtained when giving NGF to rats with injured cholinergic neurons. NGF administration almost completely prevented the degeneration of septal cholinergic neurons that normally follows transection of the septohippocampal pathway (Table 1). The findings provide further evidence that NGF does not affect central dopaminergic neurons and confirm the high degree of specificity of NGF's effect on cholinergic neurons. Similar to the negative results obtained with NGF on dopaminergic neurons, intracerebral injections of insulin failed to prevent the loss of dopaminergic neurons after transections of the nigrostriatal pathway (Table 1).

Several studies provide indirect evidence for the existence of a neurotrophic factor for dopaminergic neurons. Heller and collaborators found that survival and biochemical differentiation of dopaminergic cells in cultures of aggregated neurons was increased when dopaminergic cells were cocultured with cells from the corpus striatum. In such cocultures, the number of dopaminergic neurons, the density of the neurites, and the evoked release of dopamine were higher than in cultures containing only nigral neurons (28). The fact that cocultures with cells from areas other than the striatum failed to be similarly effective suggested that striatal cells exert the selective trophic influence on dopaminergic cells. Similar effects of striatal cells on dopaminergic neurons were described by Prochiantz and collaborators, who used cultures of dissociated neurons (29). The trophic effect of striatal cells in these cultures required cell–cell contact between nigral and striatal neurons. Isolated membranes from striatal tissue were equally effective as living striatal cells. These findings were taken to suggest that a membrane-bound molecule expressed by striatal target cells mediates the trophic actions on dopaminergic neurons. More recently, Tomozawa and Appel (30) reported the partial purification of a peptide isolated from striatal tissue that promoted survival and differentiation of dopaminergic neurons in cultures of dissociated nigral cells. Ferrari and collaborators (31) characterized a small protein producing similar trophic effects.

The isolation of a neurotrophic factor for dopaminergic neurons represents a major challenge of today's neurological research. A factor able to promote survival, function, and neurite elongation of dopaminergic neurons would be of obvious importance in the context of Parkinson's disease. Application of such a factor might retard the degeneration and stop or attenuate the progression and clinical manifestations of the disease process.

NGF AND TRANSPLANTATION IN PARKINSON'S DISEASE

In experimental animals, behavioral deficits caused by the loss of nigrostriatal dopaminergic neurons are compensated for by transplanted dopaminergic neurons from fetal brains (32). Similar beneficial effects were obtained with transplant from adrenal medullary cells (33). The catecholamine-releasing cells from the adrenal medulla are ontogenetically related to sympathetic neurons and respond, during early development, to nerve growth factor. When grown in cell culture, adrenal medullary cells can be induced by nerve growth factors to produce neurons and transform themselves into neuron-like cells (34). Adrenal medullary cells were transplanted in recent clinical trials that were reported to be beneficial by some investigators but not by others (35,36). It is not clear whether adrenal medullary cells of adult humans respond to NGF. If they are found to express NGF receptors, exposing adrenal medullary neurons to NGF before implantation into the brain might improve their chances for survival and growth in the host.

CONCLUSIONS

Nerve growth factor is one of the series of proteins called neurotrophic factors that promote survival and function of neurons. NGF acts as a neurotrophic factor for peripheral sympathetic and sensory neurons and for the cholinergic neurons of the basal forebrain. These cholinergic neurons respond to NGF during the entire life span. NGF is able to prevent the degeneration of cholinergic neurons in animals with experimental lesions and to stimulate the growth of cholinergic fibers into the denervated areas. NGF does not affect dopaminergic neurons of the substantia nigra that are affected in Parkinson's disease. At present, there is indirect evidence only for the existence of neurotrophic factor for mesencephalic dopaminergic neurons. No such factor has been purified or characterized so far. Adrenal medullary cells respond to NGF during development. NGF might therefore help these cells to survive and grow after transplantation into the brain.

Acknowledgment: The author was supported by the National Parkinson Foundation, Miami, FL, and by a grant from the National Institutes of Health (NS22933).

REFERENCES

1. Levi-Montalcini, R. (1987): The nerve growth factor 35 years later. *Science*, 237:1154–1162.
2. Thoenen, H., and Edgar, D. (1985): Neurotrophic factors. *Science*, 229:238–242.
3. Appel, S. H. (1981): A unifying hypothesis for the cause of amyotrophic lateral sclerosis, parkinsonism, and Alzheimer's disease. *Ann. Neurol.*, 10:499–505.
4. Heumann, R., Korsching, S., Bandtlow, C., and Thoenen, H. (1987): Changes of nerve growth factor synthesis in nonneuronal cells in response to sciatic nerve transection. *J. Cell. Biol.*, 104:1623–1631.
5. Konkol, R. J., Mailman, R. B. Bendeich, E. G., Garrison, A. M., Mueller, R. A., and Breese, G. R. (1982): Evaluation of the effects of nerve growth factor and anti-nerve growth factor on the development of central catecholaminergic neurons. *Brain Res.*, 144:277–285.
6. Gnahn, H., Hefti, F., Heumann, R., Schwab, M., and Thoenen, H. (1983): NGF-mediated increase of choline acetyltransferase (ChAT) in the neonatal forebrain; evidence for a physiological role of NGF in the brain? *Dev. Brain Res.*, 9:45–52.
7. Korsching, S., Auburger, G., Heumann, R., Scott, J., and Thoenen, H. (1985): Levels of nerve growth factor and its mRNA in the central nervous system of the rat correlate with cholinergic innervation. *EMBO J.*, 4:1389–1393.
8. Shelton, D. L., and Reichardt, L. F. (1984): Expression of the nerve growth factor gene correlates with the density of sympathetic innervation in effector organs. *Proc. Natl. Acad. Sci. U.S.A.*, 81:7951–7955.
9. Hefti, F., Hartikka, J., Salvatierra, A., Weiner, W. J., and Mash, D. C. (1986): Localization of nerve growth factor receptors in cholinergic neurons of the human basal forebrain. *Neurosci. Lett.*, 69:37–41.
10. Springer, J. E., Koh, S., Tayrien, M. W., and Loy, R. (1987): Basal forebrain magnocellular neurons stain for nerve growth factor receptor: correlation with cholinergic cell bodies and effects of axotomy. *J. Neurosci. Res.*, 17:111–118.
11. Hefti, F., Dravid, A., and Hartikka, J. (1984): Chronic interventricular injections of nerve growth factor elevate hippocampal choline acetyltransferase activity in adult rats with partial septo-hippocampal lesions. *Brain Res.*, 293:305–309.
12. Hefti, F., Hartikka, J., Eckenstein, F., Ganhn, H., Heumann, R., and Schwab, M. (1985):

Nerve growth factor (NGF) increases choline acetyltransferase but not survival or fiber growth of cultured septal cholinergic neurons. *Neuroscience*, 14:55–68.

13. Hefti, F. (1986): Nerve growth factor (NGF) promotes survival of septal cholinergic neurons after fimbrial transsections. *J. Neurosci.*, 6:2155–2162.
14. Williams, L. R., Varon, S., Peterson, G. M., et al. (1986): Continuous infusion of nerve growth factor prevents basal forebrain neuronal death after fimbria fornix transection. *Proc. Natl. Acad. Sci. U.S.A.*, 83:9231–9235.
15. Will, B., and Hefti, F. (1985): Behavioral and neurochemical effects of chronic intraventricular injections of nerve growth factor in adult rats with fimbria lesions. *Behav. Brain Res.*, 17:17–24.
16. Fischer, W., Wictorin, K., Bjorklund, A., Williams, L. R., Varon, S., and Gage, F. H. (1987): Amelioration of cholinergic neuron atrophy and spatial memory impairment in aged rats by nerve growth factor. *Nature* (Lond.): 329:65–68.
17. Manthorpe, M., Skaper, S. D., Williams, L. R., and Varon, S. (1986): Purification of adult rat sciatic nerve ciliary neuronotrophic factor. *Brain Res.*, 367:282–286.
18. Barde, Y. A., Davies, A. M., Johnson, J. E., Lindsay, R. M., and Thoenen, H. (1987): Brain-derived neurotrophic factor. In: *Progress in Brain Research*, Vol. 71, edited by F. J. Seil, E. Herbert and B. M. Carlson, pp. 185–189. Elsevier, Amsterdam.
19. Wagner, J. A., and D'Amore, P. A. (1986): Neurite outgrowth induced by an endothelial cell mitogen isolated from retina. *J. Cell. Biol.*, 103:1363–1367.
20. Gloor, S., Odink, K., Guenther, J., Nick, H., and Monard, D. (1986): A glia-derived neurite promoting factor with protease inhibitory activity belongs to the protease nexins. *Cell*, 47:687–693.
21. Gurney, M. E., Heinrich, S. P., Lee, M. R., and Yin, H. S. (1987): Molecular cloning and expression of neuroleukin, a neurotrophic factor for spinal and sensory neurons. *Science*, 234:566–574.
22. Smith, R. G., Vaca, K., McManaman, J., and Appel, S. H. (1986): Selective effects of skeletal muscle extract fractions on motoneuron development in vitro. *J. Neurosci.*, 6:439–447.
23. Morrison, R. S. (1987): Fibroblast growth factors: potential neurotrophic agents in the central nervous system. *J. Neurosci. Res.*, 17:99–101.
24. Morrison, R. S., Kornblun, H. I., Leslie, F. M., and Bradshaw, R. A. (1987): Trophic stimulation of cultured neurons from neonatal rat brain by epidermal growth factor. *Science*, 238:72–75.
25. Recio-Pinto, E., Rechler, M. M., and Ishii, D. N. (1986): Effects of insulin, insulin-like growth factor-II, and nerve growth factor on neurite formation and survival in cultured sympathetic and sensory neurons. *J. Neurosci.*, 6:1211–1219.
26. Kligman, D., and Marshak, D. R. (1985): Purification and characterization of a neurite extension factor from ovine brain. *Proc. Natl. Acad. Sci. U.S.A.*, 82:7136–7139.
27. Rogers, S. L., Letourneau, P. C., Palm, S. L., McCarthy, J., and Furcht, L. T. (1983): Neurite extension by peripheral and central nervous system neurons in response to substratum-bound fibronectin and laminin. *Dev. Biol.*, 98:212–220.
28. Shalaby, I. A., Kotake, C., Hoffmann, P. C., and Heller, A. (1983): release of dopamine from coaggregate cultures of mesencephalic tegmentum and corpus striatum. *J. Neurosci.*, 3:1565–1571.
29. Denis-Donini, S., Glowinski, J., and Prochiantz, A. (1983): Specific influence of striatal target neurons on the in vitro outgrowth of mesencephalic dopaminergic neurites: a morphological quantitative study. *J. Neurosci.*, 3:2292–2299.
30. Tomozawa, Y., and Appel, S. H. (1986): Soluble striatal extracts enhance development of mesencephalic dopaminergic neurons in vitro. *Brain Res.*, 399:111–124.
31. Ferrari, G., Soranzo, C., Skaper, S. D., et al. (1987): Chemical and biological characterization of a striatal-derived neuronotrophic factor (SDNF): comparison with other neuronotrophic factors. *Proc. Soc. Neurosci.*, 13:1611.
32. Brundin, P., Nilsson, O. G., Strecker, R. E., et al. (1986): Behavioral effects of human fetal dopamine neurons grafted in a rat model of Parkinson's disease. *Exp. Brain Res.*, 65:235–240.
33. Freed, W. J., Morihisa, H. M., Spoor, E., et al. (1981): Transplanted adrenal chromaffin cells in rat brain reduce lesion-induced rotational behavior. *Nature (Lond)*, 292:351–352.

34. Naujoks, K. W., Korsching, S., Rohrer, H., and Thoenen, H. (1982): Nerve growth factor-mediated induction of tyrosine hydroxylase and of neurite outgrowth in cultures of bovine adrenal chromaffin cells: dependence of developmental stage. *Dev. Biol.*, 92:365–379.
35. Lindvall, O., Backlund, E. O., Farde, L., et al. (1987): Transplantation in Parkinson's disease: two cases of adrenal medullary grafts to the putamen. *Ann. Neurol.*, 22:457–468.
36. Madrazo, I., Drucker-Colin, R., Diaz, V., Martinez-Mata, J., Torres, C., and Becerril, J. (1987): Open microsurgical autografts of adrenal medulla to the right caudate nucleus in two patients with intractable Parkinson's disease. *N. Engl. J. Med.*, 316:831–834.

Parkinsonism and Aging, edited by
Donald B. Calne et al., Raven Press, Ltd.,
New York © 1989.

Oxygen Toxicity Protecting Enzymes in Aging and Parkinson's Disease

R. J. Marttila and U. K. Rinne

Department of Neurology, University of Turku, SF-20520 Turku, Finland

Human tissues, including the brain, are continuously exposed to toxicity from reduced oxygen species. Most of the oxygen used by cells is reduced to water by the cytochrome oxidase system. However, part of the oxygen receives one electron at a time, the results then being superoxide radical, hydrogen peroxide and hydroxyl radical. These species, if not eliminated efficiently, may cause harmful effects in cells. Cell damage may occur through lipid peroxidation, denaturation of proteins, or DNA modifications (1).

The hypothesis linking oxygen toxicity with the aging process of nervous tissue mainly derives on one hand from the high oxygen consumption by the brain, implying also a high level of exposure to reduced oxygen species, and on the other hand from the high amount of unsaturated lipids susceptible to oxidant toxicity in the brain (2). Similarly, imbalance between the production of reduced oxygen species and the intracellular scavenging capacity has been suggested as being involved in the degeneration of dopamine neurons in Parkinson's disease (3). This review focuses upon the role of oxygen toxicity protecting enzymes in both of these conditions, i.e., aging of the nervous tissue and Parkinson's disease.

OXYGEN TOXICITY PROTECTING ENZYMES

Enzymatic defense against reduced oxygen species involves a cooperative action of several enzymes. The major defense against the toxicity of superoxide radicals is conferred by superoxide dismutase (SOD). This enzyme catalyzes the dismutation of the superoxide radical to hydrogen peroxide. Two types of the enzyme occur in human cells: cytosolic copper–zinc SOD and mitochondrial manganese SOD (4). The resulting hydrogen peroxide does not qualify as a free radical, whereas a highly toxic hydroxyl radical is produced when hydrogen peroxide reacts with transition metals, such as iron or copper (5). The enzymes scavenging hydrogen peroxide, catalase and glutathione peroxidase (GSH-PX), therefore act in concert with SOD. Catalase, mostly located in the peroxisomes (6), decomposes hydrogen peroxide to water, whereas GSH-PX removes hydrogen peroxide by using it to oxidize the reduced glutathione. The resulting oxidized glutathione is reconverted by glutathione reductase (GSSG-RD) to reduced glutathione. Both GSH-PX and GSSG-RD are cytosolic enzymes, but are also present in mitochondria (7,8). In the brain tissue, the major protection both against hydrogen peroxide and against lipid peroxides is probably conferred by GSH-PX (3,5).

SOD, GSH-PX, GSSG-RD, and catalase activities are known to be present in the brain tissue of different animal species and humans. In experimental animals, the distribution of SOD activity in different brain areas has been found to be uniform (9), or some concentration has been noted in the pons, substantia nigra, striatum, and hypothalamus (10–12). In humans, the regional distribution of SOD appears to be relatively even between different brain regions (13–16). GSH-PX activity in the rat brain has been noted to be somewhat higher in the striatum and substantia nigra than in other brain regions (12,17), and a similar, although very slight, regional difference has also been seen in GSSG-RD activity (12). In human brains, the distributions of GSH-PX and GSSG-RD have not exhibited any substantial regional differences (16,18,19). The highest catalase activity in the rat brain has been detected in the hypothalamus and substantia nigra (20), whereas the distribution in the human brain does not indicate marked regional differences (16).

AGING

In experimental animals, cytosolic copper–zinc SOD activity has been reported as remaining unaltered (9,21) or as decreasing with age (22), or as behaving differently in various brain regions (12). Particulate manganese SOD, however, appears to increase with age (9,21,22). Cytosolic GSH-PX activity has been found to remain unaltered (7), to increase (12), or to decrease with age (23). Mitochondrial GSH-PX in the rat brain has been observed to increase in aging animals (7). As for GSH-PX, similarly conflicting results have been obtained for age-related changes in GSSG-RD activity (7,12,21). Catalase may remain stable during aging (7,21).

In our study of the oxygen-protecting enzymes in the human brain (16), altogether 21 brain regions were dissected from the brains of five men of various ages dead by violence or by myocardial infarction. The activities of SOD, catalase, GSH-PX, and GSSG-RD were determined both in the cytosolic and particulate fractions of the brain tissue samples. To study the effect of aging on the enzyme activities, the combined activities of all of the brain regions of the individual cases were analyzed by linear regression in relation to the age of the individuals. The SOD and catalase activities in the cytosolic fraction decreased significantly with age, whereas the particulate activities remained unchanged. The activities of GSH-PX and GSSG-RD behaved differently; the cytosolic activity remained stable, whereas the particulate activities decreased with advancing age. We also analyzed the activities of oxygen toxicity protecting enzymes in human cerebrospinal fluid (Marttila et al., unpublished results). In 55 patients with various neurological disorders, measurable activities of SOD and GSH-PX were constantly observed in cerebrospinal fluid (CSF), whereas detectable levels of GSSG-RD or catalase could not be measured. Neither SOD or GSH-PX activities in the CSF had any correlation with age.

Available data from experimental animals and our results on human brain tissue suggest that age-related modifications may occur in enzymatic protection against oxygen toxicity. Due to the limited number of studies available, no definite pattern of these modifications has as yet emerged. Furthermore, it is not known whether these changes contribute to the aging process or whether they result from the aging of the nervous tissue. In addition, the brain tissue is composed of two types of cells, neurons and glial cells. The partition of the oxygen toxicity protecting enzymes between neurons and glia is largely unknown and nothing is known about whether these enzymes exhibit different age-related changes in different cell types in the brain.

PARKINSON'S DISEASE

Relatively few studies have addressed the integrity of oxygen toxicity protecting enzymes in Parkinson's disease. Ambani et al. (24) studied peroxidase and catalase activities in seven Parkinson's disease brains and found decreased peroxidase and catalase activities in the substantia nigra and striatum. Based on a study of two Parkinson's disease brains and using amyotrophic lateral sclerosis (ALS) patients as controls, Mizuno (25) reported an increased total SOD activity in the parkinsonian frontal cortex and putamen. This increase appeared to be due to manganese SOD. GSH-PX activity was slightly increased in the putamen, whereas catalase did not exhibit any significant changes. This study did not include the substantia nigra. More recently, Kish et al. (19) reported a 20% decrease in GSH-PX activity in the Parkinson's disease frontal cortex, putamen, globus pallidus, and substantia nigra. However, SOD, catalase, GSH-PX, and GSSG-RD activities in the erythrocytes of Parkinson's disease patients have been observed to be comparable to those in control erythrocytes, suggesting that there is no generalized defect in enzymatic oxygen toxicity protection (26).

Our studies of oxygen toxicity protecting enzymes in Parkinson's disease (27) have shown that the activities of oxygen toxicity protecting enzymes

(SOD, GSH-PX, GSSG-RD, and catalase) appear to be unaltered in parkinsonian peripheral blood lymphocytes and granulocytes, thus further substantiating that there is no generalized defect in any of these enzymes in Parkinson's disease. Furthermore, we did not find any alterations in the activities of SOD or GSH-PX in parkinsonian cerebrospinal fluid. We also studied the enzyme activities in 11 Parkinson's disease brains including 12 different brain regions: the frontal and temporal cortex, centrum semiovale, cerebellum, nucleus ruber, thalamus, caudate nucleus, putamen, pallidum, amygdala, basal nucleus of Meynert, and substantia nigra. The activities of GSH-PX and GSSG-RD and of catalase, both in the cytosolic and particulate fractions, were comparable to the normal brain. However, in the parkinsonian brain, there was a significant increase of cytosolic SOD activity; the increase was observed in the temporal cortex, nucleus ruber, and thalamus, where the enzyme activities were increased by 27 to 50% over the control values. The increase, however, was concentrated in the substantia nigra and basal nucleus, where a 55 to 96% increase in cytosolic SOD activities was found. The particulate SOD activities were not altered in the parkinsonian brain.

If the increase of SOD-like activity in the parkinsonian brain is due to an increase in the actual enzyme protein, it then appears to be due to cytosolic copper–zinc SOD, since the particulate activities, mainly due to manganese SOD, were not altered. In that case, the enzyme activity could derive either from neuronal or glial cells. However, the number of glial cells in the Parkinson's disease substantia nigra does not differ from that in age-matched control brains (28). Furthermore, at least in the canine or rat brain, astrocytes do not exhibit copper–zinc SOD immunoreactivity (29), which means that astrocyte-derived SOD is unlikely to explain increased SOD activity in the parkinsonian brain.

Since these results were obtained using the xanthine oxidase–cytochrome c method (30), another possible cause for the increased SOD activity is the presence of a compound with SOD-like activity or a redox-cycling compound interfering with cytochrome reduction. Many compounds are known to mimic SOD activity (31,32), including melanin (33) and catecholamines (3). Dopamine scavenges superoxide radicals and could possibly result in an increase of brain SOD-like activity in levodopa-treated patients. However, the highest dopamine values in levodopa-treated patients are found in the putamen and caudate nucleus (34), yet the SOD activity in those nuclei was unaltered. Interaction by melanin could result in an increase of SOD-like activity in the substantia nigra, but is unlikely to be involved, since other unpigmented regions, such as the basal nucleus, temporal cortex, and thalamus, also exhibited increased SOD activity. Iron chelates, such as citrate–Fe^{3+}, exhibit SOD-like activity by directly scavenging superoxide and by inhibiting cytochrome reduction (32). Since the iron content in the parkinsonian brain is increased (35), particularly ferric iron (36), iron-induced increase of SOD-like activity is possible. However, the presence of an unknown compound with SOD-like activity or with redox-cycling properties in the parkinsonian brain is also possible. Compatible with such an assumption is the observation of low reduced glutathione content in Parkinson's disease substantia nigra (37), which may indicate the presence of a toxic substance that can be conjugated with reduced glutathione by glutathione transferase, thereby leading to a decrease of glutathione content in the substantia nigra (38).

CONCLUSIONS

Data from animal and human studies suggest that the enzymatic defense against oxygen toxicity in the brain exhibits age-related modifications, either reflecting the effects of aging or directly participating in the progression of the aging process. However, the basic biology of the elimination of toxic oxygen species in brain tissue is not adequately known, and in particular it is uncertain whether there are any differences in various neuronal populations or in the glial cells during aging. In Parkinson's disease, there appears to be no generalized defect in the enzymatic defense against oxygen toxicity. In parkinsonian brain tissue, the activities of catalase, glutathione peroxidase, or glutathione reductase do not exhibit any substantial alterations, whereas an increased superoxide dismutase activity has been observed in the substantia nigra and basal nucleus. This may depend on the increase of the actual enzyme protein, or be a result of the presence of a compound either with superoxide dismutase-like activity or with redox-cycling properties.

Acknowledgment: Our studies reviewed here have been supported by the Medical Research Council of the Academy of Finland (Project 09/338).

REFERENCES

1. Freeman, B. A., and Crapo, J. D. (1982): Free radicals and tissue injury. *Lab. Invest.*, 47:412–426.
2. Harman, D. (1983): Free radical theory of aging: consequences of mitochondrial aging. *Age*, 6:86–94.
3. Cohen, G. (1983): The pathobiology of Parkinson's disease: biochemical aspects of dopamine neuron senescence. *J. Neural Transm.* 19(suppl):89–103.
4. Weisiger, R. A., and Fridovich, I. (1973): Mitochondrial superoxide dismutase. Site of synthesis and intramitochondrial localization. *J. Biol. Chem.*, 248:4793–4796.
5. Halliwell, B., and Cutteridge, J. M. C. (1985): Oxygen radicals and the nervous system. *Trends Neurol. Sci.*, 8:22–26.
6. Gaunt, G. L., and De Duve, C. (1976): Subcellular distribution of *d*-amino acid oxidase and catalase in rat brain. *J. Neurochem.*, 26:749–759.
7. Vitorica, J., Machado, A., and Satrustegui, J. (1984): Age-dependent variations in peroxide-utilizing enzymes from rat brain mitochondria and cytoplasm. *J. Neurochem.*, 42:351–356.

8. Mbemba, F., Houbion, A., Raes, M., and Remacle, J. (1985): Subcellular localization and modification with ageing of glutathione, glutathione peroxidase and glutathione reductase activities in human fibroblasts. *Biochim. Biophys. Acta*, 838:211–220.

9. Danh, H. C., Benedetti, M. S., and Dostert, P. (1983): Differential changes in superoxide dismutase activity in brain and liver of old rats and mice. *J. Neurochem.*, 40:1003–1007.

10. Thomas, T. N., Priest, D. G., and Zemp, J. W. (1976): Distribution of superoxide dismutase in rat brain. *J. Neurochem.*, 27:309–310.

11. Ledig, M., Fried, R., Ziessel, M., and Mandel, P. (1982): Regional distribution of superoxide dismutase in rat during postnatal development. *Dev. Brain Res.*, 4:333–337.

12. Mizuno, Y., and Ohta, K. (1986): Regional distribution of thiobarbituric acid-reactive products, activities of enzymes regulating the metabolism of oxygen free radicals, and some of the related enzymes in adult and aged rat brains. *J. Neurochem.*, 46:1344–1352.

13. Loomis, T. C., Yee, G., and Stahl, W. L. (1976): Regional and subcellular distribution of superoxide dismutase in brain. *Experientia*, 32:1374–1376.

14. Marklund, S. L. Oreland, L., Perdahl, E., and Winblad, B. (1983): Superoxide dismutase activity in brains from chronic alcoholics. *Drug Alcoh. Dependence*, 12:209–215.

15. Marklund, S. L., Adolfson, R., Gottfries, C. G., and Winblad, B. (1985): Superoxide dismutase isoenzymes in normal brains and in brains from patients with dementia of Alzheimer type. *J. Neurol. Sci.*, 67:319–325.

16. Marttila, R. J., Röyttä, M., Lorentz, H., and Rinne, U. K. (1988): Oxygen toxicity protecting enzymes in the human brain. *J. Neural Transm.*, 74:87–95.

17. Brannan, T. S., Maker, H. S., Weiss, C., and Cohen, G. (1980): Regional distribution of glutathione peroxidase in the adult rat brain. *J. Neurochem.*, 35:1013–1014.

18. Ansari, K. A., Bigelow, D., and Kaplan, E. (1985): Glutathione peroxidase activity in surgical and autopsied human brains. *Neurochem. Res.*, 10:703–711.

19. Kish, S. J., Morito, C., and Hornykiewicz, O. (1985): Glutathione peroxidase activity in Parkinson's disease brain. *Neurosci. Lett.*, 58:343–346.

20. Brannan, T. S., Maker, H. S., and Raes, I. P. (1981): Regional distribution of catalase in the adult rat brain. *J. Neurochem.*, 36:307–309.

21. Roy, D., Pathak, D. N., and Singh, R. (1983): Effect of centrophenoxine on the antioxidative enzymes in various regions of the aging rat brain. *Exp. Gerontol.*, 18:185–197.

22. Vanella, A., Geremia, E., D'Urso, G., et al. (1982): Superoxide dismutase activities in aging rat brain. *Gerontology*, 28:108–113.

23. Hothersall, J. S., El-Hassan, A., McLean, P., and Greenbaum, A. L. (1981): Age-related changes in enzymes of rat brain. 2. Redox system linked to NADPH and glutathione. *Enzyme*, 26:271–276.

24. Ambani, L. M., Van Woert, M. H., and Murphy, S. (1975): Brain peroxidase and catalase in Parkinson disease. *Arch. Neurol.*, 32:114–116.

25. Mizuno, Y. (1984): Studies on the pathogenesis of degenerative neurological disorders. *Clin. Neurol.*, 24:118–124.

26. Poirier, J., and Barbeau, A. (1987): Erythrocyte antioxidant activity in human patients with Parkinson's disease. *Neurosci. Lett.* 75:345–348.

27. Marttila, R. J., Lorentz, H., and Rinne, U. K. (1988): Oxygen toxicity protecting enzymes in Parkinson's disease. Increase of superoxide dismutase-like activity in the substantia nigra and basal nucleus. *J. Neurol. Sci.*, 86:321–331.

28. Bogerts, B., Häntsch, J., and Herzer, M. (1983): A morphometric study of the dopamine-containing cell groups in the mesencephalon of normals, Parkinson patients, and schizophrenics. *Biol. Psychiatry*, 18:951–969.

29. Thaete, L. G., Crouch, R. K., Nakagawa, F., and Spicer, S. S. (1986): The immunocytochemical demonstration of copper–zinc superoxide dismutase in the brain. *J. Neurocytol.*, 15:337–343.

30. Kirby, T. W., and Fridovich, I. (1982): A picomolar spectrophotometric assay for superoxide dismutase. *Anal. Biochem.*, 127:435–440.

31. Gulyaeva, N. V., Obidin, A. B., and Marinov, B. S. (1987): Modulation of superoxide dismutase by electron donors and acceptors. *FEBS Lett.*, 211:211–214.

32. Minotti, G., and Aust, S. D. (1985): Superoxide-dependent redox cycling of citrate Fe^{3+}: evidence for a superoxide dismutaselike activity. *Arch. Biochem. Biophys.*, 253:257–267.

33. Korytowski, W., Hintz, P., Sealy, R. C., and Kalyanarman, B. (1985): Mechanism of

dismutation of superoxide produced during autoxidation of melanin pigments. *Biochem. Biophys. Res. Commun.* 131:659–665.

34. Rinne, U. K., Sonninen, V., Riekkinen, P., and Laaksonen, H. (1974): Postmortem findings in parkinsonian patients treated with L-dopa: biochemical considerations. In: Yahr MD, ed. *Current Concepts in the Treatment of Parkinsonism*, edited by M. D. Yahr, pp. 211–233. Raven Press, New York.
35. Earle, K. M. (1968): Studies on Parkinson's disease including x-ray fluorescent spectroscopy of formalin fixed brain tissue. *J. Neuropathol. Exp. Neurol.*, 27:1–14.
36. Riederer, P., Sotic, E., Rausch, W. D., and Hebenstreit, G. (1988): Tyrosine hydroxylase, dopamine, and energy metabolism: role in Parkinson's disease and aging. In: *Parkinsonism and Aging*, edited by D. B. Calne, et al., New York, Raven Press, pp. 69–74.
37. Perry, T. L., Godin, D. V., and Hansen, S. (1982): Parkinson's disease: a disorder due to nigral glutathione deficiency? *Neurosci. Lett.*, 33:305–310.
38. Perry, T. L., and Yong, V. W. (1986): Idiopathic Parkinson's disease, progressive supranuclear palsy and glutathione metabolism in the substantia nigra of patients. *Neurosci. Lett.*, 67:269–274.

Parkinsonism and Aging, edited by
Donald B. Calne et al., Raven Press, Ltd.,
New York © 1989.

Kynurenines, Glia, and the Pathogenesis of Neurodegenerative Disorders

Robert Schwarcz, Carmela Speciale, and Waldemar A. Turski

Maryland Psychiatric Research Center, Baltimore, Maryland 21228

Neurodegenerative diseases of the basal ganglia present an opportunity for research into the etiology of movement disorders. Since there can be little doubt that the symptomatic presentation of diseases such as Parkinson's disease or Huntington's disease (HD) is intimately associated with the selective neuronal death observed in these illnesses, investigative efforts increasingly focus on the *mechanisms* by which nerve cells die in the course of the disease process. To this end, neuroscientists studying the brain's dopaminergic system and its role in Parkinson's disease have used toxins such as 6-hydroxydopamine and, more recently, N-methyl-4-phenyl-1,2,3,6-tetrahydropyridine (MPTP), which have the ability selectively to ablate monoaminergic neurons in experimental animals. The specific nature of the neuronal degeneration precipitated by the parenteral or intracerebral injection of these and related toxins has led to the suggestion that similar mechanisms may underlie the loss of nerve cells in both Parkinson's disease and its animal models (1). Consequently, the production of an endogenous 6-hydroxydopamine-related compound has been speculatively linked to the pathogenesis of idiopathic parkinsonism (2).

A similar reasoning may apply to the etiology of the striatal cell loss that is invariably observed in HD. In 1976, Coyle and Schwarcz reported that intrastriatal injection in rats of the powerful neuroexcitant kainic acid, isolated from the seaweed *Diginea simplex*, leads to the degeneration of striatal neurons (3). Notably, the observed lesion was restricted to neuronal cell bodies, did not affect transversing or afferent nerve fibers, and appeared to cause little if any damage to nonneuronal elements (4). Thus, kainate-induced nerve cell loss in the striatum closely mimicked the neuropathological and neurochemical features of HD (3,5). Due to the structural analogy of kainic acid and endogenous acidic amino acids such as glutamate and aspartate, and based on Olney's concept linking the neuroexcitatory and neurotoxic potency of this family of compounds (6), the idea was born that a pathological overabundance of such an endogenous "excitotoxin" may be causing selective cell destruction in HD (7). By the same argument, it was hypothesized that specific antagonists acting at excitatory amino acid receptors [most prominently, the *N*-methyl-D-aspartate (NMDA) receptor] (8,9) may become of therapeutic value because of their suspected ability to prevent the precipitation of nerve cell death (10).

KYNURENINES: FOCUS ON QUINOLINIC AND KYNURENIC ACID

Of the many brain metabolites that have so far been tested for their excitotoxic potential (11), quinolinic acid (QUIN), known for decades as a product of tryptophan catabolism in the periphery (12), has certainly emerged as the most interesting one. For reasons that are not fully understood, the lesions caused by intrastriatally injected QUIN provide the most accurate HD model available so far. Thus, the survival of medium-sized aspiny neurons containing somatostatin, neuropeptide Y, and NADPH–diaphorase and of acetylcholinesterase-positive large aspiny neurons in HD neostriatum is faithfully replicated by QUIN-lesions of the rat striatum (13,14). Moreover, in remarkable analogy to the presumed late onset of neuronal loss in HD (5), QUIN is far less toxic to the developing than to the adult rat striatum (15). The most likely explanation for the remarkable selectivity of QUIN's toxic effects lies in the developmentally and regionally heterogeneous distribution of neuronal NMDA receptors, the site that seems to be exclusively responsible for the mediation of QUIN's excitatory (16) and neurodegenerative (15) effects. However, other factors, such as the poorly understood contribution of afferent fibers (11) and heterogeneity in the function of kynurenic acid (KYNA; see below), may play important roles in determining the specificity of QUIN-induced neuronal loss.

KYNA, discovered in the 1920s as a constituent of mammalian urine (17), has recently gained prominence as a rather nonselective (broad spectrum) antagonist at excitatory amino acid receptors. Thus, KYNA is able to block the excitatory, convulsive, and neurotoxic actions of QUIN (18,19) but has also been shown to antagonize the actions of kainate and quisqualate, prototypical agonists at non-NMDA receptors in the brain (20,21). The blockade of QUIN effects is of particular interest in view of the close metabolic relationship that exists between QUIN and KYNA in the periphery (Fig. 1). Thus, a yin-yang principle, which conceptually links neurodegeneration to *either* a hyperfunctional QUIN system *and/or* a deficient KYNA system, has been postulated to exist in pathological brain tissue (11).

Whereas the pharmacological and physiological profiles of the actions of both QUIN and KYNA on central neurons are still subject to extensive investigations, we have begun to unravel the intricacies of kynurenine biochemistry in the brain. Both QUIN and KYNA have been unequivocally identified as regular constituents of the human brain (22,23), novel tech-

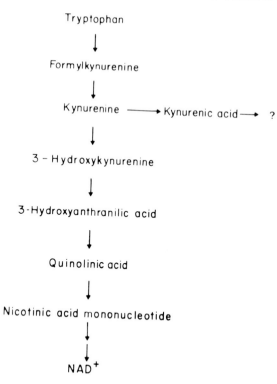

Tryptophan

Formylkynurenine

Kynurenine ⟶ Kynurenic acid ⟶ ?

3 - Hydroxykynurenine

3-Hydroxyanthranilic acid

Quinolinic acid

Nicotinic acid mononucleotide

NAD$^+$

FIG. 1. Kynurenine pathway.

niques have been developed to assess the cellular localization and catalytic properties of some of the enzymes of the brain kynurenine pathway, and first successful attempts have been made to elucidate the function of brain kynurenines following bioprecursor administration.

CELLULAR UPTAKE OF L-KYNURENINE

As the common precursor of both QUIN and KYNA (Fig. 1), L-kynurenine (KYN) occupies an important strategic position in the regulation of its metabolic products. Work from Gál's laboratory had indicated that 60% of brain KYN derives from the periphery under physiological conditions, whereas the rest is probably produced by intracerebral conversion from tryptophan (24). However, until very recently, there existed no information regarding the fate of KYN following its entry into the brain. Using [³H]KYN and tissue slice preparations, cellular uptake of KYN has now been demonstrated (25). Notably, rat brain slices appear to have a more than five times higher ability to concentrate KYN from their environment than slices prepared from peripheral tissues. Moreover, only cerebral tissue exhibits a slow sodium-dependent KYN-uptake process in addition to a rapid, sodium-independent

ase (3HAO) and quinolinic acid phosphoribosyltransferase (QPRT), the immediate anabolic and catabolic enzymes of QUIN, respectively, have been extensively studied in both rat and human brain tissue. In both species, there exists a pronounced regional heterogeneity of enzyme activities (34–37). Kinetic analyses show a far higher V_{max} value for 3HAO than for QPRT while the K_m's for their respective substrates are virtually identical (in the low micromolar range). This implies that *in vivo* 3HAO must be under stringent regulatory control, exerted either at the level of substrate availability or by direct modulation of the enzyme by Fe^{2+} or any of a series of potential endogenous factors (34), in order to avoid the rapid accumulation of neurotoxic quantities of QUIN.

Early observations on differences in the regional distribution of rat brain 3HAO and QPRT activities have recently been complemented by immunohistochemical data obtained at the light and electron microscopic level with antibodies raised again the purified rat liver enzymes (38,39). Taken together, these studies revealed that (a) both 3HAO and QPRT are preferentially localized in nonneuronal elements in the brain; (b) 3HAO, as judged by its extensive colocalization with glial fibrillary acidic protein, is probably an almost exclusively astroglial enzyme; (c) QPRT, too, is in part contained in astrocytes but can frequently also be detected in oligodendroglia-like structures and in punctate elements in or on the surface of neuronal perikarya; and (d) 3HAO is an exclusively cytosolic enzyme, whereas QPRT frequently appears to be associated with the lysosomal element within the cell.

A glial localization of both enzymes can also be inferred from lesion studies, again taking advantage of the selective neurodegenerative effects of intrastriatally injected ibotenic acid. As shown in Table 3, substantial increases in 3HAO and QPRT activities, the former more dramatic than the latter, were observed in lesioned striata 7 days after surgery.

Studies in two human neurodegenerative disorders demonstrate that the cellular distribution of 3HAO and QPRT observed in the rat brain is likely to parallel their localization in the human brain. Thus, cerebral tissue obtained postmortem from HD victims showed pronounced increases in 3HAO

TABLE 3. *Effect of striatal ibotenic acid injections (40 μg/2 μl) on local QUIN metabolism*

	Injected striatum	Contralateral striatum
3HAO (pmol/h/mg protein)	2741 ± 305*	628 ± 47
QPRT (fmol/h/mg protein)	99.9 ± 16.7*	44.0 ± 5.3

Animals (N = 5–6) were killed 7 days after surgery. 3HAO and QPRT activities were measured as detailed in refs. 34 and 35. Data (mean ± SEM) from contralateral striata were not statistically different from those determined in naive control rats. * $p < 0.01$ vs. contralateral striatum (paired t test).

activity as compared to well matched control brains (36). The higher ability to produce QUIN was particularly dramatic in the caudate nucleus and putamen, the two areas that suffer the heaviest neuronal loss in HD (5). However, most other brain regions examined also demonstrated increases in the activity of QUIN's biosynthetic enzyme. While it is not entirely clear at present if a genetic component exists that may be in part responsible for the phenomenon, the animal data described above suggest that the large (approximately fourfold) increases in 3HAO activity in areas of the HD brain that undergo severe neurodegeneration and concomitant astrogliosis (5) are related to the presence of the enzyme in glia. Notably, QPRT activity was found to be unchanged in the caudate and putamen of HD brains, thus suggesting differential cellular localization of QUIN's metabolic enzymes (and a nonneuronal origin of QPRT) in the human brain (37).

As yet unpublished data, obtained in collaboration with Drs. F. Javoy-Agid and Y. Agid (Paris), indicate that a similar selective increase in 3HAO activity can be discerned in brain specimens of patients dying from progressive supranuclear palsy (PSP). The elevations are confined to the caudate nucleus and globus pallidus, two areas with pronounced neurodegeneration in PSP (40), but are far less dramatic than in HD, increasing to 160 and 170% of controls, respectively (manuscript in preparation). As in the case of HD, there is reason to believe that the biochemical change noted should be interpreted as secondary to the selective loss of nerve cells in PSP.

SYNOPSIS: GLIA-DERIVED KYNURENINES AND NERVE CELL LOSS

Taken together, the individual pieces of evidence clearly point to a central role of glial cells in the neurobiology of the kynurenines. Several essential aspects of the puzzle remain to be elucidated, however, before a comprehensive attempt can be made to understand the metabolism and possible function of QUIN, KYNA, and biologically related compounds. To list the most pressing questions, it is mandatory to examine in detail (a) the regulation of KYN production, the mechanisms(s) responsible for its penetration from the periphery into the brain, and the processes modulating its accumulation by brain cells; (b) the sequestration of intracellular KYN along the kynurenine pathway to QUIN or via a transaminase step to KYNA; (c) the possibility of alternative biosynthetic mechanisms for the production of both QUIN and KYNA in the brain; (d) the conditions that exert regulatory control over the liberation of QUIN and KYNA from their cellular confinement and thus determine their extracellular presence and access to neuronal excitatory amino acid receptors; and (e) possible changes that may take place in the cerebral QUIN/KYNA system in association with central nervous system development, aging, or disease states.

Interactions between neurons and glia are increasingly being recognized as much more than the original master–slave relationship that had defined the role of glial cells as that of providing structural support, nurture, and electrical insulation. Thus, it now appears that glial cells constitute important elements of central neurotransmission and are instrumental for controlling the extracellular milieu with regard to ions and neurotransmitters (41). In addition, the buffering capacity of glial cells can be envisioned to serve a protective function in the early stages following excitotoxin-initiated neuronal insults so that glia may in fact be responsible for the reversible nature of excitotoxic damage during the initial period of neurodegeneration (42). Study of brain kynurenines add a novel facet to neuron–glia interactions with regard to cell death since it now appears that glial cells produce and harbor compounds that can determine the survival of adjacent nerve cells. The precise nature of the role of QUIN and/or KYNA in this scenario will certainly be at the focus of intensive investigation in the near future.

Clearly, the thorough investigation of brain kynurenines would be greatly facilitated by the availability of pharmacological agents that specifically influence selected aspects of their biological function. In addition to the merit of such drugs for tackling basic research issues, they can also be envisioned to be of therapeutic value in case a dysfunction of the QUIN/KYNA system is found to be linked to the precipitation of nerve cell death in humans. Conceptually, it may make little difference at which level of metabolism the pharmacological intervention takes place, i.e., any compound that is capable of lowering the extracellular levels of QUIN (e.g., a selective 3HAO inhibitor) and/or increasing the extracellular levels of KYNA will evoke substantial interest regarding their clinical potential. Drugs that exert beneficial influence on brain kynurenine metabolism may indeed constitute therapeutic agents that are superior to the much heralded NMDA-receptor antagonists (43), since they can be expected to circumvent an indiscriminate interference with NMDA receptors which are increasingly recognized for their role in *normal* brain function (44). Thus, drugs designed to modulate QUIN/KYNA dysfunction in the brain may hold great promise for the treatment of any of the disease entities that have been speculatively linked to excitotoxic mechanisms (11,43). It can be hoped that the first generation of such compounds will become available in the not too distant future.

Acknowledgment: This work was in part supported by USPHS grants NS 16102 and NS 20509. We thank Mrs. J. Burgess for excellent secretarial assistance.

REFERENCES

1. Jonsson, G. (1980): *Annu. Rev. Neurosci.*, 3:1169–1187.
2. Cohen, G., Dembiec, D., Mytilineou, C., and Heikkila, R. E. (1976): In: *Advances in Parkinsonism*, edited by W. Birkmayer and O. Hornykiewicz, Basel, Editiones Roche, pp. 251–257.
3. Coyle, J. T., and Schwarcz, R. (1976): *Nature (Lond.)*, 263:244–246.

4. Coyle, J. T., Molliver, M. E., and Kuhar, M. J. (1978): *J. Comp. Neurol.*, 180:301–324.
5. Chase, T. N., Wexler, N. S., and Barbeau, A., eds. (1979): *Huntington's Disease: Advances in Neurology*, Vol. 23, New York, Raven Press.
6. Olney, J. W. (1974): In: *Heritable Disorders of Amino Acid Metabolism*, edited by W. L. Nyhan, New York, Wiley, pp. 501–512.
7. Coyle, J. T., Schwarcz, R., Bennett, J. P., and Campochiaro, P. (1977): *Prog. Neuropsychopharmacol.*, 1:13–30.
8. Watkins, J. C., Evans, R. H. (1981): *Annu. Rev. Pharmacol. Toxicol.*, 21:165–204.
9. McLennan, H. (1983): *Prog. Neurobiol.*, 20:251–271.
10. Schwarcz, R., Fuxe, K., Hökfelt, T., Andersson, K., and Coyle, J. T. (1979): In: *Dopaminergic Ergot Derivatives and Motor Function*, edited by K. Fuxe and D. B. Calne, Oxford, Pergamon, pp. 115–126.
11. Schwarcz, R., Foster, A. C., French, E. D., Whetsell, W. O., Jr., and Köhler, C. (1984): *Life Sci.*, 35:19–32.
12. Henderson, L. M., and Hirsch, H. M. (1949): *J. Biol. Chem.*, 181:667–675.
13. Beal, M. F., Kowall, N. W., Ellison, D. W., Mazurek, M. F., Swartz, K. J., and Martin, J. B. (1986): *Nature (Lond.)*, 321:168–171.
14. Ferrante, R. J., Beal, M. F., Kowall, N. W., Richardson, E. P., Jr., and Martin, J. B. (1987): *Brain Res.*, 411:162–166.
15. Foster, A. C., Collins, J. F., and Schwarcz, R. (1983): *Neuropharmacology*, 22:1331–1342.
16. Stone, T. W., and Perkins, M. N. (1981): *Eur. J. Pharmacol.*, 72:411–412.
17. Späth, E. (1921): *Monatsh. Chem.*, 42:89–95.
18. Perkins, M. N., and Stone, T. W. (1982): *Brain Res.*, 247:183–187.
19. Foster, A. C., Vezzani, A., French, E. D., and Schwarcz, R. (1984): *Neurosci. Lett.*, 48:273–278.
20. Ganong, A. H., Lanthorn, T. H., and Cotman, C. W. (1983): *Brain Res.*, 273:170–174.
21. Herrling, P. L. (1985): *Neuroscience*, 14:417–426.
22. Wolfensberger, M., Amsler, U., Cuénod, M., Foster, A. C., Whetsell, W. O., Jr., and Schwarcz, R. (1983): *Neurosci. Lett.*, 41:247–252.
23. Turski, W. A., Nakamura, M., Todd, W. P., Carpenter, B. K., Whetsell, W. O., Jr., and Schwarcz, R. (1988): *Brain Res.*, 454:164–169.
24. Gál, E. M., and Sherman, A. D. (1978): *J. Neurochem.* 30:607–613.
25. Speciale, C., Turski, W. A., Brookes, N., and Schwarcz, R. (1987): *Soc. Neurosci. Abstr.*, 13:464.17.
26. Schwarcz, R., Hökfelt, T., Fuxe, K., Jonsson, G., Goldstein, M., and Terenius, L. (1979): *Exp. Brain Res.*, 37:199–216.
27. Björklund, H., Olson L, Dahl, D., and Schwarcz, R. (1986): *Brain Res.*, 371:267–277.
28. Joseph, M. H. (1978): *J. Chromatogr.*, 146:33–41.
29. Turski, W. A., Gramsbergen, J. B. P., Traitler, H., and Schwarcz, R. (1989): *J. Neurochem.* (in press).
30. Webb, J. L. (1966): *Enzyme and Metabolic Inhibitors*, Vol. II, New York, Academic Press, pp. 358–359.
31. Turski, W. A., and Schwarcz, R. (1988): *Exp. Brain Res.*, 71:563–567.
32. Battie, C., and Verity, M. A. (1981): *J. Neurochem.*, 36:1308–1310.
33. Kawai, J., Okuno, E., and Kido, R. (1988): *Enzyme*, 39:181–189.
34. Foster, A. C., White, R. J., and Schwarcz, R. (1986): *J. Neurochem.*, 47:23–30.
35. Foster, A. C., Zinkand, W. C., and Schwarcz, R. (1985): *J. Neurochem.*, 44:446–454.
36. Schwarcz, R., Okuno, E., White, R. J., Bird, E. D., and Whetsell, W. O., Jr. (1988): *Proc. Natl. Acad. Sci. U.S.A.* (in press).
37. Foster, A. C., Whetsell, W. O., Jr., Bird, E. D., and Schwarcz, R. (1985): *Brain Res.*, 336:207–214.
38. Okuno, E., Köhler, C., and Schwarcz, R. (1987): *J. Neurochem.*, 49:771–780.
39. Köhler, C., Okuno, E., Flood, P. R., and Schwarcz, R. (1987): *Proc. Natl. Acad. Sci. U.S.A.* 84:3491–3495.
40. Steele, J. C. (1972): *Brain*, 95:693–704.
41. Schoffeniels, E., Franck, G., Hertz, L., and Tower, D. B., eds. (1978): *Dynamic Properties of Glial Cells*, Oxford, Pergamon Press.
42. Foster, A. C., Gill, R., and Woodruff, G. N. (1987): *Soc. Neurosci. Abstr.*, 13:287.6.
43. Schwarcz, R., and Meldrum, B. (1985): *Lancet*, 2:140–143.
44. Barnes, D. M. (1988): *Science*, 239:254–256.

Parkinsonism and Aging, edited by
Donald B. Calne et al., Raven Press, Ltd.,
New York © 1989.

Aging and Gene Expression in the Mammalian Brain: Normal and Pathological Changes

Caleb Finch, James Goss, Steven Johnson, Steven Kohama, Patrick May, Jeffrey Masters, Sharon Millar, David Morgan, Nancy Nichols, Heinz Osterburg, and Giulio Pasinetti

Andrus Gerontology Center and the Department of Biological Sciences, University of Southern California, Los Angeles, California 90089-0191

This synopsis of recent work from our laboratory focuses on questions of gene expression in the brain during aging and in two age-related neurological diseases, Parkinson's and Alzheimer's disease. A long-standing view holds that nondividing cells such as neurons are predisposed to senescent involution. While it is true that few of the central neurons in mammals are formed *de novo* after puberty or can regenerate after injury (1,2), we question whether senescent involution generally occurs in most neurons. For example, two neurosecretory systems show no evidence of general failure up through the average lifespan in humans: the LHRH neurons that maintain sustained elevations of pituitary gonadotropins long beyond menopause (3) and the vasopressinergic neurons that show progressively increased sensitivity to osmotic stimulae in elderly men (4). At the molecular level, an analysis of whole brain RNA from male rats across their lifespan did not detect changes in the levels of messenger RNA (polyA + mRNA isolated from polyribosomes) or in its nucleotide sequence complexity, which assays the number of different types of mRNA species (5). On the other hand, many other types of neurons show statistically significant trends for degenerative changes during aging, particularly in the hippocampus, cerebral cortex, and in monoaminergic projection systems (6,7). The changes include alterations in dendritic structure, loss of receptors, decreases in cell body RNA, and, to an unknown extent, death of neurons. Future studies may reveal how many of these changes occur in all individuals.

We are trying to identify the mechanisms of age-related change that predispose to neuronal dysfunctions and loss during aging. At least two major classes of phenomena can now be identified that may share important features: (I) the *deafferentation syndromes* (consequent to decreased input of afferent systems) and (II) *steroid-induced neuron damage*. Details of the most recent findings are not given here because some journals require that data in submitted manuscripts not be simultaneously published.

DEAFFERENTATION SYNDROMES

Microspectrophotometric observations of postmortem brain from elderly normal individuals and from those with age-related neurological diseases often show nucleolar shrinkage or loss of cell body RNA in large neurons (8–10), e.g., in the substantia nigra (Parkinson's) or basal cholinergic nuclei and hippocampus. The nucleolar shrinkage in the remaining neurons of the substantia nigra in parkinsonism was particularly puzzling, because lesions of this pathway induce hyperactivity of the remaining neurons in young rats, as judged by increased synthesis and release of dopamine at the terminals of increased synthesis of TH (tyrosine hydroxylase) (11–14).

We have produced a lesion model that demonstrates the parkinsonian atrophy of nigral neurons, yet which also shows the enhanced synthesis at the remaining terminals (G. Pasinetti et al.). Adult male rats were given unilateral 6-hydroxydopamine (6-OHDA) injection into the substantia nigra, and sacrificed 9 months later. Measurements of striatal catecholamines showed major depletion of dopamine (DA) on the lesioned side, but increased DOPAC/DA ratios; this indicates increased release of DA at the remaining striatal terminals, as expected from the compensatory responses of the nigrostriatal terminals (see above). To our knowledge, the maintenance of this compensatory increase for such a long portion (35%) of the rodent lifespan had not been indicated before.

The cell bodies of these lesioned neurons, however, showed an opposite response to 6-OHDA lesions; they were atrophied just as seen in parkinsonism. In these measurements, dopaminergic neurons were identified by immunocytochemistry with antisera to rat TH. The cell bodies, nuclei, and nucleoli of TH-immunoreactive neurons were about 30% smaller than in the contralateral (non-lesioned) side. The smaller nucleoli imply decreased synthesis of ribosomes, which would be consistent with the gross loss of neuronal RNA reported in the substantia nigra during Parkinsonism (9).

To establish the extent of change in neuron RNA, we examined two messenger RNA populations using *in situ* hybridization: TH mRNA and β-tubulin mRNA. For these measurements, brain sections were prepared for ICC (immunocytochemistry) to TH, followed by hybridization to cRNA (complementary) antisense strand probes made in a transcription vector. This approach allows us to assay specific mRNA in identified dopaminergic neurons. The loss of TH mRNA was larger than for β-tubulin.

These results pose some interesting questions. In regard to increased dopamine metabolism, the opposite changes of the TH mRNA in its cell body and of DA synthesis and release at its striatal terminals imply a dichotomous regulation. Is the efficiency of TH mRNA translation increased several-fold to compensate for reduced mRNA at a time when more DA is synthesized and released per neuron? The greater deficit of TH mRNA than tubulin mRNA is also interesting, and illustrates that even during neuron cell body atrophy with nucleolar shrinkage, some mRNAs are relatively unaffected. We plan to include additional mRNA in these studies to ascertain the extent of coordinate regulation of mRNA for cytoskeletal proteins, housekeeping enzymes, and specialized cell functions.

Several mechanisms for these changes can be considered. It is possible that 6-OHDA has long-lasting toxic effects that cause damage to even the remaining neuron cell bodies, while allowing the terminals to manage some compensation. Alternatively, there may be transynaptic effects through the striatonigral pathways containing γ-aminobutyric acid (GABA) and substance P, which influence the nondopaminergic neurons of the substantia nigra pars reticulata (15). We hypothesize that the net reduction of DA release after 6-OHDA lesions causes changes in the striatonigral afferents. This perspective may apply to age-related loss of striatal RNA in aging rodents (16,17) and the age-related slowing of striatal DA turnover (18,19). We hypothesize that the slowed release of DA would cause decreased RNA synthesis in striatal neurons, particularly in the medium spiny I neurons that atrophy in parkinsonism (20). According to this view, some neurotransmitters may be linked to neurotrophic factors. The reversal of cholinergic neuron atrophy in the striatum and basal forebrain of 2-year-old rats by infusion of NGF (21) indicates an extensive role of neurotrophic factors, but need not result from primary deficiencies of such factors. We suggest that many other examples of age-related neuron atrophy could be interpreted as the result of deafferentation syndromes. Apparently, similar atrophy of basal forebrain cholinergic neurons also can be induced by decortication (22). Moreover, lesions that kill 30% of basal forebrain cholinergic nuclei in rats cause very slowly evolving neurodegenerative transynaptic cascades that lead to neuronal degeneration in the entorhinal cortex and hippocampus (23); these changes give a striking model for neuronal atrophy in these same pathways during Alzheimer's disease (24). We need more detailed knowledge about the changes in specific RNA and protein species in order to establish if neuron atrophy has the same final common regulatory pathway, e.g., in aging, diseases like parkinsonism with major neuron loss, or after experimental deafferentation. Finally, we also note the potential bearing of these results on the choice of drugs used to treat parkinsonism. It will be important to learn how various drug treatments influence the levels and translation of TH mRNA, and it may be possible to increase the translatable pool of TH mRNA.

On the other hand, deafferentation may cause compensatory *increases* in macromolecular biosynthesis in other types of neurons. In the hippocampus, during normal aging and during Alzheimer's disease, there is dendritic growth in the molecular layer of granule cells in the dentate gyrus of the hippocampal formation (25,26). These densely packed neurons receive major input from the pyramidal neurons of the entorhinal cortex; by histochemical criteria, the same sprouting reactions are induced in young rats by lesions of the entorhinal cortex. In this case, the deafferented granule cells increase in size during Alzheimer's disease (26).

We are developing molecular approaches to study the genomic basis for these phenomena. The strategy involves (a) cloning of mRNA from the Alzheimer hippocampus; (b) selecting those that are increased ($AD+$); and (c) identifying which of the $AD+$ clones represent sequences associated with reactive synaptogenesis by cross-screening with hippocampal RNA from rats after entorhinal cortex lesions. The results, though preliminary, are encouraging.

First, we were able to obtain high molecular weight poly(A)RNA from postmortem human hippocampus and cortex, with no obvious differences between Alzheimer's disease brains or age-matched controls (27,28). After processing more than 50 pairs of samples, we concluded that the postmortem interval is not crucial (0–24 hr) but that other factors such as premorbid hypoxia or wasting conditions may be more important. To great satisfaction, we found that poly(A)RNA from the Alzheimer brain is relatively intact in favorably undegraded specimens and can be cloned effectively with conventional procedures that yielded double stranded cDNA of average size 1.5 kb (range of 0.5–5.0 kb) (27). A library of recombinants was made in the cloning vector lambda gt10 and yielded 61 plaques that showed ≥2-fold change in Alzheimer's disease through differential plaque hybridization screening procedures. The $AD+$ clones isolated so far fall into two classes: a substantial number (80%) that cross-hybridized to each other, demonstrating extensive homology. On the basis of the partial sequence available at this moment, they contain coding sequences for glial fibrillary acidic protein (GFAP). Blot hybridization indicates threefold increases of mRNA for GFAP in hippocampus and cortical regions that degenerate in Alzheimer's disease, but no changes in the cerebellum (29,30). We appear to have isolated a nearly full length clone for GFAP that contains the entire coding sequence. By reference to mouse GFAP data in GenBank, this human GFAP clone has an 83% identical base sequence. More about GFAP below.

Another class of clones being isolated from the hippocampal library is not related to GFAP. One clone (pADHc9) detects an interesting regional change in RNA prevalence. On Northern blots, this clone hybridizes to a 2,000 nucleotide RNA that is selectively increased in the hippocampus, but not in cortex regions that usually show extensive degeneration during Alzheimer's disease (frontal, occipital, or temporal cortex). Such regionally selective changes suggest that there are RNA changes that are markers for responses of particular cell types to neurodegeneration. This clone is being investigated further to establish its cell types of origin and possible relation to reactive synaptogenesis. The limited amount of base sequence data obtained so far (0.4 kb) does not have homologues to other sequences in GenBank. These results show the possibility of isolating clones from human brain that can detect regionally specific changes in Alzheimer's disease and possibly in normal aging. With such approaches, it will be plausible to ask detailed mechanistic questions about changes in neuron gene expression with aging and with Alzheimer's disease.

The increased prevalence of GFAP mRNA in the hippocampus and several cortex regions of Alzheimer's brain is consistent with reports of increased numbers of fibrous astrocytes (31,32). We note that the Alzheimer's disease cerebellum did not show such increases of GFAP mRNA relative to age-matched controls. An unexpected feature came to light in comparing individual brains: marked GFAP mRNA elevations were strongly correlated in senescent male C57BL/6J mice (28–34 months old) that showed a wasting condition (33). Gross pathologic examination identified the presence of tumors in some mice. Thus, major physiologic disturbances can trigger elevations of astrocyte mRNA as well as the well-established reactive astrocytosis that follows from local neuron injury or death. In studies of postmortem human brain, it will be important to identify premorbid conditions that elevated GFAP mRNA, since the abundant class mRNA can dominate differential screening procedures.

STEROID-INDUCED CHANGES

Another class of age-related changes in the brain involves chronic effects of steroids. Under some conditions, endogenous or exogenous estrogens and glucocorticoids appear to cause irreversible changes on selective targets in the adult rodent brain. As shown in an extensive series of studies from this laboratory (34–37), ovarian steroids cause irreversible changes in the regulation of estrous cycles and control of gonadotropins. In these studies, inbred mice are ovariectomized at various ages to remove ovarian steroids and then another set of ovaries is replaced at later ages. Through this approach we showed that exposure to endogenous ovarian steroids is responsible for a variety of hypothalamic-associated age changes: the transition from short (4d) to longer estrous cycles (35), reduction in the sensitivity of negative and positive feedback by estradiol of LH regulation (37,38), and increased numbers of reactive astrocytes in the arcuate nucleus of the hypothalamus (39). Although the later change implies neuronal damage, there is no strong evidence for neuron loss at this time: for example, the numbers of luteinizing hormone–releasing hormone (LHRH) neurons in the mouse hypothalamus are unchanged at least up to a nearly average lifespan (40), which is long after major neuroendocrine impairments. The absence of hypothalamic LHRH neuron loss despite major impairments in the regulation of LH is consistent with the maintained output of LH in postmenopausal women (see introduction) and demonstrates that there can be major functional changes in the aging brain without necessarily losing neurons that are known to be crucial, as is the case for LHRH neurons; here the defect appears to be in the responsiveness of the LHRH neurons to afferent stimulae, rather than in their ability to produce LHRH. Efforts continue to identify the location of damaged neurons that could account for the ovary-dependent neuroendocrine age changes.

Estradiol appears to be the steroid responsible for these changes. We recently showed that estradiol given to ovariectomized mice at physiologic doses through the drinking water for 12 weeks induces permanent impairments in estrous cycles when ovaries are replaced (41). Virtually all of the female reproductive neuroendocrine age changes that can be retarded by ovariectomy are prematurely induced in young rodents by chronic exposure to estrogen (34). Attempts to use molecular cloning techniques for isolating estrogen responsive genes were initially encouraging (42), but have not given consistent enough data to pursue.

Adrenal steroids also interact with brain aging, at least in the hippocampus. Studies by Landfield (43,44) and by Sapolsky (45) indicate that age-related damage to hippocampal pyramidal neurons in rats can be reduced by adrenalectomy or intensified by chronic exposure to high levels of corticosterone. To approach this phenomenon, we are studying corticosteroid-responsive hippocampal mRNAs that show rapid and large scale changes, e.g., as shown by translation products on two-dimensional gel electrophoresis (46). Three clones have been characterized so far (47). Clone *pCR16* corresponds to a poly(A)RNA that increases rapidly (<24 hr) after corticosterone treatment in granule and pyramidal layers of the hippocampus of young rats; limited sequence data do not identify homologues. Two other clones that also corresponded to rapid large scale RNA responses proved to be well-known corticosteroid responsive genes: glycerol-3-phosphate dehydrogenase (in oligodendroglia) and glutamine synthetase (in astrocytes). We are impressed by the prominence of reactive glial changes during aging and are considering ways in which glial astrocytes could be more mechanistically important in aging than as a response to neuronal injury.

SUMMARY

This summary of recent work describes our efforts to identify the distal physiological mechanisms that cause age-related changes in cell function during normal aging and in parkinsonism, Alzheimer's disease, and other age-related neurodegenerative conditions. We are using molecular genetics techniques to obtain new markers for studying the mechanisms of neuro-degeneration in terms of gene expression. One outcome of these studies might be a detailed sequence of changes in gene expression during chronic and acute phases of neurodegeneration, such as has been shown for bacteria during lytic and lysogenic infections by bacteriophage. By analogy, we may be able to define the steps by which insults to neurons from virus, toxins, steroids, or transynaptic influences cause different gradations of changes with different time courses. Ultimately, genomic information will be decoded to reveal why some neurons are at high risk for degeneration and why others appear to be highly resistent and survive to the end of life, barring accidental death from stroke or mechanical trauma. We suspect that many aspects of cell aging in the brain and elsewhere are not intrinsic to the differentiated state of particular cells, but represent the influence of extrinsic factors from the environment or from other cells in the body (48–50). If so, many of the common degenerative changes of age should be open to clinical intervention as well as to understanding at a fundamental level.

Acknowledgment: This research was supported by grants from the NIH, the Office of Naval Research, ADRA, the French Foundation, AFAR, and the John D. and Katherine T. MacArthur Foundation.

REFERENCES

1. Jacobson, M. (1978): *Developmental Neurobiology*, 2nd ed., New York, Holt, Rinehart and Winston.
2. Rakic, P. (1985): *Science*, 227:1054–1056.
3. Scaglia, H., Medina, M., Pinto-Ferreira, A. L., Vasques, G., Gual, C., and Perez-Palacios, G. (1976): *Acta Endocrinol.*, 81:673–679.
4. Robertson, G. L., and Rowe, J. (1980): *Peptides*, 1(suppl. 1):158–162.
5. Colman, P. D., Kaplan, B. B., Osterburg, H. H., and Finch, C. E. (1980): *J. Neurochem.*, 34:335–345.
6. Flood, D. G., Buell, S. J., Horwitz, G. J., and Coleman, P. D. (1987): *Brain Res.*, 402:205–216.
7. Morgan, D. G., May, P. C., and Finch, C. E. (1987): *J. Am. Geriatr. Soc.*, 35:334–345.
8. Doebler, J. A., Marksbery, W. R., Anthony, A., and Rhoads, R. E. (1987): *J. Neuropathol. Exp. Neurol.*, 46: 28–39.
9. Mann, D. M. A., and Yates, P. O. (1983): *Mech. Aging Dev.*, 21:193–203.
10. Mann, D. M. A., Yates, P. O., and Marcyniuk, B. (1984): *Neuropathol. Appl. Neurobiol.*, 10:185–207.
11. Agid, Y., Javoy, F., and Glowinski, J. (1973): *Nature (Lond.)*: 245:150–151.
12. Hefti, F., Melamed, E., and Wurtman, R. (1980): *Brain Res.*, 195:123–137.
13. Zigmond, M. J., and Striker, E. M. (1984): *Life Sci.*, 35:5–18.
14. Stachowiak, M. K., Keller, R. W., Striker, E. M., and Zigmond, M. J. (1987): *J. Neurosci.*, 7:1648–1654.
15. Saji, M., and Reis, D. J. (1987): *Science*, 235:66–69.
16. Chaconas, G., and Finch, C. E. (1973): *J. Neurochem.*, 21:1469–1473.
17. Shaskan, E. G. (1977): *J. Neurochem.*, 28:509–516.
18. Finch, C. E. (1973): *Brain Res.*, 52:261–276.
19. Osterburg, H. H., Donahue, H. G., Severson, J. A., and Finch, C. E. (1981): *Brain Res.*, 224:337–352.

20. McNeil, T., Brown, S. A., Shoulson, I., Lapham, L., Eskin, T., and Rafols, J. (1987): *Basal Ganglia II*, New York, Plenum Press, pp. 475–482.
21. Fischer, W., Wictorin, K., Bjorklund, A., Williams, L. R., Varon, S., and Gage, F. H. (1987): *Nature (Lond.)*, 329:65–68.
22. Pearson, R. C. A., Gatler, K. C., and Powell, J. P. S. (1983): *Brain Res.*, 261:321–326.
23. Arendash, G. W., Millard, W. J., Dunn, A. J., and Meyer, E. M. (1987): *Science*, 238:95.
24. Hyman, B. T., Van Hoesen, G. W., Damasio, A. R., and Barnes, C. L. (1984): *Science*, 225:1168–1170.
25. Geddes, J. W., Monaghan, D. T., Cotman, C. W., Lott, I. T., Kim, R. C., and Chui, H. C. (1985): *Science*, 230:1179–1181.
26. Flood, D. G., Buell, S. J., Horwitz, G. J., and Coleman, P. D. (1987): *Brain Res.*, 402:205–216.
27. May, P. C., Johnson, S. A., Masters, J. N., Lampert-Etchells, M., and Finch, C. E. (1987): *Proc. Neurosci. Soc.*, 17.
28. Johnson, S. A., Morgan, D. G., and Finch, C. E. (1986): *J. Neurosci. Res.*, 16:267–280.
29. Morgan, D. G., Johnson, J. R., and Finch, C. E. RNA metabolism in Alzheimer's disease: selective increase in GFAP RNA (in preparation).
30. May, P. C., Johnson, S. A., Masters, J. N., Lampert-Etchells, M., and Finch, C. E. Cloning of poly(A)RNA sequences differentially expressed in Alzheimer's disease hippocamus (in preparation).
31. Schecter, R., Yen, S. H. C., and Terry, R. D. (1981): *J. Neuropathol. Exp. Neurol.*, 40:95–107.
32. Mancardi, G. L., Liwnicz, B. H., and Mandybur, T. I. (1983): *Acta Neuropathol.*, 61:76–80.
33. Goss, J. R., Morgan, D. G., and Finch, C. E. (1987): *Proc. Neurosci. Soc.*, 17.
34. Finch, C. E., Felicio, L. S., Mobbs, C. V., and Nelson, J. R. (1984): *Endocrinol. Rev.*, 5:467–497.
35. Felicio, L. S., Nelson, J. F., and Finch, C. E. (1986): *Dev. Comp. Immunol.*, 10:85–91.
36. Telford, N., Mobbs, C. V., Sinha, Y. N., and Finch, C. E. (1986): *Neuroendocrinology*, 43:135–142.
37. Mobbs, C. V., Cheyney, D., Sinha, Y. N., and Finch, C. E. (1984): *Biol. Reprod.*, 30:556–563.
38. Mobbs, C. V., Cheyney, D., Sinha, Y. N., and Finch, C. E. (1985): *Endocrinology*, 116:813–820.
39. Schipper, H., Brawer, J. R., Nelson, J. F., Felicio, L. S., and Finch, C. E. (1981): *Biol. Reprod.*, 25:413–419.
40. Hoffman, G. E., and Finch, C. E. (1986): *Neurobiol. Aging*, 7:45–48.
41. Kohama, S., May, P., and Finch, C. E. (1986): *Proc. Neurosci. Soc.*, 16.
42. Masters, J. N., Nichols, J. R., and Finch, C. E. (1986): *Endocrine Soc. Abstr.* 284.
43. Landfield, P. W., Waymire, J. C., and Lynch, G. (1978): *Science*, 202:1098–1102.
44. Landfield, P. W., Sundberg, D. K., Smith, M. S., et al. (1980): *Peptides*, 1(suppl. 1):185–196.
45. Sapolsky, R. M., Krey, L. C., and McEwen, B. S. (1985): *J. Neurosci.*, 5:1222–1227.
46. Nichols, N. R., Masters, J. N., May, P. C., Millar, S. L., and Finch, C. E. (1986): *Proc. Neurosci. Soc.*, 12:691.
47. Masters, J. N., Nichols, J. R., and Finch, C. E. (1987): *Proc. Neurosci. Soc.*, 17.
48. Finch, C. E. (1976): *Q. Rev. Biol.*, 51:49–83.
49. Finch, C. E. (1987): *Modern Biological Theories of Aging*, edited by H. Warner, New York, Raven Press, pp. 261–306.
50. Finch, C. E. (1987): *Gerontologist* (in press).

Parkinsonism and Aging, edited by
Donald B. Calne et al., Raven Press, Ltd.,
New York © 1989.

Does Aging Contribute to Aggravation of Parkinson's Disease?

Y. Agid, J. Blin, A. M. Bonnet, B. Dubois, F. Javoy-Agid,
M. Ruberg, and *D. Sherman

*INSERM U. 289 and Clinique de Neurologie et Neuropsychologie, Hôpital de la
Pitié-Salpêtrière, and *Institut de Biologie Physico-Chimique, Paris, France*

Loss of nigrostriatal dopaminergic neurons in Parkinson's disease fulfills the criteria of a degenerative disorder of the central nervous system (1): neuronal loss is relatively selective (2), it occurs progressively over a long period of time (3,4), and parkinsonian symptoms appear only after a certain threshold of dopaminergic denervation has been reached (4,5). This characteristic cell degeneration has been postulated to be "multi-factorial in origin, resulting from environmental factors acting on genetically susceptible individuals" (6). However, since the incidence of Parkinson's disease increases in the later decades of life, the cause of the disorder has been suggested to be linked in some way with the aging of the nervous system (7).

The essential question is whether neuronal degeneration develops against a background of normal aging or if aging contributes to cell death. Experimental evidence that aging renders nigral dopaminergic neurons more sensitive to the neurotoxin MPTP has been obtained in animals (8). Moreover, epidemiological studies have shown that the prevalence of Parkinson's disease increases with age (9–11). In other studies, however, the age-specific prevalence of Parkinson's disease reached a maximum in patients 60 to 70 years of age and declined thereafter (12–14). The incidence of the disease also decreases after a certain point during normal aging, indicating that aging does not play a major role in the genesis of Parkinson's disease, and, indeed, in spite of a dramatic increase in the percentage of the normal population living on into old age, the mean age at onset of idiopathic Parkinson's disease reported during the past century has remained around 54 to 58 years (15). A decrease in the prevalence of the disease among the very old would be expected to follow a decline in its incidence in the sixth or seventh decade. It may also, however, indicate a higher mortality rate for parkinsonians compared to other persons in this age group. If it can be asked whether aged parkinsonians are more fragile than their undiseased contemporaries, the role of aging in the progression of the disease in affected patients must also be determined.

This question has been addressed in two retrospective investigations. In the first study, the severity of the parkinsonian syndrome was assessed in two groups of patients who had suffered from Parkinson's disease for similar periods of time, but whose symptoms had appeared at different ages. In the second study, the degree of dopaminergic denervation in the striatum was evaluated postmortem in patients with early and late onset of the disease.

STUDY ONE—INFLUENCE OF AGE AT ONSET OF THE DISEASE ON PARKINSONIAN MOTOR SYMPTOMS

Patients with idiopathic Parkinson's disease (criteria for inclusion are in ref. 16) were divided into two groups that had similar disease durations (7.7 ± 0.5 years), but differed with respect to their age when their symptoms first appeared. The early onset group (n = 69) was under 50 years of age (43.9 ± 0.6 years); the late onset group (n = 69) was over 60 years (65.8 + 0.6 years). Approximately 22 years, then, separated the two groups of patients, both with respect to age at which the disease manifested itself and the moment at which their motor scores were determined, for purposes of the study. Both early and late onset (or younger and older) patients had also received levodopa for similar lengths of time (6.4 ± 0.5 and 6.6 ± 0.6 years, respectively) and at doses (669 ± 46 and 730 ± 44 mg/day, respectively) that did not differ significantly. The patients' motor handicap was evaluated using the modified Columbia scale, with each item scored from 0 (no symptom) to 4 (maximal severity), the highest possible score being 92. Both baseline and treated scores were determined for each patient, as previously reported (17). Briefly, the baseline score was calculated after cessation of treatment when motor disability reached a stable level (18 h to 7 days). The treated score, considered to reflect nondopaminergic brain lesions, was determined after levodopa treatment was reinstated, at the time when therapeutic efficacy became maximal for each patient. The difference between the baseline score (without levodopa) and the treated score (with levodopa) was taken as an index of the deficiency in dopaminergic transmission (17,18).

Both the early and late onset groups had similar baseline scores, but the treated score was higher in late onset patients (Fig. 1), indicating greater residual handicap under medication. The levodopa sensitive score (difference between baseline and treated score) was greater in the younger (early onset) than in the older group, suggesting that a greater part of their motor disability was amenable to dopamine replacement therapy than in the older, late onset patients. A similar result was obtained when the percentage of clinical improvement resulting from levodopa treatment was calculated (data not shown). The subscores on the parkinsonian disability scale followed the

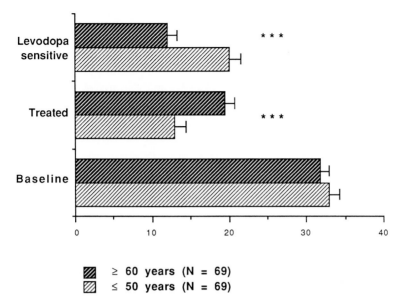

FIG. 1. Parkinsonian global motor score in patients with young and late onset of the disease (see the text). Results are means ± SEM. *** $p < 0.001$.

same trend. Although the baseline subscores were similar in both groups of patients (Fig. 2), the treated scores for gait, postural stability, rigidity, tremor, and akinesia were more severe in patients with late onset of the disease compared to those with early onset (Fig. 3). The levodopa-sensitive subscores (and the percentage of improvement—not shown) for gait, rigidity, tremor, and akinesia were significantly greater in younger than in older patients (Fig. 4). In summary, then, after similar periods of evolution, young and late onset patients were disabled to the same extent, but the latter derived less benefit from treatment.

This observation must be treated with caution, however. Parkinsonian motor scores with and without levodopa are only approximate indices of the functional state of dopaminergic transmission in the brain. This subject has been discussed at length elsewhere (17). It may be objected, in particular, that parkinsonian motor disability is often variable after interruption of levodopa therapy or when the benefit of treatment is at its acme, but in this study the patients were scored when it was certain that the parkinsonian symptoms were stable over time. The notion that the treated score and the difference between the baseline and treated score reflect, respectively, the severity of nondopaminergic and dopaminergic lesions may also be questioned. However, pharmacological data from experimental studies on animals corroborate the data concerning the extent of loss of dopaminergic and nondopaminergic neurons in the brains of parkinsonian patients (16).

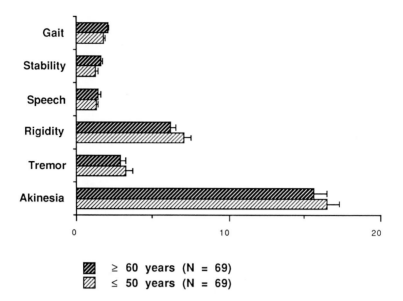

FIG. 2. Parkinsonian baseline subscores after cessation of levodopa treatment in patients with young and late onset of the disease. Results are means ± SEM.

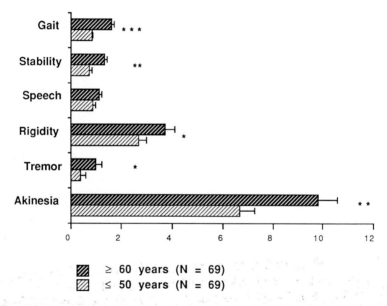

FIG. 3. Parkinsonian treated subscores after reinstoration of levodopa treatment in patients with young and late onset of the disease. Results are means ± SEM. *$p < 0.05$; **$p < 0.01$; ***$p < 0.001$.

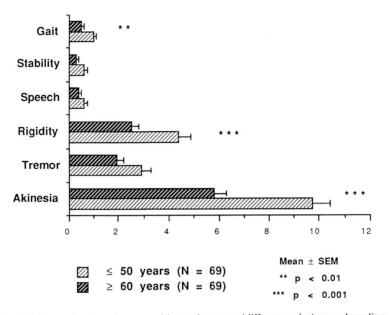

FIG. 4. Parkinsonian levodopa-sensitive subscores (difference between baseline and treated subscores) in patients with young and late onset of the disease. Results are means ± SEM. $**p < 0.01$; $***p < 0.001$.

The observation that the parkinsonian motor score appears to be independant of age of onset but that symptoms in late onset patients respond less well to levodopa has often been made with respect to the global parkinsonian score, and is also verifiable for each of the principal symptoms of the disease, all of which remain more severe under maximally effective levodopa treatment in later onset patients (Fig. 3). These same symptoms seem to respond better to treatment in younger patients. This raises two questions. Does levodopa ''work'' less well in older patients, and if so why? Do older patients have different symptoms, e.g., a greater proportion of symptoms that do not derive from dopaminergic lesions, and therefore cannot be ameliorated by treatment?

If one accepts that the evaluation of parkinsonian disability with and without levodopa effectively reflects the extent, respectively, of dopaminergic and nondopaminergic lesions in the brains of the patients, it follows that patients whose disease began earlier will have more severe dopaminergic lesions. This would explain the severity of the classical triad of symptoms (akinesia, rigidity, and tremor), which can be produced experimentally by lesions of the nigrostriatal dopaminergic pathway (19), as well as the good response to levodopa, and the existence of adverse reactions provoked by levodopa (on–off phenomena, levodopa-induced abnormal involuntary movements) observed primarily in this type of patient (20,21). Patients whose disease began late, on the other hand, would have supplementary nondo-paminergic lesions but less severe dopaminergic lesions. This would explain their lesser response to levodopa, particularly that of axial symptoms such as gait disorder, postural instability, and speech disorders, known to respond poorly to levodopa (17), and the relative infrequency of levodopa-associated side effects. Many questions subsist as to the nature of the nondopaminergic lesions, and their relationship to the nigrostriatal dopaminergic system in the control of movement. Are these lesions independent of the pathological process, and related to aging? Or do they have the same origin as those caused by idiopathic Parkinson's disease?

STUDY TWO—INFLUENCE OF AGE AT ONSET OF PARKINSON'S DISEASE ON STRIATAL DOPAMINERGIC DEFICIENCY, A STUDIED POSTMORTEM WITH DIHYDROTETRABENAZINE BINDING

One way of evaluating the influence of aging on the degeneration of do-paminergic neurons in the substantia nigra is to compare the degree of de-struction of the nigrostriatal dopaminergic pathway in parkinsonian patients whose disease began at an early age and in those whose disease began later. This type of study is not evident to perform, however, because of technical difficulties in using the available markers of dopaminergic neurons. The ideal would be to count the dopaminergic neurons in the substantia nigra of young and old parkinsonian subjects, but the large number of anatomical samples that would be necessary for such a study render it impracticable. Postmortem assay of dopamine concentrations in the striatum (22) is more manageable, but the data are quite imprecise, given the rapid decrease in monoamine concentrations after death (23). A new marker of monoaminergic terminals, tritiated α-dihydrotetrabenazine ([^{3}H]TBZOH), which inhibits uptake of monoamines by chromaffin granules in the adrenal medulla and all mon-oaminergic synaptic vesicles in the nervous system, is preferable to mon-oamine assay as an index of monoaminergic innervation because the binding sites are remarkably stable postmortem, thereby reducing scatter in the re-sults (24). Although [^{3}H]TBZOH binding reflects the sum of monoaminergic innervations (dopaminergic, noradrenergic, and serotoninergic), it is never-theless a good index of dopaminergic innervation in the human caudate nu-cleus, where noradrenaline concentrations are negligible and serotonin levels 20 times less than those of dopamine (25).

In order to evaluate the rate of loss of dopaminergic innervation in the striatum of patients with Parkinson's disease, [^{3}H]TBZOH binding was mea-sured in the caudate nucleus of 54 patients with Parkinson's disease selected on the basis of a clinical history compatible with the diagnosis of Parkinson's disease and the presence of Lewy bodies in the substantia nigra of the pa-tients on anatomopathological examination. The mean age at death was 73

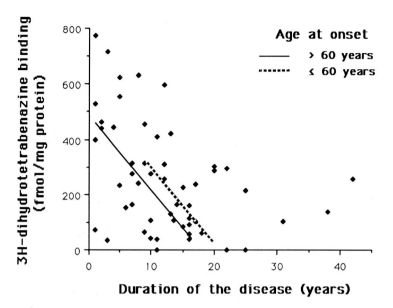

FIG. 5. [3H]-Dihydrotetrabenazine binding in the caudate nucleus of parkinsonian patients with young and late onset of the disease as a function of the duration of the disease. The correlation was calculated in the 45 patients whose disease duration was less than 20 years.

± 1 years, and the mean duration of the disease was 12.5 ± 1.2 years. All patients had received long-term levodopa treatment (18.9 ± 1.5 years), with a mean daily dose at time of death of 515 ± 52 mg. The brain dissection and assay procedures have previously been described (24).

As shown in Fig. 5, the binding of [3H]TBZOH in the caudate nucleus decreased with the duration of the disease. The correlation was highly significant ($r = 0.50$, $p < 0.001$) in the patients whose disease duration was less than 20 years ($n = 45$). In most patients whose disease lasted 20 years or more ($n = 9$), the density of [3H]TBZOH binding fell considerably, but not as much as in a large number of patients with much shorter disease durations.

When parkinsonian patients with a duration of the disease of less than 20 years were subdivided into subgroups according to their age at onset of the disease (52.7 ± 1.2 and 71.5 ± 1.4 years), the slopes of the regression lines for the two groups were similar (Fig. 5). Although the pattern of progression of the disease determined in this study was necessarily an approximation, since it was determined by comparing different individuals affected by the disease for different lengths of time, the data suggest that aging does not change the rate at which dopaminergic neurons degenerate in Parkinson's disease, at least in patients with disease durations under 20 years. Inspection of the regression lines in Fig. 5 also suggests that, for equivalent durations of the disease, patients in the early onset group have higher levels of [³H]TBZOH binding, and presumably less severe loss of dopaminergic lesions, than the late onset patients. Furthermore, the observation that loss of dopaminergic innervation in the striatum was somewhat less severe in patients with the longest disease durations (30 to 40 years) might indicate that the rate of neuronal death was even slower in these patients, or that certain dopaminergic neurons were more resistant to the disease in patients of this type. It must also be noted that the duration of the disease was different in patients with earlier or later ages at onset: consistently greater than 10 years for the former, from 1 to 16 years for the latter, but in the range of 10 to 15 years of evolution; [³H]TBZOH binding, and by inference dopaminergic innervation of the caudate nucleus, declined in parallel in the early and late onset groups.

It may be concluded, then, from the decrease in [³H]TBZOH binding in the caudate nucleus that degeneration of dopaminergic neurons in Parkinson's disease occurs at the same rate in all patients regardless of the age at which the disease became manifest, and that aging does not accelerate neuronal death in the nigrostriatal system.

CONCLUSION

Comparison of motor scores *in vivo* and striatal denervation *in vitro* in patients with early and late onset Parkinson's disease has shown that there is no simple response to the question of the role of age in the evolution of brain lesions in this affection. This may be summarized as follows: (a) The degeneration of nigrostriatal dopaminergic neurons is not aggravated by the age at which the disease appears in most cases of idiopathic Parkinson's disease, and in certain cases (notably those with very long evolution) neuronal death might even be slower. It remains to be determined whether these cases can be distinguished as a clinical entity. (b) Although the parkinsonian motor score was found to be identical for a given duration of evolution, regardless of whether the disease begins early or late, the late onset forms of the disease are characteristically less reactive to levodopa (in particular with respect to axial signs), and therefore probably by the presence of more severe nondopaminergic lesions than in the early onset forms. Both of the above studies tend to suggest that dopaminergic lesions are also more severe in late onset groups compared to early onset groups after equivalent periods of evolution of the disease. This also hints that the two groups may be separate clinical entities, but more studies, both postmortem and *in vivo*, are needed to substantiate the conclusions.

REFERENCES

1. Agid, Y., and Blin, J. (1987): Nerve cell death in degenerative diseases of the central nervous system: clinical aspects. *CIBA Found. Symp.* 126. 3–19.

2. Ehringer, H., and Hornykiewicz, O. (1960): Verteilung von Noradrenalin und Dopamin (3-hydroxytyramin) im Gehirn des Menschen und ihr Verhalten bei Erkrankungen des extrapyramidalen Systems. *Wien Klin. Wocheschr.*, 38:1236–1239.

3. McGeer, P. L., McGeer, E. G., and Suzuki, J. S. (1977): Aging and extrapyramidal function. *Arch. Neurol.*, 34:33–35.

4. Scherman, D., Desnos, C., Darchen, F., Javoy-Agid, F., and Agid, Y. (1988): Striatal dopamine deficiency in Parkinson's disease: role of aging. *Ann. Neurol.* (in press).

5. Riederer, P., and Wuketich, S. (1976): Time course of nigrostriatal degeneration in Parkinson's disease. *J. Neural Transm.*, 38:271–276.

6. Barbeau, A., Roy, M., Cloutier, T., Plasse, L., and Paris, S. (1986): Environmental and genetic factors in the etiology of Parkinson's disease. *Adv. Neurol.*, 45:299–306.

7. Calne, D. B., Duvoisin, R. C., and McGeer, E. (1984): Speculations on the etiology of Parkinson's disease. *Adv. Neurol.*, 40:353–360.

8. Langston, J. W., Irvin, J., Forno, L. S., and Delanney, L. E. (1987): Parkinson's disease, aging and MPTP: clinical and experimental observations. In: *Recent Developments in Parkinson's Disease*, edited by S. Fahn, C. D. Marsden, D. Calne, and M. Goldstein, Vol. 2, pp. 59–74. Macmillan Healthcare Information, Florham Park.

9. Nobrega, F. T., Glattie, E., Kurland, L. T., and Okazaki, H. (1967): Genetics and epidemiology of Parkinson's disease. In: *Progress in Neurogenetics*, edited by A. Barbeau and J. R. Brunette, pp. 474–485. Excerpta Medica, Amsterdam.

10. Harada, H., Nishikawa, S., and Takahashi, K. (1983): Epidemiology of Parkinson's disease in a Japanese city. *Arch. Neurol.*, 40:151–154.

11. Mutch, W., (1986): Dingwall-Fordyce, I., Downie, A. W., Paterson, J. G., and Roy, S. K. Parkinson's disease in a Scottish city. *Br. Med. J.*, 292:534–536.

12. Gudmundsson, K. R. A. (1967): *Acta Neurol. Scand.*, 33(suppl. 43):353–360.

13. Martilla, R. J., and Rinne, U. K. (1964): Dementia in Parkinson's disease. *Acta Neurol. Scand.*, 27:237–240.

14. Rosati, G., Granieri, E., Pinsa, J., et al. (1980): The risk of Parkinson's disease in mediterranean people. *Neurology*, 30:250–255.

15. Koller, W., O'Hara, R., Weiner, W., et al. (1986): Relationship of aging to Parkinson's disease. *Adv. Neurol.*, 45:317–321.

16. Agid, Y. Biochemistry of Parkinson's disease: a critical review 30 years later. Raven Press, New York (in press).

17. Bonnet, A. M., Loria, Y., Saint-Hilaire, M. H., Lhermitte, F., and Agid, Y. (1987): Does long-term aggravation of Parkinson's disease result from non-dopaminergic lesions? *Neurology*, 37:1539–1542.

18. Esteguy, M., Bonnet, A. M., Kefalos, J., Lhermitte, F., and Agid, Y. (1985): Le test á la L-DOPA dans la maladie de Parkinson. *Rev. Neurol.*, 141:413–415.

19. Langston, J. W. (1985): MPTP neurotoxicity: an overview and characteristics of phases of toxicity. *Life Sci.*, 36:201–206.

20. Gershanik, O., Heikkila, R. E., and Duvoisin, R. C. (1983): Behavioral correlates of dopamine receptors activation. *Neurology*, 33:1489–1492.

21. Quinn, N., Critchley, P., and Marsden, C. D. (1987): Young onset Parkinson's disease. *Movement Disorders*, 1:65–68.

22. Bernheimer, H., Birkmayer, W., Hornykiewicz, O., Jellinger, K., and Seitelberger, F. (1973): Brain dopamine and syndromes of Parkinson's and Huntington: clinical, morphological and neurochemical correlation. *J. Neurol. Sci.*, 20:415–455.

23. Sloviter, R. S., and Connor, J. D. (1976): Post-mortem stability of norepinephrine, dopamine and serotonin in rat brain. *J. Neurochem.*, 29:1129–1131.

24. Scherman, D., Raisman, R., Ploska, A., and Agid, Y. (1988): [^{3}H] Dihydrotetrabenazine, a new in vitro monoaminergic probe in human brain. *J. Neurochem.*, 47:331–339.

25. Scatton, B., Javoy-Agid, F., Rouquier, L., Dubois, B., and Agid, Y. (1983): Reduction of cortical dopamine, noradrenaline, serotonine and their metabolism in Parkinson's disease. *Brain Res.*, 275:321–328.

Parkinsonism and Aging, edited by
Donald B. Calne et al., Raven Press, Ltd.,
New York © 1989.

Is Parkinson's Disease Related to Aging?

Erik Ch. Wolters and Donald B. Calne

*Belzberg Laboratory of Clinical Neuroscience, Department of Medicine,
Division of Neurology, U.B.C. Health Sciences Centre Hospital,
Vancouver, British Columbia, Canada V6T 1W5*

While Parkinson's disease is clearly not simply a consequence of aging, a number of factors point to age-related attrition of dopaminergic nigral neurons as a factor that may contribute to the appearance and progression of symptoms. Observations suggesting a role for both aging and an environmental factor in the etiology for Parkinson's disease include the following: (a) the normal accelerating decay of indices of dopaminergic integrity in late life; (b) the faster progress of Parkinson's disease in late life; (c) the latency often encountered between exposure to environmental factors causing parkinsonism (e.g., encephalitis lethargica, Guamanian environment, and MPTP) and the onset of symptoms; (d) the familial clustering of Parkinson's disease that develops at the same time rather than the same age; (e) the predilection of Parkinson's disease for late life; and (f) the geographic distribution of Parkinson's disease.

DECAY OF INDICES OF DOPAMINERGIC INTEGRITY

Age-related attrition in the central nervous system is a selective process. There can be no doubt that dopaminergic cells of the substantia nigra undergo this attrition during the course of aging (1,2), as is also the case for cholinergic cells of the basal forebrain (3), and for motor neurons in the spinal cord (4). A decrease in enzymes involved in dopamine synthesis occurs with advancing age: tyrosine hydroxylase and dopa decarboxylase fall precipitously during the first 20 years of life and more slowly thereafter (1,5). Concentrations of dopamine decline with age (6,7). Postmortem (8) and PET studies (9) imply a fall in dopamine receptors. However, reports conflict on whether neuronal loss is more rapid in early life or senescence.

The major weight of current knowledge points to a faster nigrostriatal degeneration in the elderly (10). Evidence derives from direct morphometric studies, showing a steady loss of neurons of 1.4% per decade up to 65 years, with an eightfold increase in later life (9) [while a former more limited study indicated a steady 7% loss per decade (3)]. Extensive analyses of postmortem dopamine concentrations also indicate a more profound decrease during the ages 60 to 90 years (6).

The extent of neuronal plasticity after an injury also seems to decline with the aging process. The potential of central nervous system (CNS) tissue to recover from injury depends on the substances and processes that support neuron survival, promote axonal sprouting, and guide the neurites to their targets (neuronotrophic factors). Neuronotrophic activity has been assayed in the fluid secreted in an artificial cavity in the entorhinal cortex of rats; more activity was detected in younger than in older rats (11).

Adult mammalian striatal extracts contain neuronotrophic activity capable of enhancing survival of mesencephalic cells *in vitro* and of augmenting specific high-affinity dopamine uptake. Its activity is increased by nigrostriatal lesions, 100% more in young compared with old animals (12).

In response to denervation, remaining undamaged neurons show extensive axonal sprouting and new synapses are formed to replace those lost in either young or old animals. However, both in cholinergic and catecholaminergic fibers, this regenerative axonal sprouting is slower and less extensive in old rats (13,14). Experimental lesions of the terminal blood supply to part of the neocortex leads to retrograde changes in cholinergic neurons of the nucleus basalis magnocellularis. One hundred twenty days after this lesion, full recovery of enzymatic activity is found in young but not in old rats (15). Ganglioside GM-1 protects young and mature but not old rats from both morphological and biochemical changes; interestingly, there is an increase in enzymatic activity in sham-operated animals (15).

In this context, it is relevant to mention that MPTP (1-methyl-4-phenyl-1,2,3,6-tetrahydropyridine) produces sustained dopamine depletion in older mice, but not in younger mice (using identical doses of MPTP and the same, intraperitoneal route of administration) (16). In conclusion, there is a decay of dopaminergic integrity in late life due to (a) age-related, localized neuronal death and (b) generalized loss of neuronal plasticity.

THE FASTER PROGRESS OF PARKINSON'S DISEASE IN LATE LIFE

It has been estimated that striatal dopamine content must fall to 20% of normal, i.e., far below the level reached in normal aging, before the symptoms of Parkinson's disease become manifest (17). In Parkinsonian patients, neuronal counts in the substantia nigra are some 20% of normal, age-matched controls (18,19).

Above this threshold, compensatory reactions maintain function: the remaining dopaminergic neurons show augmented activity, as indicated by an increase in the ratio of homovanillic acid to dopamine in the striatum, and the rise in concentration of postsynaptic dopamine receptors (20).

As a result of the compensatory rise in dopamine turnover, a vicious cycle of increasing damage to dopaminergic cells has been proposed, perhaps mediated by the formation of free radicals (21). The production of these highly toxic free radicals in the course of metabolizing catecholamines may be one of the causes of accelerating neuronal decay over the decades. The antioxidant capacity of the cell may also decrease slowly with time, such that it becomes much more vulnerable to the assault of free radicals (22).

Electrolytic lesions of the rat forebrain bundle in the lateral hypothalamic area or microinfusions of 6-hydroxydopamine along the mesotelencephalic dopaminergic projection induce sensorimotor impairment, but only when the subsequent striatal dopamine depletion is 75 to 90%; recovery of function occurs in younger rats, but in older animals the deficit is persistent. In younger animals whose functional impairment had improved, significant (unilateral) deterioration takes place in late life (23).

In young adult rats that had partially recovered from unilateral nigrostriatal damage, sedative drugs reinstated full contralateral impairment (24). Unilateral damage to dopamine systems early in life left the animals asymmetrically vulnerable to nonspecific deleterious influences such as aging or sedative drugs.

In clinical terms, the rate of spread and the rate of loss of mobility are faster in patients whose Parkinson's disease starts in later life (25). The progress of the disease in the average 65-year-old patient is some four times greater than for a patient aged 35 years. This conclusion is based upon observations of the natural history of the disease in the pre-levodopa era (25).

Consistent with these findings, Calne and Lees (25a) have noted that in patients with postencephalitic parkinsonism, whose deficit has been relatively stable during many years, a progression of their neurological impairment occurs in late life. The progressive rate of normal age-related selective neuronal death, together with the toll to be paid for the increased compensatory mechanisms and the generalized loss of neuronal plasticity in aging, may account for this faster progression of parkinsonism in late life.

This finding is reminiscent of the postpoliomyelitis syndrome, where new, slowly progressive, predominantly focal muscle weakness can occur decades after the initial infection and in the absence of evidence of continuing poliomyelitis virus infection (26).

LATENCY BETWEEN TOXIC INSULT CAUSING PARKINSONISM AND SYMPTOMS

In accord with the recurrence or exacerbation of neurological deficits in later life, parkinsonian symptoms may develop after a latent period when damage to the nigrostriatal system is inadequate to produce overt symptoms.

Latent periods have been reported, lasting from a few years to several decades, between exposure to infective, traumatic, or neurotoxic factors and the appearance of parkinsonian features.

In the epidemic of encephalitis lethargica, for example, there was a substantial cohort of patients whose parkinsonism appeared 5 to 20 years after their acute disease (27). Pugilist's encephalopathy, which is a progressive parkinsonism–dementia syndrome, may develop over 20 years after giving up boxing (28).

The etiology of the amyotrophic lateral sclerosis (ALS)–parkinson–dementia complex of Guam has been suggested to involve consumption of food products derived from the *Cycas circinalis* (29). The occurrence of this illness in Chamorro migrants has been reported after periods of absence from Guam of 1 to 34 years (30).

In clinically normal subjects exposed to MPTP, positron emission tomography showed a partial reduction of striatal accumulation of fluorodopa (31). The damage to the striatonigral system was apparently not sufficient to produce parkinsonism. With the passage of time, however, some asymptomatic patients exposed to MPTP have developed symptoms of early parkinsonism (32).

AGE OF ONSET IN FAMILIAL CLUSTERS

Simultaneous environmental exposure within a family exposed to a risk factor for Parkinson's disease should lead to the relatively simultaneous appearance of parkinsonian symptoms. Recently, evidence has been reported implicating an environmental origin for at least some of the familial patterns (33).

In six families, case histories conformed to the expected pattern for environmental causation: the affected family members all had onset of clinical symptoms at approximately the same time, with age differences at the time of onset averaging about 25 years between children and parents (33). There are two reports of this familial pattern, indicating an environmental cause (33,34). In another cluster of familial Parkinson's disease, however, symptoms in parents and children seem to have developed at similar ages (35).

PREDILECTION OF PARKINSON'S DISEASE FOR LATE LIFE

The overall prevalence in Europe and North America is in the region of 1 to 1.5 in 1,000. Incidence rates for Parkinson's disease vary greatly with age, in a way that is consistent with the normal accelerating decay of dopaminergic integrity in life. After the fourth decade, the incidence rate increases about tenfold so that by about 75 years of age, there are 120 to 140 new cases per 100,000 per year (36,37).

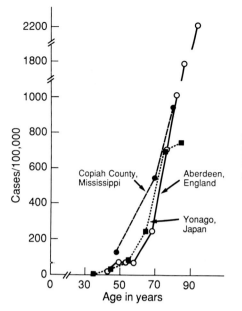

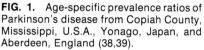

FIG. 1. Age-specific prevalence ratios of Parkinson's disease from Copiah County, Mississippi, U.S.A., Yonago, Japan, and Aberdeen, England (38,39).

Age-specific prevalence ratios for Parkinson's disease generally also show consistently increasing figures with increasing age, into the ninth decade (38,39) (see Fig. 1).

After age 75 years, incidence figures may not be reliable because the elderly who develop signs of parkinsonism are less likely to seek medical care. They are often living in extended care facilities, and there are clinical and physiological similarities between senescence and parkinsonism (40). There have been reports of a decline in the incidence rate after 70 to 75 years of age in epidemiologic studies (41,42). The percentage of U.S. population above 65 years in age increased from 4.7 (1920) to 11.6% (1982) while the incidence of Parkinson's disease remained more or less constant in Rochester, Minnesota (43).

GEOGRAPHIC DISTRIBUTION OF PARKINSON'S DISEASE

In the quest for an environmental cause of disease, an uneven geographic distribution is important. It has been suggested that prevalence rates for Parkinson's disease are lower in regions situated nearer the equator (39,44). Relatively high rates have been found in rural or remote, nonindustrialized areas in comparison with more densely populated regions (45). Attempts have been made to correlate this geographic distribution of Parkinson's disease with exposure to putative etiologic agents: heavy metals (particularly chromium), pesticides, well water, and industrial pollutants such as those deriving from the forestry industry (46,47).

The geographical distribution of Parkinson's disease has been studied in Swedish counties over the period 1977–1984. The findings were in accordance with the expectations: a lower prevalence rate was found in the southern part and in higher population densities (46). A north–south gradient in the utilization of levodopa has been reported for Spanish counties (48).

Comparing the average annual age-adjusted Parkinson's disease death rates in the U.S. with the multiple sclerosis (MS) mortality data and MS case/control ratios, Lux and Kurtzke (49) found higher death rates in the northern tier of states. Of the states lying generally below the latitude of 37–38° north (= southern tier), none showed a mortality rate greater than the national average.

In order to minimize variability in levels of case ascertainment, a standard procedure (using a door-to-door survey technique and uniform diagnostic criteria) was implemented among a biracial U.S. population (black and white) and in populations in Nigeria and the People's Republic of China. There were no substantial differences in age-adjusted prevalence ratios of blacks and whites in the United States. However, blacks in Nigeria have a much lower prevalence ratio of Parkinson's disease than blacks or whites in the United States (38). The differences in prevalence figures in U.S. and Nigerian blacks are too large to be explained by possible variations in survival; the disparity is likely to reflect a difference in incidence rates (38).

In a recent study on the epidemiology of Parkinson's disease in Natal (50), the disorder was less frequent in blacks, as compared with whites and Indians. These conclusions derived from records of the use of levodopa, and from the number of neurological consultations in three major Durban hospitals. The prevalence is also lower in Japan and China (38). These observations support the concept of an environmental etiologic factor.

EVIDENCE AGAINST AGING PLAYING A ROLE IN THE PRODUCTION OF PARKINSONIAN DEFICITS

The most cogent argument against aging playing a role in the production of parkinsonian deficits derives from the histological appearance of more active cell disruption in the substantia nigra of parkinsonian brains compared to age-matched controls (51). To account for this, it may be argued that following subclinical damage the excessive, compensatory activity of remaining neurons compromises their own survival and accelerates their demise. Alternatively, the concept of a "slow toxin" can be invoked (52). Here the notion proposed is that exposure to a toxin might impair the "life expectation" of a group of neurons, which would die collectively after a period of years or decades. The time interval between exposure and cell death can be construed as aging, although it is perhaps not "normal" aging since changes occur over time because of a specific environmental event or series of events.

Finally, it is appropriate to acknowledge that there are controversial aspects of certain reports that we have quoted as evidence in support of aging having a role in the evolution of parkinsonian symptoms. For example, it has been argued that Parkinson's disease may not progress more rapidly in elderly subjects (53). In areas where conflicting observations have been made, it is clearly desirable to obtain further information and perhaps the most valuable attribute of an hypothesis is its ability to provoke the design of new experiments and the acquisition of new clinical, pathological, and epidemiological findings.

REFERENCES

1. McGeer, P. L., McGeer, E., and Suzuki, J. S. (1977): *Arch. Neurol.*, 34:33–35.
2. Mann, D. M. A. (1984): In: *The Neurobiology of Dopamine Systems*, edited by W. Winlow and R. Markstein, Manchester, England, University Press, pp. 87–103.
3. McGeer, P. L., McGeer, E. G., Suzuki, J., Dolman, C. E., and Nagai, T. (1984): *Neurology*, 34:741–745.
4. Tomlinson, B. E., and Irving, D. (1977): *J. Neurol. Sci.*, 34:213–219.
5. Cote, L. J., and Kremzner, L. T. (1983): *Adv. Neurol.*, 38:19–30.
6. Carlsson, A., and Winblad, B. (1976): *J. Neural. Transm.*, 38:271–276.
7. Carlsson, A., Nyberg, P., and Winblad, B. (1984): In: *Brain Monoamines in Normal Aging and Dementia*, edited by P. Nyberg, Umeo, Umeo University Med. Diss., pp. 53–84.
8. Severson, J. A. Marcusson, J., Winblad, B., and Finch, C. E. (1982): *J. Neurochem.*, 39:1623–1631.
9. Wong, D. F., Wagner, J. H. N., Danaals, R. F., et al. (1984): *Science*, 226:1393–1396.
10. Calne, D. B., and Peppard, R. F. (1987): *Can. J. Neurol. Sci.,* 14:424–427.
11. Nieto-Sampedro, M., Lewis, E. R., Cotman, C. W., et al. (1982): *Science*, 17:860–861.
12. Dal Toso, R., Presti, D., Benvegnu, D., et al. (1986): In: *Molecular Aspects of Neurobiology*, edited by R. L. Montalcini, Berlin, Springer, pp. 198–201.
13. Cotman, C. W., and Scheff, S. W. (1979): *Physiol. Cell Biol. Aging*, 8:109–120.
14. Scheff, S. W., Benardo, L. S., and Cotman, C. W. (1980): *Brain Res.*, 199:21–38.
15. Cuello, A. C., Stephens, P. H. Maysinger, D., Tagari, P., and Garofalo, L. (1987): In: *Neuroplasticity: A New Therapeutical in the CNS Pathology*, edited by R. Masland, A. Portera-Sanchez, and G. Toffano, Padua, Liviana Press, 75–84.
16. Ricaurte, G. A., Langston, J. W., Irwin, I., DeLanney, L. E., and Forno, L. S. (1985): *Soc. Neurosci. Abstr.*, 11:631.
17. Berheimer, H., Birkheimer, W., Hornykiewicz, O., Jellinger, K., and Seitelberger, F. (1973): *J. Neurol. Sci.*, 20:415–455.
18. Mann, D. M. A., and Yates, P. O. (1983): *Mech. Ageing Dev.*, 21:193–203.
19. Gibb, W. R. G., and Lees, A. J. (1987): *Acta Neuropathol.*, 73:195–201.
20. Hornykiewicz, O. (1986): In: *The Neurobiology of Dopamine Systems*, edited by W. Winslow and R. Markstein, Manchester, England, University Press, pp. 319–330.
21. Barbeau, A. (1984): *Can. J. Neurol. Sci.*, 11:24–28.
22. Langston, J. W., Irwin, I., and Ricaurte, G. A. (1987): *Pharmacol. Ther.*, 32:19–49.
23. Schallert, T. (1983): *Behav. Neurosci*, 97:159–164.
24. Schallert, T. (1987): *Ann. N.Y. Acad. Sci.*, 515:108–119.
25. DeJong, J. D., and Burns, B. D. (1967): *J. Can. Med. Assoc.*, 97:49–56.
25a. Calne, D. B., and Lees, A. J. (1988): *Can. J. Neurol. Sci.*, 15:135–138.
26. Dalakas, M. C. (1986): *Muscle Nerve*, 9(5S):108.
27. Duvoisin, R. C., and Yahr, M. D. (1965): *Arch. Neurol.*, 12:227–239.

locomotor dysfunction in animals grazing on the plant (15,20). The highly poisonous inner portion (female gametophyte or kernel) of the cycad seed once served as an important source of food and topical medicine for the Chamorro people of the Mariana Islands (21). After removing the husk, the whitish kernel was either crushed and applied to skin wounds as a poultice or, in preparation for eating, repeatedly soaked in water for a varying period (approximate range: 2–30 days), during which the poisonous principles were leached out to differing extents. These practices were very common during World War II, when rice and medicine were unavailable to the beleaguered Guamanian people of Guam and Rota but, in subsequent years, as Chamorros acculturated to the practices of the continental United States, use of cycad seed for food and medicine declined—as did the incidence of ALS (12,21). The cycad hypothesis was proposed in the early 1960s but fell into disfavor some years later for two principal reasons: cycads were found not to be eaten either in the Kii peninsula or New Guinea foci of ALS/P–D, and nonprimate laboratory animals repeatedly exposed to cycad components failed to develop a paralytic disorder. In 1986, we reawakened interest in the cycad hypothesis with the experimental induction of a motor-system disease in primates fed β-N-methylamino-L-alanine (BMAA) (22, see also refs. 17 and 23), an unusual amino acid with excitant properties found in *Cycas* seed. Detailed examination of published and unpublished literature on cycad toxicity and the epidemiology of Guam ALS/P–D demonstrated the plausibility of the cycad hypothesis (21), a view that was subsequently adopted and reiterated by others investigating the disease (24). These advances were followed a few months later by our discovery that cycad seed was used for medicinal purposes in the ALS/P–D foci of Irian Jaya and Kii Peninsula (Hobara) (25,26). There is now concrete evidence to demonstrate significant human cycad exposure in all three high-incidence foci of western Pacific ALS/P–D.

Oral or percutaneous exposure to the kernel of the raw seed of various *Cycas* spp. is the single factor that presently links the three geographically separate disease foci. Auyu people living in affected villages of Irian Jaya consider the fresh cycad kernel an optimal medicine for the topical treatment (at all ages) of various skin lesions, including large open sores (tropical ulcers). For this purpose, scrapings of the juicy kernel are crushed by hand, the resulting pulp immersed in the poisonous milky exudate, and the sodden mass applied directly to the lesion on a leaf, which is then strapped into position. The pulp is replaced daily until the skin is healed. On a single occasion at the age of 15 years, one 29-year-old male with ALS of recent onset told of applying the preparation for 1 month to a 5 to 10-cm diameter open lesion on the ankle. This practice is likely to be declining since the Auyu, who only 40 years ago were a Stone Age people subsisting as forest-dwelling hunter–gatherers, now live in organized villages and have increasing access to Indonesian medicine (25). Similarly, on Guam, the traditional

Chamorro practice of treating wounds topically with crushed cycad seed in coconut oil (27)—said to have been widely used during World War II—has probably died out in the intervening years of Americanization. Use of folk medicine has also declined in Japan, although a resurgence of interest now seems to be underway. In the Hobara region of the Kii Peninsula, where ALS/P–D has been common (8), the mature seed of *Cycas revoluta* Thunb. is stocked by certain pharmacies that fill prescriptions written by practitioners of folk medicine. Daily use of an aqueous oral steepe prepared from 3–10 g of cycad seed is used for the treatment of various ailments. Reportedly, cycad seed may also be used to induce abortion, to predict the future, and to achieve eternal youth (26). Field studies are needed in the Hobara and Kozagawa foci of ALS to ascertain a direct link between oral medicinal use of cycad seed and the later development of neurodegenerative disease. Additionally, laboratory studies are required to determine the chemical composition of seed of *Cycas* spp. implicated in western Pacific ALS/P–D, as a function both of differential kernel maturity and time following kernel maceration.

CYCADISM IN HUMANS AND ANIMALS

The effects of cycad poisoning in humans and in grazing animals are strikingly similar. Signs of acute toxicity in humans commence 12 to 40 h after ingestion of improperly detoxified cycad components. Nausea and vomiting develop suddenly, hepatomegaly and convulsions then appear, and the subject loses consciousness and usually dies (27). The disease in grazing animals is also marked by hepatotoxicity, enterotoxicity, and death. Rapid twitching of the eyelids, nostrils, lips, and jaw muscles with periodic tremors of the body are reported in sheep, and muscle fasciculation has been noted in poisoned heifers. Animals that survive acute cycad poisoning develop some weeks later a locomotor disorder associated with weakness and wasting of the hindlimbs. Initially, there is a staggering, weaving gait, with crossing of the legs, incoordination, and "ataxia." More severe forms are characterized by posterior motor weakness, dragging of extended hindlegs, and, occasionally, a stringhalt-like action of the hocks. Function of bladder, anus, and tail is unimpaired. The few pathological reports of this condition in cattle describe degeneration of long, presumably motor tracts in the lumbar region, with changes in the fasciculus gracilis and dorsal spinocerebellar tracts in the cervical area (20). Urgently needed are studies of the brains of long-surviving animals to determine whether the pathological changes are reminiscent of those seen in humans with western Pacific ALS/P–D.

Experimental study of the chemical and toxic properties of cycads has a long history (27). Most work during the past quarter century has centered on the azoxyglucoside cycasin and its metabolite methylazoxymethanol, a

potent heptatotoxin and carcinogen held responsible for the acutely poisonous properties of cycads. Although specific data are unavailable, rodents
appear to be far more susceptible to the carcinogenic properties of cycads
than do grazing animals that develop the locomotor disorder described above
(A. Seawright, personal communication). A neurotoxic principle in *Cycas
circinalis* seed was predicted from the observation that motor neuron degeneration and arm weakness developed in a single macaque fed for several
months with cycad flour reportedly free of cycasin (29). Never confirmed
nor refuted, this remarkably relevant study predated by many years the
discovery in *Cycas* seed of the nonprotein convulsant amino acid α-amino-
β-methylaminopropionic acid (30), now known as BMAA (17). However,
interest in BMAA was short-lived because repeated administration of sub-
convulsive doses to rodents failed to elicit a locomotor disorder (31). Similar
difficulties were experienced with the chemically related compound β-*N*-
oxalylamino-L-alanine (BOAA), a potent excitatory amino acid isolated from
the legume *Lathyrus sativus*, an established cause of the upper-motor-neuron
disorder lathyrism (32).

In 1981, we began a series of clinical and experimental studies to examine
more closely the neurotoxic properties of BOAA and BMAA and to assess
their possible roles in lathyrism and western Pacific ALS/P–D, respectively.
Initial clinical investigations of lathyrism in India and Bangladesh (33) established the clinical criteria for an animal model of the human disease. An
early phase of lathyrism was subsequently induced in macaques by prolonged feeding of fortified diets consisting either of *Lathyrus sativus* (LS)
or of *Cicer arietinum* (a nontoxic legume) plus LS extract or BOAA (34).
The central etiologic role of BOAA in lathyrism was thereby established.
Studies were then performed in mouse central nervous system (CNS) tissue
in situ and in culture to compare and contrast the pharmacological properties
of BOAA and BMAA (35–37). The *Cycas* neurotoxin (BMAA) proved less
potent than BOAA, but both promptly induced postsynaptic edema and
dark shrunken neurons in CNS explants, a pattern pathognomonic for potent
glutamate agonists. Recent receptor-binding studies suggest that BOAA is
most active at the quisqualate of A2 receptor (38), a subclass of neuronal
membrane receptors responding to the putative excitatory transmitters glutamate and aspartate. By contrast, the excitotoxic properties of BMAA are
blocked dose-dependently by antagonists (AP7, MK 801) for the *N*-methyl-
D-aspartate (NMDA) or A1 receptor (17,36,37). Unlike the proposed relationship between BOAA and the quisqualate receptor, direct activation of
the NMDA receptor is unlikely to occur since BMAA lacks the dicarboxylic
acid structure of a glutamate agonist, is unable at low concentrations to
displace binding of specific NMDA ligands (38), elicits delayed-onset convulsions after intracerebroventricular or intraperitoneal injection in rats (36),
and induces neurotoxic damage in CNS explants at relatively high concentrations (35,37). The action of BMAA may occur via a metabolite, by in-

terrupting a metabolic pathway associated with an endogenous excitant amino acid, or through some other indirect NMDA-linked mechanism.

The distinctive pharmacological properties of the *Cycas* and *Lathyrus* amino acids possibly account for their radically different effects in repeatedly dosed primates. Whereas BOAA elicits a pyramidal disorder analogous to human lathyrism (34), BMAA induces signs suggestive of pyramidal, extra-pyramidal, and behavioral dysfunction that, in combination, show an interesting parallel to ALS/P–D (17,23). In the majority of animals tested to date, the forelimbs were affected first, with wrist-drop clumsiness, tremor, and difficulty picking up small objects. Muscle weakness and loss of muscle bulk followed. Many animals displayed unilateral and bilateral extensor hindlimb posturing, with or without leg crossing (a primate sign associated with impairment of corticospinal function), a stooped posture, unkempt coat, and tremor and weakness of lower extremities. More prolonged administration of BMAA led to periods of immobility with an expressionless face and blank stare, a crouched posture, and a bradykinetic, shuffling, bipedal gait performed with legs flexed and rump close to the ground. Additional clinical features included reduction or loss of aggressive behavior, disinterest in the environment, changes in the normal diurnal pattern of vigilance, urinary incontinence, altered vocalization, slowed mastication, and a whole-body tremor. Electrophysiological examination revealed decrements of the entire motor pathway (cortex to muscle), and neuropathological study showed a hierarchy of regional motoneuronal susceptibility: motor cortex (most affected), spinal cord (less affected), and substantia nigra (mostly unaffected). The most striking changes were found in giant Betz (and other pyramidal) cells, which underwent central chromatolysis, neurofilament accumulation, and changes reminiscent of chronic cell degeneration. Isolated, large anterior horn cells of the spinal cord were similarly affected but to a lesser degree, and the pars compacta of the substantia nigra from one animal that had received BMAA for 13 weeks showed isolated neuritic swellings. In sum, therefore, the neuropathology reflected the early clinical dominance of motor neurons and the subsequent appearance of signs suggestive of additional extrapyramidal dysfunction.

Although there is an interesting and potentially important relationship between chronic BMAA toxicity in primates and human ALS/P–D, it must be emphasized that the experimental disorder lacks certain crucial features of the human disease, including plentiful paired helical filaments, degeneration of the nigrostriatal pathway, pronounced nerve-fiber loss in spinal cord and motor nerves, and denervation atrophy of striated muscles. It is noteworthy, however, that the experimental pathological changes developed over weeks (as compared with years or decades in humans), and that animals were not exposed to whole cycad seed, to other environmental factors (e.g., aluminum) proposed as causally related to ALS/P–D, or to the combined effects of toxic damage and age-related attrition of CNS-susceptible neurons

common trait of many neurotoxins. To answer this question, we recently began evaluating a number of other neurotoxins known to affect various aminergic systems within the brain. Age-related effects were assessed by comparing the neurotransmitter depletions induced by these compounds in young mature (6- to 8-week old) and older (8- to 10-month old) mice. These two age groups were chosen because it was in this model that the age-related effects of MPTP were first noted.

Amphetamine

We first studied methamphetamine, a compound that produces nigrostriatal axonal degeneration and persistent depletions of caudate dopamine and its metabolites (2–4). Examining this toxin was of interest because methamphetamine may damage nigrostriatal neurons by inducing the conversion of endogenous dopamine to 6-hydroxydopamine (5), a process that has itself been suggested to be involved in "neuronal aging." No significant difference in the degree of methamphetamine-induced dopamine depletion was observed between the young and the older animals (6).

These results provided the first suggestion that MPTP might be relatively unique among aminergic neurotoxins, and led to an additional series of experiments to determine why one systemically administered neurotoxin should be age-related and another one not. Whether or not older neurons become more sensitive to the effects of systemically administered toxins is complicated by a variety of factors (e.g., distribution or biotransformation) that might alter the amount reaching the central nervous system (CNS). For this reason we examined several neurotoxins that are effective when introduced directly into the brain, via the intracerebroventricular (ICV) route of administration. By avoiding the peripheral system and presenting the toxin directly to the CNS, alterations in neuronal sensitivity could be directly assessed.

6-Hydroxydopamine

Initial studies utilized 6-hydroxydopamine (6-OHDA), a compound that has proved useful as an experimental toxin in the study of Parkinson's disease (7). This compound damages both noradrenergic and dopaminergic neurons in the CNS after ICV administration. The dose-related, dopamine-depleting effects of 6-OHDA in mice of three different ages were examined: 2-month, 8- to 12-month, and 18- to 24-month-old mice. Similar to methamphetamine, we observed no age-related increase in the toxicity of 6-OHDA (8). This result is particularly interesting because evidence obtained by other investigators has indicated that the toxicity of 6-OHDA is due, at least in part, to the production of oxidative stress (for review, see ref. 9).

The autoxidation of 6-OHDA generates hydrogen peroxide and other highly reactive oxy-radicals that are thought to produce cellular damage by oxidizing critical substituents or proteins. Thus, this experiment also provided a test of the hypothesis that, with aging, neurons become increasingly susceptible to the affects of oxidative stress (10). This experiment suggested that they do not.

5,7-Dihydroxytryptamine

We next examined the dose-related, amine-depleting effects of the neurotoxin 5,7-dihydroxytryptamine (5,7-DHT) in old and young mice (11). This compound selectively damages serotonergic and noradrenergic neurons after ICV administration (12–14). Here again we found that aging failed to alter the noradrenergic-depleting effects of 5,7-DHT while, somewhat unexpectedly, actually offering some degree of protection against its actions on serotonergic systems.

Several lines of evidence suggest that oxidative stress also plays an important role in the ability of 5,7-DHT to damage noradrenergic neurons (10,15,16). Hence, the lack of an age-related increase in 5,7-DHT-induced noradrenergic toxicity provides additional evidence for the conclusion that the ability of neurons to withstand oxidative stress does not diminish with age. Regarding the effects of 5,7-DHT on serotonin, our results show that the capacity of the nervous system to counteract the neurochemical events responsible for the effects of this neurotoxicant may actually improve rather than decline with increasing age.

Thus, of the toxins we have studied to date, only MPTP clearly demonstrates an increasing capacity to exert its neurotoxic effects as the nervous system ages. Given our findings with 6-OHDA and 5,7-DHT, this effect seems unlikely to be explained by the notion that aging neurons are in some general or nonspecific way more susceptible to injury from a toxic insult. In particular, the results do not support the idea that older neurons are more susceptible to the damaging effects of oxidative stress.

WHY DO THE EFFECTS OF MPTP INCREASE WITH AGE?

The results presented above suggest that, rather than being a general consequence of neuronal aging, the age-dependent effects of MPTP are the exception rather than the rule. If other neurotoxins are not age-dependent, what is it about MPTP that accounts for this rather special attribute? Two hypotheses borrowed from classical pharmacology should be considered. First, the age-related effects of MPTP could be due to a toxicodynamic process (i.e., increased sensitivity of aged neurons to MPTP and/or its metabolites). If toxicodynamic factors were at play, our data with 6-OHDA and

5,7-DHT would suggest that MPTP is not acting through a mechanism that involves oxidative stress (this, in fact, may be true; see ref. 17 for review). Alternatively, the age-related effects of MPTP could be due to toxicokinetic factors (i.e., factors that result in the increased delivery of greater amounts of the toxin to its target site).

Our early data suggested that toxicodynamic factors might be responsible for the age-related effects of MPTP. In these experiments, when the dose of MPTP was adjusted so that similar levels of MPP+ (the putative toxic metabolite of MPTP) were achieved in the striatum of both young and older animals at *1 hour* (to do this, it was necessary to give twice the dose to younger animals), greater depletions of striatal dopamine were measured in older animals 1 week later (6). However, we later conducted additional studies that included later time points; these experiments showed that the levels of MPP+ continued to increase for another 1 to 2 hr in the older animals, and thus the total exposure of striatum to MPP+ over time (area under the curve) was greater (18). These latter results pointed towards a toxicokinetic effect.

To study this question directly, we employed the ICV route of administration, thereby circumventing peripheral factors related to the distribution and elimination of systemically administered MPTP and its metabolites. These studies were possible because ICV-administered MPP+ selectively depletes striatal dopamine in a manner similar to systemically administered MPTP. Further, by injecting MPP+ rather than MPTP directly into the CNS compartment, differences in production of MPP+ from MPTP within the brain, which might vary with age, were avoided.

This model, therefore, allowed us to eliminate "upstream" variables in order to concentrate on several possibilities for age-related differences. We could determine if there was any change in the removal of MPP+ from the CNS compartment (i.e., MPP+ might be rapidly biotransformed to a nontoxic metabolite or more rapidly eliminated from the CNS compartment in younger animals). Thus, studies were carried out to see if MPP+ was further biotransformed into other metabolites and to determine if the kinetics of elimination for ICV-administered MPP+ from the CNS differed between young and old mice. In the first set of experiments, [^{3}H]- and [^{14}C]-labeled, ICV-administered MPP+ was found not to be biotransformed, but rather was found to be eliminated directly (19). The ICV paradigm was further supported by a parallel set of experiments showing that the rate of elimination of MPP+ from the CNS compartment was similar regardless of whether it reached the brain after systemic administration of MPTP or after direct injection of MPP+ (20). A final series of experiments showed that there were no differences in the rate of elimination of MPP+ from the CNS compartment in young or older animals.

With these data in hand, it became possible to assess directly the toxicodynamic hypothesis by comparing the dopamine-depleting effects of ICV-administered MPP+ in old and young animals. Somewhat unexpectedly, these experiments showed that there was no difference in the degree of dopamine depletion (and hence, presumably, the degree of damage to nigrostriatal neurons) between young and older animals (21). These data strongly indicated that toxicodynamic factors are not responsible for the increasing vulnerability of the nigrostriatal system to MPTP with age. This fairly compelling evidence against the toxicodynamic hypothesis, combined with the knowledge that (a) MPP+ is not further metabolized and (b) there are no differences in the rate of elimination of MPP+ from the CNS compartment between young and older animals, indicates that "upstream" metabolic factors are at work. By upstream, we mean the biologic events that lead to the delivery of MPTP/MPP+ to nigrostriatal neurons after MPTP gains entrance to the body.

THE MAO CONNECTION

The first suspect on the list of upstream factors is the enzyme monamine oxidase (MAO). MAO is one of the few substances that has been shown to increase in the brain during the aging process. In rats (22) and humans (23,24), the increased enzyme activity appears exclusively due to the B form of the enzyme, the activity of the A form remaining essentially unchanged. In humans, the increase in activity appears to occur predominantly after the fifth decade of life, with the largest increases seen in the eighth and ninth decades (23,24). The observation that it is the B form of the enzyme that increases with age may be of critical importance, in view of the seminal observation that MAO-B is responsible for the biotransformation of MPTP to the putative toxin MPP+ (25).

The obvious question is whether or not this increased MAO-B activity, by enhancing the transformation of MPTP to MPP+, is responsible for the age-dependent effects of MPTP. There is evidence to support this conclusion (18,26). For example, we have found that in homogenates prepared from the brains of older mice, the rate of conversion of MPTP to MPP+ is 20 to 40% greater than in those prepared from younger animals (18). Additionally, *in vivo* there is a direct relationship between age and the concentrations of MPP+ in the mouse striatum after the administration of equivalent doses of MPTP (18).

However, as attractive as this "unitary" MAO hypothesis is to explain the age-enhanced effects of MPTP, the fact that both increase with age does not prove a cause-and-effect relationship. Further, the parallel is not an exact one. For example, although striatal MAO-B activity increases about 30% in C57B1/6 between 2 and 10 months of age (11), striatal MPP+ concentrations in the *in vivo* experiments described above increased more than twofold between these same ages. We therefore turned to another neurotoxin to further study the "MAO hypothesis."

STUDIES ON A NORADRENERGIC NEUROTOXIN

If increasing MAO-B activity is responsible for the age-dependent effects of MPTP, one might expect that the effects of other neurotoxins that are dependent on MAO-B for activation might increase with age as well. Recently, it has been reported that the effects of the noradrenergic neurotoxin *N*-(2-chloroethyl)-*N*-ethyl-2-bromobenzylamine (DSP-4) are prevented by deprenyl (a selective MAO-A inhibitor) but not by clorgyline (a selective MAO-A inhibitor) (27). These results were interpreted as suggesting that, similar to MPTP, DSP-4 is bioactivated by MAO-B. To test the hypothesis that other MAO-B–dependent neurotoxins are more effective in older animals, the norepinephrine-depleting effects of DSP-4 were tested in young mature and older mice (11); however, no differences in hippocampal norepinephrine were found between age groups.

At first, this result seemed to contradict the MAO hypothesis. However, *ex vivo* studies in rats have demonstrated that deprenyl (at a dose of 10 mg/kg) inhibits the uptake of [^{3}H]norepinephrine by 30 to 50% (28,29), and noradrenergic uptake blockers, such as desipramine, are known to block the amine-depleting effects of DSP-4 (30,31). These earlier studies suggested the possibility that the protective actions of deprenyl were due not to MAO-B inhibition but rather to reuptake blockade. To evaluate this alternate explanation, the time course of MAO inhibition produced by deprenyl was determined and compared with the duration of its protective effects against DSP-4 toxicity. It was found that DSP-4 produced large depletions of norepinephrine at time points when MAO-B activity remained almost completely inhibited by deprenyl. In additional studies carried out *in vitro*, DSP-4 was not metabolized by MAO. These findings suggest that the protective effects of deprenyl are not due to MAO-B inhibition, and further that MAO appears unlikely to be involved in the mechanism of action of DSP-4. Rather, deprenyl may be protecting against the amine-depleting effect of DSP-4 by blocking the catecholaminergic reuptake system. The latter hypothesis still requires experimental verification. Because DSP-4 does not appear to be bioactivated by MAO-B, the fact that its effects do not increase with age cannot be used to argue against the MAO hypothesis. However, the inability of DSP-4 to produce age-related alterations, similar to 5,7-DHT, again suggests that older norepinephrine-containing neurons do not become more sensitive to the effects of these toxins.

While it still seems likely that MAO plays a role in mediating the age-related effects of MPTP, other factors are probably involved as well. For example, there may be enhanced delivery of the toxin to the CNS if the liver begins to fail to oxidize MPTP to MPP+ with age; such a decline would allow more of the lipophilic MPTP to cross the blood–brain barrier. Other factors, as yet undetermined, may also be at work in causing a shift in the burden of the neurotoxin to the CNS.

IMPLICATIONS AND PARKINSON'S DISEASE

At a broader level, this work may provide insights about the relationship between Parkinson's disease and aging. If these neurotoxins are teaching us anything, it is that we are not dealing with a problem of enhanced susceptibility of neurons to toxic insult. In fact, the studies with 5,7-DHT and 6-OHDA challenge the venerable concept that neurons become increasingly sensitive to oxidative stress as they age. We conclude, therefore, that a declining capacity to tolerate oxidative stress is unlikely to play a role in age-related degeneration of nigrostriatal neurons, whether they be due to the normal aging process or to the factors that cause Parkinson's disease. This is not to say that oxidative stress does not play a role, as there may be other factors that enhance oxidative stress, eventually overcoming normal defense mechanisms. However, our data suggest that a *failing defense* is not the key.

A second conclusion that can be drawn from this body of work is that if exogenous neurotoxins do play a role in Parkinson's disease, MPTP represents the best model when it comes to the study of the relationship between aging and the process of neuronal degeneration. None of the other neurotoxins that we have studied to date, including DSP-4, 6-OHDA, methamphetamine, and 5,7-DHT, were found to display age-related effects. These observations once again suggest the exceptional usefulness of MPTP in the study of Parkinson's disease.

Finally, we may be developing a broader framework in the use of neurotoxins to study neurodegenerative disease. Perhaps these diseases are due to changes in the biodisposition of exogenous neurotoxins that, with aging, lead to greater delivery of these toxins to the brain. At least that is what is suggested by the MPTP model. If so, this hypothetical construct represents a change in the conventional wisdom that older neurons somehow become more susceptible to insult as they age. Only time will tell whether or not this new model will hold up under critical testing, but at least it represents a new research direction for the future.

One caveat must be put forward regarding this body of experimental work, however, and that relates to the age of the animals studied in most of these experiments. As has been noted throughout, animals were studied at 6 to 8 weeks of age (young animals) and 8 to 10 months of age (older animals). Using 1 month in the life of a mouse as the approximate equivalent of 3 human years in terms of the normal aging process, the young animals used in these studies would be roughly equivalent to 6-year-old humans, and the older animals approximately the equivalent of 30-year-old humans. Thus these investigations focused primarily on the period between youth and full maturity. There are several implications. First, it will be critical to extend these studies to older animals (ideally at least 20 months of age or older). If the age-related changes discussed in this article plateau in mice after the age of 8 to 10 months, it will suggest that we are probing *development* more than aging. However, such results could also have implications for Parkinson's disease.

Although Parkinson's disease is rare in subjects below age 40, most of investigators believe the disease may have a very long preclinical phase, possibly dating back to the teens or twenties. Indeed, a recent study of sibling pairs with Parkinson's disease suggests that this time period may coincide exactly with the time of likely exposure to an exogenous causative agent (Ali Rajput, personal communication). Perhaps this work will lead us in a new direction, suggesting that Parkinson's disease is more of a developmental disease than an aging disease. By this, we mean to suggest that the nervous system must achieve a certain degree of maturity to become susceptible to the one or more exogenous agents responsible for the disease. After that, it may be a matter of either additional exposure or perhaps a self-sustaining process of neuronal degeneration initiated by a time-limited exposure to a neurotoxin during a period of susceptibility. This concept of long-latency toxins has gained additional credibility from recent work with the amyotrophic lateral sclerosis–Parkinsonism–dementia complex of Guam (32,33), suggesting that it may (a) be mediated by a neurotoxin and (b) require many years for the toxic insult to gain clinical expression.

Acknowledgments: The authors thank David Rosner and Pamela Schmidt for their help in the preparation of this manuscript. Dr. Finnegan is a recipient of The 1987–1988 Lillian Schorr Research Fellowship from the Parkinson's Disease Foundation, New York, New York. This work was supported in part by the United Parkinson Foundation, the Parkinson's Disease Foundation, and the National Institute of Aging (ROI AG07348-01).

REFERENCES

1. Langston, J. W. (1987): *Trends in Pharmacological Science*, 8:7–8.
2. Seiden, L. S., Fischman, M. W., and Schuster, C. R. (1975): *Drug Alcohol Depend.*, 1:215–219.
3. Ellison, G., Eison, M. S. Huberman, H. S., and Daniel, F. (1978):201:276–278.
4. Ricaurte, G. A., Guillery, R. W., Seiden, L. S., Schuster, C. R., and Moore, R.Y. (1982): *Brain Res.*, 235:93–103.
5. Seiden, L. S., and Vosmer, G. (1984): *Pharmacol. Biochem. Behav.*, 21(1):29–31.
6. Ricaurte, G. A., Irwin, I., Forno, L. S. DeLanney, L. E., Langston, E., and Langston, J. W. (1987): *Brain Res.*, 403:43–51.
7. Kostrzewa, R., and Jacobowitz, D. (1974): *Pharmacol. Rev.*, 26:199–287.
8. Ricaurte, G. A., DeLanney, L. E., Finnegan, K. T., Irwin, I., and Langston, J. W. (1988): *Brain Res.*, 438:395–398.
9. Jonsson, G. (1980): *Ann. Rev. Neurosci.*, 3:169–187.
10. Cohen, G. (1986): *Adv. Neurol.*, 45:119–125.
11. Finnegan, K. T., DeLanney, L. E., Irwin, L., Ricaurate, G. A., and Langston, J. W. (1988): *Soc. Neurosci. Abstracts*, 14(1):774.
12. Baumgarten, H. G., and Lachenmayer, L. (1972): *Z. Zellforsch.*, 135:399–414.
13. Baumgarten, H. G., Bjorklund, A., Lachenmayer, L., and Nobin, A. (1973): *Acta Physiol. Scan.*, 391:1–19.

14. Jacoby, J. G., Lytle, L. D., and Nelson, M. F. (1974): *Life Sci.*, 14:909–919.
15. Allis, B., and Cohen, G. (1977): *Eur. J. Pharmacol.*, 43:269–272.
16. Cohen, G., and Heikkila, R. E. (1978): *Ann. N.Y. Acad. Sci.*, 305:74–84.
17. Langston, J. W., and Irwin, I. (1986): *Clin. Neuropharmacol.*, 9:485–507.
18. Langston, J. W., Irwin, I., and DeLanney, L. E. (1987): *Life Sci.*, 40:749–754.
19. Langston, J. W., Irwin, I., and DeLanney, L. E. (1988): *9th International Symposium on Parkinson's Disease*, p. 85.
20. Irwin, I., DeLanney, L. E., Di Monte, D., and Langston, J. W. (1988): *MPTP—Sardinia '88 Degeneration and Regeneration Process in CNS*, p. 13.
21. Irwin, I., Ricaurte, G. A., DeLanney, L. E., and Langston, J. W. (1988): *Neurosci. Lett.*, 87:51–56.
22. Benedetti, M. S., and Keane, P. E. (1980): *J. Neurochem.*, 35:1026–1032.
23. Robinson, D. S., Nies, A., Davis, J. N., Bunney, W. E., Davis, J. M., Colblurn, R. W., Bourne, H. R., et al. (1972): *Lancet*, 1:290–291.
24. Fowler, C. J. Oreland, L., Marcusson, J., and Winblad, B. (1980): *Arch. Pharmacol.*, 311:263–272.
25. Chiba, K., Trevor, A. J., and Castagnoli, N. (1984): *Biochem. Biophys. Res. Commun.*, 120:574–578.
26. Jarvis, M. F., and Wagner, G. C. (1985): *Neuropharmacology*, 24:581–583.
27. Gibson, C. (1987): *Eur. J. Pharmacol.*, 141:135–138.
28. Knoll, I., and Maygar, K. (1972): *Adv. Biochem. Psychopharmacol.*, 5:393–408.
29. Knoll, J. (1983): *Acta Neurol. Scand.*, 68:57–80.
30. Ross, S. B. (1976): *Br. J. Pharmacol.*, 58:521–527.
31. Jonsson, G., Hallman, H., and Sundstrom, E. (1982): *Neuroscience*, 7:2895–2907.
32. Spencer, P. S., Nunn, F. B., Hugon, J., Ludolph, A. C., Ross, S. M., Roy, D. N., and Robertson, R. C. (1987): *Science*, 237:465–564.
33. Calne, D. B., McGeer, E., Eisen, A., and Spencer, P. (1986): *Lancet*, 1067–1070.

Parkinsonism and Aging, edited by
Donald B. Calne et al., Raven Press, Ltd.,
New York © 1989.

MR Imaging in Parkinson's Disease and Aging

C. W. Olanow, *R. C. Holgate, †R. Murtaugh, and †C. Martinez

*Departments of Neurology and †Radiology, University of South Florida, Tampa, Florida 33606 and *Department of Radiology, Medical University of South Carolina, Charleston, South Carolina 29425*

High field strength magnetic resonance (MR) imaging can be used for *in vivo* mapping of the distribution of brain iron (1). The accumulation of brain iron is associated with decreased signal intensity on T2-weighted high field strength MR images (Fig. 1) and is roughly proportional to the intensity of the signal attenuation. These areas of signal attenuation occur in precisely the distribution of ferric iron as demonstrated by Perl's stain and in proportion to the known quantitative deposition of ferric iron in specific brain regions (2). Similar patterns of ferric iron distribution have been reported in nonhuman primates and rats (3). We have previously reported on the results of high field strength MR scans in patients with Parkinson plus syndromes (4). These patients consistently demonstrate signal attenuation indicative of increased iron in the posterolateral portion of the putamen (Fig. 2). By contrast, we have found that patients with clinical features of idiopathic Parkinson's disease are more likely to have normal MR scans, although some demonstrate a narrowing of the region of high signal between the red nucleus and the substantia nigra or a "smudging" such that there is a lack of distinction between these two nuclear groups (Fig. 3). Occasionally, patients with clinical features suggestive of idiopathic Parkinson's disease have increased iron in the posterolateral putamen (5). We hypothesize that this group of patients is more likely to have a poor response to drug therapy, an accelerated course of disease, and to evolve into a Parkinson plus syndrome. While the mechanism responsible for increased iron deposition has not yet been defined and the significance of iron deposition remains unknown, our studies indicate that iron distribution as evidenced by signal attenuation on MR scan serves as a marker to distinguish patients with atypical parkinsonism or Parkinson plus syndromes from those with typical idiopathic Parkinson's disease and may predict their subsequent course and response to treatment.

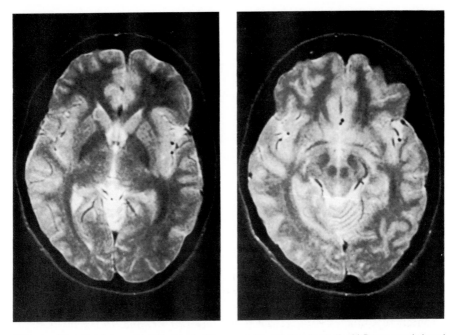

FIG. 1.   High field strength MR scan in 20-year-old control patient. **(Left)** Decreased signal consistent with iron accumulation in the medial portion of the globus pallidus. Note the relative lack of signal attenuation in the putamen. **(Right)** Signal attenuation consistent with iron accumulation in the red nucleus and substantia nigra.

In assessing this finding in an individual patient, it is essential to know the pattern of iron accumulation associated with normal aging. In normal adults, discrete areas of decreased signal intensity on T2 scan compatible with increased iron are present in specific brain regions—notably the globus pallidus, red nucleus, pars reticularis of the substantia nigra, and dentate nucleus of the cerebellum (Fig. 1). Iron in these regions increases as part of the normal aging process (2). This normal accumulation of iron, particularly in the putamen, raises the potential for confusion in identifying abnormal patterns as might be seen in patients with Parkinson plus syndromes. To better distinguish iron accumulation related to normal aging from that observed in pathologic states such as Parkinson plus syndromes, we have evaluated MR scans performed in a control population comprised of patients in sequential age groups.

SUBJECTS AND METHODS

The control group was selected from a group of ''normal'' patients at the University of South Florida and the Medical University of South Carolina

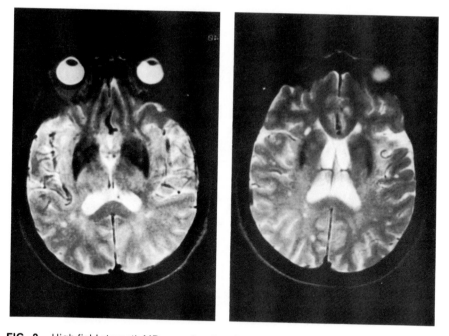

FIG. 2. High field strength MR scan showing signal attenuation in patient with Parkinson plus syndrome. Note the prominent signal attenuation in the region of the putamen that exceeds that in globus pallidus in both **left** and **right**.

who were referred for MR scan either as controls for this study or with a history of a normal neurological examination and complaints such as dizziness, orbital disease, headaches, to rule out multiple sclerosis, etc. All MR scans were performed on a high field strength (1.5 T) MR system (General Electric). Both T1- and T2-weighted spin–echo (SE) pulse sequences were used. Determinations were primarily made on the T2 series, which was obtained using a TR of 2,500–2,800 ms and TE of 80 ms (SE2500–2,800/80). An image matrix of 256 × 256 and a single signal average (two excitations) were routinely used for axial images. Images with intermediate weighting using a TR of 2,500–2,800 ms and a TE of 40 ms (SE2,500–2,800/40) were obtained concurrently with the SE2,500–2,800/80 millisecond images as part of an asynchronous multisection multiple SE pulse sequence. Slice thickness of 5 mm was routinely used and software enabling flow compensation was employed in most cases. Visual analysis of MR images was performed by at least two investigators, who were unaware of the clinical history or age of the patient. Iron scores were evaluated on T2-weighted images using a quantitative scoring system (Table 1). Iron scores were graded for the globus pallidus, putamen, caudate, substantia nigra, red nucleus, dentate nucleus, thalamus, cortex, white matter, cerebellum, and brainstem. Attempts were made to evaluate iron scores using similar window settings in all patients.

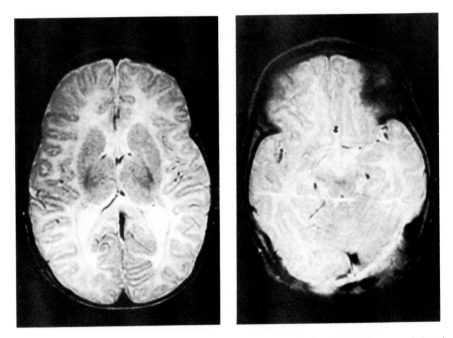

FIG. 4.   High field strength MR scan in normal 3-month-old infant. **(Left)** Decreased signal in posterior portion of the posterior limb of the internal capsule. No signal attenuation indicative of iron accumulation can be detected in the region of the globus pallidus or putamen. Note the increased signal in cerebral white matter associated with a relative lack of myelination in this age group. **(Right)** No definite attenuation of signal in the region of the red nucleus or substantia nigra.

served until approximately the third or fourth decade. Levels increase at a relatively slow rate until the seventh decade, when iron levels begin to increase at a more rapid rate. Changes are most pronounced in the posterolateral portion of the putamen often in a relatively thin border along the most extreme lateral portion of the putamen. In no instance in the control population did any subject demonstrate an attenuation of signal in the putamen that exceeded that in the globus pallidus. A comparison of the rate of accumulation of iron in the globus pallidus and putamen is illustrated (Fig. 6). No consistent pattern of iron accumulation was detected in other brain regions. Changes related to myelination of the nervous system were observed with aging in a pattern identical to that previously described (6).

DISCUSSION

Serial MR studies of iron accumulation in normal aging have been performed as a means of trying to differentiate those changes associated with normal aging from those related to the pathological accumulation of iron.

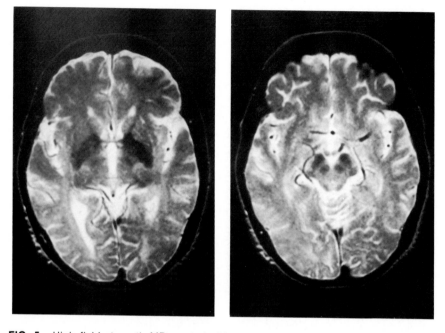

FIG. 5. High field strength MR scans in 80-year-old control patient. **(Left)** Prominent signal attenuation in the region of the globus pallidus. Signal attenuation is also noted along the lateral border of the putamen but is less pronounced than in the globus pallidus. **(Right)** Signal attenuation in the red nucleus and substantia nigra.

The relationship between iron accumulation in the globus pallidus and putamen in different age groups is relatively constant and differs markedly from that observed in patients with Parkinson plus syndromes. Signal attenuation is more pronounced in the globus pallidus than in any portion of the putamen in almost all normal individuals. In a few aged individuals, signal attenuation in the putamen approaches and may even equal that noted in the globus pallidus but in no normal control individual that we have observed does signal attenuation in the putamen exceed that in the globus pallidus. This contrasts with changes we have described in patients with Parkinson plus syndromes (particularly the multisystem atrophies including OPCA, Shy–Drager syndrome, and striatonigral degeneration), where in virtually every case signal attenuation in the posterolateral portion of the putamen is more pronounced than that in the globus pallidus and serves as a marker of this disease process (Fig. 2).

Changes in the substantia nigra and red nucleus suggestive of Parkinson's disease are more difficult to differentiate from changes due to normal aging than is the case with the Parkinson plus syndrome. Occasionally, "smudging" with a loss of distinction between the red nucleus and substantia nigra

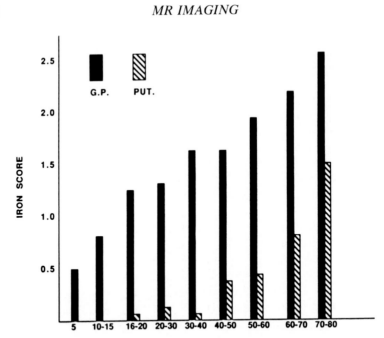

FIG. 6. Comparison of iron score in globus pallidus and putamen in different age groups.

can be observed in normal controls presumably as a result of technical factors. On an individual scan, "smudging" must be interpreted with caution.

Our earlier studies have demonstrated that the finding of increased iron in the posterolateral portion of the putamen in patients with parkinsonism is associated with a rapid rate of disease progression and a poor response to drug therapy (4,5). The majority of these patients either have or evolve into a Parkinson plus syndrome. We postulate that the accumulation of iron in the putamen reflects damage to striatal dopamine receptors, rendering them unresponsive to dopamine replacement therapy. The finding that iron in the putamen of control subjects approaches but does not usually equal or ever exceed that found in the globus pallidus allows distinction between aging patients and those with pathological accumulation of iron as seen in Parkinson plus syndromes. This contrasts with Parkinson's disease patients, where the pathology and occasionally the MR changes are in the substantia nigra. In these patients, iron distribution in the putamen is normal, presumably reflecting the preservation of striatal dopamine receptors and the capacity to respond to dopamine replacement therapy. The finding of increased iron in the putamen of occasional patients with what appears to be idiopathic Parkinson's disease raises the possibility that these patients will evolve into a Parkinson plus syndrome. It is now well appreciated that as many as 20% or more of patients who have Parkinson syndromes have or will develop a Parkinson plus syndrome. Early on, these patients may be difficult to differentiate from those with idiopathic Parkinson's disease and it is possible that MR changes in the putamen will serve as a marker to permit differentiation of this population of patients from those with idiopathic Parkinson's disease.

How iron enters the brain is unknown, since iron does not normally cross the blood–brain barrier. Transferrin receptors have been identified in the brain, but these are remote from sites of iron accumulation (7). It has been proposed that iron may be relayed to those remote regions by axonal flow. This may be the basis of iron accumulation with normal aging, but it is unclear how this would account for iron accumulation under pathological conditions. Preliminary observations suggest that there may be an increased number of infarctions or capillary dilations in the striatum of patients with Parkinson plus syndromes compared to those with Parkinson's disease or controls and it is possible that iron leaks into the striatum as a consequence of the resulting breakdown in the blood–brain barrier. Perhaps more likely is the possibility that iron accumulates as the result of neuronal degeneration. This would be supported by the finding of iron accumulation in the striatum of patients with a number of different degenerative processes including chorea, amyotrophic lateral sclerosis (ALS), and Alzheimer's disease. The accumulation of iron in these patients might reflect the underlying neuronal degeneration with the resultant clinical picture a function of the specific neurons involved. If this hypothesis is correct, the accumulation of iron in normal individuals may be a reflection of neuronal dropout that occurs in association with normal aging. If so, however, it is not clear why this should be confined to specific brain regions, particularly those that are high in concentration of GABAergic neurons.

Finally, it is well established that iron plays a role in facilitating oxidation reactions with the consequent release of free radicals (8). Iron is a transition metal that can provide an electron to either oxygen or hydrogen peroxide and promote the release of free radicals. The more iron that is present, the more likely oxidation reactions are to occur. Conversely, in the absence of iron or other transition metals, oxidation reactions are slowed or even halted (9). It is thus interesting to speculate upon whether the accumulation of iron is in some way related to the pathogenesis of disease processes such as parkinsonism or perhaps even normal aging.

Whether increased iron is simply a marker for a degenerative process or contributes to the pathogenesis of disease processes and normal aging is unknown. Studies of aging, however, make it clear that iron does not accumulate in the putamen to the extent it does in patients with Parkinson plus syndromes and that such accumulation as determined by MR scan is pathological. While iron accumulation can be seen in the putamen in a number of different conditions, this finding in patients with Parkinson features strongly suggests that the patient has or will develop a Parkinson plus syndrome and consequently will experience an accelerated rate of disease pro-

porting the hypothesis that the putamen is more closely involved in the regulation of movement than is the caudate (25). We have studied a group of patients with slightly more advanced disease, i.e., patients with significant clinical asymmetry but with bilateral involvement (26). In this group, we observed a slight symmetric decrease in caudate [^{18}F] activity and a more marked depression in putamen radioactivity accumulation. The putamen reduction was most marked contralateral to the major clinical motor deficit. The observation in these studies that the putamen is affected more than the caudate is consistent with pre-existing neurochemical data concerning the distribution of dopamine depletion in Parkinson's disease (24). Leenders et al. (27) have suggested that there is impaired capacity of the striatum to retain radioactivity after 6-FD administration, implying an impaired vesicular storage mechanism in nigrostriatal dopaminergic neuronal terminals in parkinsonian patients.

MPTP

The association between 1-methyl-4-phenyl-1,2,3,6-tetrahydropyridine (MPTP) and the clinical features of parkinsonism is well established (28–30). Langston et al. have identified a series of patients with MPTP-induced parkinsonism (31) as well as a large group of subjects who had received intravenous injections of MPTP without the development of extrapyramidal signs or symptoms. These asymptomatic subjects provide an ideal patient group to validate the concept that exposure to a toxin can produce subclinical damage to the nigrostriatal pathway. This is crucial to the hypothesis proposed by Calne and Langston (32) that Parkinson's disease results from the combination of subclinical damage to the substantia nigra induced by an environmental agent, following by the normal age-related loss of additional nigral neurons.

We have used the 6-FD/PET technique in order to seek evidence of subclinical nigrostriatal pathway damage in these asymptomatic individuals (33,34). We found a progressive decrease in 6-FD-derived striatal radioactivity from normal subjects through those exposed to MPTP to patients with Parkinson's disease. We were unable to establish a dose–response effect with certainty since quantitation of individual MPTP dosage was crude at best. There was, however, a rough correlation between the number of exposures to MPTP and the degree of striatal abnormality (34). These results have been interpreted as supporting the hypothesis that exposure to an environmental toxin may give rise to subclinical damage to the nigrostriatal pathways. By following these patients, we hope to acquire further information concerning the relationship between the development of clinical symptoms and the PET findings.

Evidence of subclinical nigrostriatal damage secondary to the administration of a low dose of MPTP has also been obtained from animal studies. Guttman and colleagues have utilized repeated unilateral carotid MPTP injections to produce an asymptomatic unilateral striatal lesion (35). By performing 6-FD/PET studies following each injection in a series, a progressive impairment of nigrostriatal function on the injected side was demonstrated, eventually culminating in the development of hemiparkinsonian symptoms.

These observations show that the 6-FD/PET technique has sufficient sensitivity not only to demonstrate abnormalities of nigrostriatal function in Parkinson's disease with its profound dopamine depletion, but also to provide evidence of a lesser degree of functional impairment preceding the development of a clinical motor deficit.

AGING

In order to assess any possible age-related effect on the striatal uptake and trapping of 6-FD derived compounds, we have developed a model for the graphical analysis of unidirectional tracer uptake data based on that of Patlak and colleagues (36,37). This model assumes that the system to be analyzed consists of a homogeneous tissue region that is perfused by a known concentration of a test substance. The tissue region may consist of any number of compartments that communicate reversibly with the blood but there must in addition be at least one compartment that the test substance enters in an irreversible manner. When the test substance is 6-FD, the irreversible compartment is formed by the decarboxylation of 6-FD to FDA and the trapping of FDA within neuronal vesicles. The original model, however, cannot be applied directly to the analysis of striatal 6-FD uptake because the major metabolite of 6-FD (3-OMFD) undergoes bidirectional transport across the blood–brain barrier, never entering the irreversible compartment. With our application of the graphical method, we have applied a correction for the presence of radioactivity due to 3-OMFD in the striatum based on the assumption that most striatal 3-OMFD comes from the blood via the neutral amino acid transport system, and that cortical 3-OMFD, arising from the same source, is present in a similar concentration to that in the striatum.

Application of this model requires that sequential measurements of tracer concentration be made in both tissue and plasma. Plasma 6-FD concentration is measured by obtaining sequential blood samples from each subject via an in-dwelling radial artery catheter during the scanning period. The total plasma radioactivity in each sample is determined with a well counter. The ratio of 3-OMFD to 6-FD and its rate of change over time is determined in each patient as described elsewhere (22). The plasma 6-FD radioactivity versus time relationship may then be determined for each patient from this ratio and the total plasma radioactivity–time curve. Sequential regional tis-

15. Chiueh, C. C., Zukowska-Grjec, Z., Kirk, K. L., and Kopin, I. J. (1983): *J. Pharmacol. Exp. Ther.*, 225:529–533.
16. Diffley, D. M., Costa, J. L., Sokoloski, E. A., Chiueh, C. C., Kirk, K. L., and Creveling, C. R. (1983): *Biochem. Biophys. Res. Commun.*, 110:740–745.
17. Chiueh, C. C., Kirk, K. L., Channing, M. A., and Kessler, R. M. (1984): *Soc. Neurosci. Abstr.*, 14:883.
18. Cumming, P., Boyes, B. E., Martin, W. R. W., et al. (1987): *J. Neurochem.*, 48:601–608.
19. Horne, M. K., Cheng, C. H., and Wooten, G. F. (1984): *Pharmacology*, 28:12–26.
20. Garnett, E. S., Firnau, G., Nahmias, C., Sood, S., and Belbeck, L. (1980): *Am. J. Physiol.*, 238:318–327.
21. Creveling, C. R., and Kirk, K. L. (1985): *Biochem. Biophys. Res. Commun.*, 130:1123–1131.
22. Boyes, B. E., Cumming, P., Martin, W. R. W., and McGeer, E. G. (1986): *Life Sci.*, 39:2243–2252.
23. Martin, W. R. W., Boyes, B. E., Leenders, K. L., and Patlak, C. S. (1985): *J. Cereb. Blood Flow Metab.*, 5(suppl. 1):S593–S594.
24. Leenders, K. L., Poewe, W. H., Palmer, A. J., Brenton, D. P., and Frackowiak, R. S. J. (1986): *Ann. Neurol.*, 20:258–261.
25. Nahmias, C., Garnett, E. S., Firnau, G., and Lang, A. (1985): *J. Neurol. Sci.*, 69:223–230.
26. Martin, W. R. W., Stoessl, A. J., Adam, M. J., et al. (1986): In: *Advances in Neurology*, Vol. 45, edited by M. D. Yahr and K. J. Bergmann, New York, Raven Press, 95–98.
27. Leenders, K. L., Palmer, A. J., Quinn, N., et al. (1986): *J. Neurol. Neurosurg. Psychiatry*, 49:853–860.
28. Burns, R. S., Chiueh, C. C., Markey, S. P., Ebert, M. H., Jacobowitz, D. M., and Kopin, I. J. (1983): *Proc. Natl. Acad. Sci.*, U.S.A., 80:4546–4550.
29. Davis, G. C., Williams, A. C., Markey, S. P., et al. (1979): *Psychiatry Res.*, 1:249–254.
30. Langston, J. W., Ballard, P., Tetrud, J. W., and Irwin, I. (1983): *Science*, 219:979–980.
31. Langston, J. W., and Ballard, P. (1984): *Can. J. Neurol. Sci.*, 11(suppl.):160–165.
32. Calne, D. B., and Langston, J. W. (1983): *Lancet*, 31:1457–1459.
33. Calne, D. B., Langston, J. W., Martin, W. R. W., et al. (1985), *Nature (Lond.)*, 317:246–248.
33. Martin, W. R. W., Stoessl, A. J., Adam, M. J., et al. (1986): In: *Imaging of Dopamine Producing a Parkinsonian Syndrome*, edited by S. P. Markey, N. Castagnoli, and I. Kopin, Orlando, FL, Academic Press, pp. 315–325.
35. Guttman, M., Yong, V. W., Kim, S. U., et al (1987): *Ann. Neurol.*, 22:172.
36. Patlak, C. S., Blasberg, R. G., Fenstermacher, J. D. (1983): *J. Cereb. Blood Flow Metab.*, 3:1–7.
37. Patlak, C. S., and Blasberg, R. G. (1985): *J. Cereb. Blood Flow Metab.*, 5:584–590.

Parkinsonism and Aging, edited by
Donald B. Calne et al., Raven Press, Ltd.,
New York © 1989.

Dopamine D_1 and D_2 Receptors in Aging, Parkinson's, and Other Neurodegenerative Diseases: An Overview

Dean F. Wong and Victor Villemagne

Division of Nuclear Medicine, Department of Radiology, The Johns Hopkins University School of Medicine and Division of Radiation Health Sciences, Department of Environmental Health Sciences, The Johns Hopkins University School of Hygiene and Public Health, Baltimore, Maryland 21205

Age-related declines in many behavioral functions, including motor activity, motivation, learning and short term memory, sexual activity, food intake, and sleep (1) have been shown in human and animal studies. Aging has also been associated with an increased frequency in the occurrence of Parkinson's disease (2,3), Huntington's disease (4), and senile dementia. It is plausible that these deficits have a neurochemical basis. *In vitro* studies of animal and human postmortem brains have shown age differences in several neurotransmitters, their associated enzymes, and their receptors (5–8). Of particular interest is the reported age-related decline of D_2 dopamine receptor density but not affinity in the striatum (9–19). With the development of specific ligands labeled with positron emitting radioisotopes, external imaging of neuroreceptors *in vivo* by positron emission tomography (PET) was made possible. PET allows noninvasive *in vivo* imaging of specific neuroreceptor ligands in normal physiological states, and also as a function of disease and therapy. We performed the first *in vivo* visualization of neuroreceptors with the imaging of D_2 dopamine and S_2 serotonin receptors in a normal adult using a potent ligand, 3-N-[^{11}C]methylspiperone ([^{11}C]NMSP) (20). We then assessed possible age and sex differences in D_2 dopamine receptors using this procedure.

AGE AND SEX DIFFERENCES

A previous study (21) included 22 male and 22 female volunteers, who were healthy as determined by medical, neurological, and neuropsychological examination. Their ages ranged from 19 to 73 years in the case of

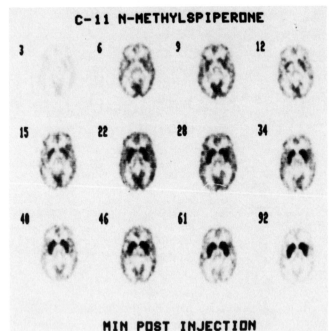

FIG. 1. PET images of the human brain at various times (3 to 92 min) after intravenous injection of [^{11}C]NMSP, at 40 mm above the canthomeatal line. This middle slice of the PET scan passes through the frontal horn and permits maximum visualization of the caudate and putamen. These images show a high accumulation of the tracer in the basal ganglia over time. (Reprinted from ref. 66 with permission.)

the males, and from 19 to 67 years for the females (mean age $\pm$ SD was 39 $\pm$ 17 years for males and 36 $\pm$ 14 years for females). A noncontrast x-ray CT scan was performed to verify the absence of pathological processes and to determine the appropriate transaxial slices for maximum delineation of the caudate, putamen, cerebellum, and the frontal cortex. For PET scans, 15 to 20 mCi of [^{11}C]NMSP was injected intravenously and multiple PET images were acquired for 90 minutes (Fig. 1). Specific binding to the D_2 dopamine receptor was then estimated by the ratio of radioactivity in the caudate to that in the cerebellum, an area of the brain where no D_2 receptors are present, while the binding to the S_2 serotonin receptor was estimated by the ratio of radioactivity in the frontal cortex to that in the cerebellum. The caudate/cerebellum ratio increased linearly with time in all of the subjects. This has been consistent in further studies, including 600 normal volunteers and patients. Under certain circumstances, the slope of the caudate/cerebellum ratio was considered to reflect the rate constant of [^{11}C]NMSP binding to the D_2 receptor (k_3). This ratio index had been previously used by other investigators, in *in vivo* rodent studies (22–25), to demonstrate the

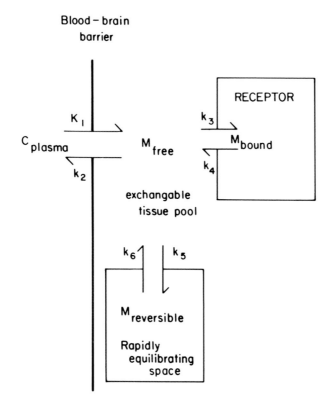

FIG. 2. Description of the three compartment model. [^{11}C]NMSP first crosses the blood–brain barrier, then binds to the D$_2$ dopamine receptors. C_{plasma}: concentration of the ligand in arterial plasma. M_{bound}: quantity of ligand bound to the D$_2$ receptors. M_{free}: quantity of drug in the exchangeable pool of the tissue. $M_{reversible}$: quantity of drug bound to the other secondary or non-D$_2$ receptors assumed to be in rapid equilibrium with the free ligand in the brain. K_1 is a clearance (from plasma) and k_2 a rate constant of escape from the brain tissue of [^{11}C]NMSP. k_3 and k_4: rate constants for, respectively, the association and dissociation of the ligand with the D$_2$ receptors. k_5 and k_6: rate constants that refer to the lower affinity or secondary rapid reversible binding, respectively, that is present in the caudate but not in the cerebellum. (Reprinted from ref. 66 with permission.)

pharmacokinetics of [^{3}H]spiperone binding and the effects of blocking drugs. Using this approach, we described an age-related decline both in the caudate/cerebellum, and in the frontal/cerebellum ratio (21). Also, the slope of the caudate/cerebellum ratio versus time changed with age in a similar manner, whereas a statistically significant difference was found between men and women in the distribution of the caudate/cerebellum ratio as a function of age.

In this initial study, using a compartmental model (Fig. 2), we argued that the ratio index reflected receptor binding, and was less related to the effect of blood flow. This interpretation depended upon a relatively low rate con-

44. Lassen, N. A., Feinberg, I., and Lane, M. H. (1960): Bilateral studies of cerebral oxygen uptake in young and aged normal subjects and in patients with organic dementia. *J. Clin. Invest.*, 39:491–500.
45. Obrist, W. D., Sokoloff, L., Lassen, N. A., Lane, M. H., Butler, R. N., and Feinberg, I. (1963): Relation of EEG to cerebral blood flow and metabolism in old age. *Electroencephalogr. Clin. Neurophysiol.*, 15:610–619.
46. Melamed, E., Lavy, S., Bentin, S., Cooper, G., and Rinot, Y. (1980): Reduction in regional cerebral blood flow during normal aging in man. *Stroke*, 11:31–35.
47. London, E. D. (1984): Metabolism of the brain. A measure of cellular function in aging. In: *Aging and Cell Function*, edited by J. E. Johnson, Jr., New York, Plenum Publishing Corporation, pp. 187–210.
48. Henry, J. M., and Roth, G. S. (1986): Solubilization of striatal D-2 dopamine receptors: evidence that apparent loss during aging is not due to membrane sequestration. *J. Gerontol.*, 41:129–135.
49. Zelnik, N., Angel, I., Paul, S. M., and Kleinman, J. E. (1986): Decreased density of human striatal dopamine uptake sites with age. *Eur. J. Pharmacol.*, 126:175–176.
50. Aquilonius, S. M., Bergstrom, K., Eckernas, S. A., et al. (1987): In vivo evaluation of striatal dopamine reuptake sites using ^{11}C-nomifensine and positron emission tomography. *Acta Neurol. Scand.*, 76:283–287.
51. Wong, D. F., Braestrup, C., and Harris, J. (1986): Assessment of D_1 and D_2 dopamine receptors in Lesch–Nyhan syndrome by positron emission tomography. *J. Nucl. Med.*, 27:1027(Abstract).
52. Farde, L., Halldin, C., Stone-Elander, S., and Sedvall, G. (1987): PET analysis of human dopamine receptor subtypes using ^{11}C-SCH 23390 and ^{11}C-raclopride. *Psychopharmacology*, 92:278–284.
53. Morgan, D. G., May, P. C., and Finch, C. E. (1986): Neurotransmitter receptors in normal human aging and Alzheimer's disease. In: *Receptors and Ligands in Psychiatry and Neurology*, edited by A. K. Sen and T. Y. Lee, New York, Cambridge University Press.
54. O'Boyle, K. M., and Waddington, J. L. (1984): Loss of striatal dopamine receptors with aging is selective for D_2 but not D_1 sites: association with increased non-specific binding of the D_1 ligand ^{3}H-piflutixol. *Eur. J. Pharmacol.*, 105:171–174.
55. Morgan, D. G., May, P. C., and Finch, C. E., (1987): Dopamine and serotonin systems in human and rodent brain: effects of age and neurodegenerative disease. *J. Am. Geriatr. Soc.*, 35:334–345.
56. Breese, G. R., Baumeister, A. A., McCrown, T. J., Emerick, S. G., Frye, G. D., and Mueller, R. A. (1984): Neonatal 6-hydroxydopamine treatment: model of susceptibility for self mutilation in the Lesch–Nyhan syndrome. *Pharmacol. Biochem. Behav.*, 21:459–461.
57. Breese, G. R., Baumeister, A. A., Napier, T. C., Frye, G. D., and Mueller, R. A. (1985): Evidence that D_1 dopamine receptors contribute to the supersensitive behavioral responses induced by L-dihydroxyphenylalanine in rats treated neonatally with 6-hydroxydopamine. *J. Pharmacol. Exp. Ther.*, 235:287–295.
58. Wong, D. F., Pearlson, G., Tune, L., et al. (1987): In vivo measurement of D2 dopamine receptor abnormalities in drug naive and treated manic–depressive patients. *J. Nucl. Med.*, 28:611.
59. Wong, D. F., Singer, H., Pearlson, G., et al. (1988): D2 dopamine receptors in Tourette's syndrome and manic–depressive illness. *J. Nucl. Med.*, 29:820.
60. Rinne, U. K., Lonnberg, P., and Koskinen, V. (1981): Dopamine receptors in the parkinsonian brain. *J. Neural Transm.*, 51:97–106.
61. Seemann, D., Danielczyck, W., Ogris, E., Jellinger, K., and Riederer, P. (1984): Dopaminergic agonists—effects on multiple receptor sites in Parkinson's disease. In: *Recent Research in Neurology*, edited by N. Callaghan and R. Galvin, London, Pitman.
62. Guttman, M., and Seeman, P. (1985): L-DOPA reverses the elevated D2 dopamine receptor density in Parkinson's disease striatum. *J. Neural Transm.*, 64:93–103.
63. Pimoule, C., Schoemaker, H., Reynolds, G. P., and Langer, S. Z. (1985): [^{3}H]SCH 23390 labeled D1 dopamine receptors are unchanged in schizophrenia and Parkinson's disease. *Eur. J. Pharmacol.*, 114:235–237.
64. Perlmutter, J. S., Kilbroun, M. R., Raichle, M. E., and Welch, M. J. (1987): MPTP-induced

up-regulation of in vivo dopaminergic radioligand–receptor binding in humans. *Neurology*, 37:1575–1579.

65. Wong, D. F., Links, J. M., Folstein, S. E., et al. (1988): Dopamine receptors in Huntington's disease: effects of partial volume correction on PET quantification *J. Comput. Assist. Tomogr.* (in press).

66. Wong, D. F., Broussolle, E. P., Wand, G., Villemagne, V., et al. (1988): In vivo measurements of dopamine receptors in human brain by positron emission tomography. In: *Central determinants of age-related declines in motor function*, Vol. 515, edited by Joseph, J. A., New York, Annals of the New York Academy of Sciences.

Parkinsonism and Aging, edited by
Donald B. Calne et al., Raven Press, Ltd.,
New York © 1989.

PET Studies in Parkinson's Disease with New Agents

K. L. Leenders

Paul Scherrer Institute, CH-5234 Villigen, Switzerland

Although the cause of Parkinson's disease has not been established yet, it is generally accepted that the main pathological feature of this condition is the lesioned dopaminergic nigrostriatal pathway. As shown in human autopsy and experimental animal studies, a lesion of this pathway results in a marked decrease of native dopamine content and diminished concentrations of related catabolic enzymes in the striatum. In recent years, it has become possible to measure *in vivo* certain aspects of human striatal dopaminergic function using radiolabeled tracers and positron emission tomography (PET). Further validation and expansion of this method may lead to elucidation of pathophysiology of movement disorders since in many of these conditions a disturbance of one or more neurotransmitter systems has been demonstrated.

Through PET studies, it will now be possible to relate changes in neurotransmitter function to clinical features. Particularly, longitudinal studies starting in an early phase of the disease and using various types of tracers seem to be promising. Cross-sectional cohort studies are less suitable due to the rather small number of patients that currently can be scanned. This is not just caused by the relatively long duration of the scanning procedures. Also, the radiochemistry is often complicated and needs to be performed immediately before a scan because of the short radioactive half-life of the radionuclides incorporated in the tracer molecules. However, data handling and analysis is the most time-consuming aspect of measuring tissue function with PET. Reduction of count measurements into manageable units and conversion of time–activity curves into meaningful pharmacological or biochemical entities is a formidable task. It seems that the developments in this field are still in an early stage. The inevitably low patient throughput per scan laboratory, in combination with the small number of PET centers worldwide, will make it understandable why accumulation of biological or clinical results with PET is a slow process.

In view of this, it is not clear which PET tracers are really "new." The

187

"old" ones, like labeled fluorodopa, have been in use for some years now but have not been exploited to their full potential yet. These tracers will certainly continue to yield new results.

POSITRON EMISSION TOMOGRAPHY (PET)

The compounds (ligands) used with PET are administered in trace amounts. A PET scanner is able to detect the uptake of these tracers into tissue like brain or heart, since a special type of radionuclide is incorporated as a "label" in the tracer molecules. These radionuclides decay by emitting a positron, e.g., oxygen-15, carbon-11, or fluorine-18. A positron is a particle with the same mass as an electron but positively charged. The main three reasons for choosing this type of radionuclide are the following: First, they are nuclides of physiological atoms, which means that their incorporation into the required tracer molecules does not change, or only slightly changes the chemical properties of the tracer. Second, the short radioactive half-life (minutes to a few hours) allows administration of tracer in a dose sufficient to obtain measurable signals while keeping the radiation dose low enough for human use. Third, the characteristic physical features accompanying positron emission are the basis of tomographical measurement of regional radioactivity.

Shortly after emission from a decaying nucleus, a positron annihilates with an electron. This results in conversion of the masses of the positron and electron into two simultaneous high energy gamma rays (511 keV) travelling into opposite directions. The construction of most PET tomographs is such that a ring of detectors surrounds the body. Simultaneous stimulation of two opposite detectors (coincidence event) by the two gamma rays resulting from emission of a positron allows exact determination of the direction from where the event took place. After collection of sufficient coincidence events ("counts") within a certain time frame (seconds to minutes), the distribution of local radioactivity in the scanned cross section (plane) can be calculated by standard tomographical reconstruction techniques. Thus, for each region in the brain, a time–activity curve can be determined in absolute units of radioactivity (microcurie per ml tissue). The buildup and washout of tracer in a certain brain tissue region become more meaningful when they can be compared with the dose delivered to the brain via the arterial system. To obtain this information, a series of blood samples is usually taken from a small indwelling radial artery cannula after administration of the tracer. From this, a so-called arterial input curve is then derived. Whether the next step, namely calculation of a pharmacological or biochemical entity related to the tracer activity, can be achieved depends on the specific properties of the tracer molecule. The mathematical models that are used for this purpose vary widely in complexity. Assumptions, validation, and problems are discussed in detail in the literature, e.g., in the handbook edited by Phelps and colleagues (1).

DOPAMINERGIC PET TRACERS

Examples of "old" and "new" tracers will be given.

Presynaptic Tracers

L-[^{18}F]fluoro-3,4-dihydroxyphenylalanine ([^{18}F]dopa)

This analogue of L-dopa can be used as a tracer for L-dopa transport from blood to brain, dopamine formation, and subsequent conversion into metabolites (in the striatum, mainly HVA and DOPAC) (2–7). Figure 1 illustrates the radioactivity distribution throughout the brain after [^{18}F]dopa administration and Table 1 summarizes the findings to date in movement disorders using [^{18}F]dopa and other tracers.

After i.v. administration, only a small fraction is taken up by the brain

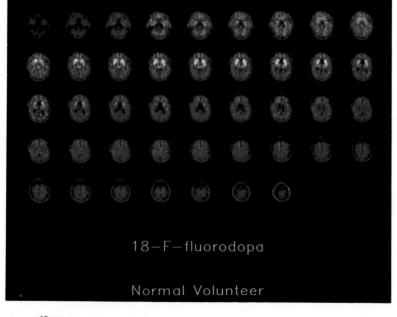

18–F–fluorodopa

Normal Volunteer

FIG. 1. L-[^{18}F]6-fluorodopa uptake in the brain of a healthy volunteer from 1 to 2 h after administration. The activity distribution is displayed from top to bottom by interpolation from 15 simultaneously measured transaxial planes. The measurements were performed using the PET tomograph at the MRC Cyclotron Unit, Hammersmith Hospital, London, U.K.

TABLE 1. *PET scan findings obtained in patients with movement disorders*

	L-[^{18}F]-fluorodopa, dopamine turnover	[^{11}C]methyl-spiperone, D$_2$ receptor density	FDG or oxygen-15 energy metabolism
Parkinson's disease	Diminished	Normal (?)	Normal or diminished
Huntington's disease	Normal	Diminished	Normal (?)
PSP	Diminished	Diminished	Diminished
Dystonia	Normal or diminished	Normal or increased (?)	Normal

because of the slow passage through the blood–brain barrier. L-Dopa transport across the blood–brain barrier is an active, energy dependent, and strictly stereoselective process in competition with other large neutral amino acids (5). [^{18}F]dopa is decarboxylated to [^{18}F]dopamine in the endothelial cells of brain capillaries and in the brain tissue itself, particularly in decarboxylase-rich regions like striatum. [^{18}F]dopamine is further metabolized into [^{18}F]HVA and [^{18}F]DOPAC, but Firnau and colleagues (3) showed that, in monkey brain the first 1 to 1.5 h after [^{18}F]dopa administration, the radioactivity in the striatum was predominantly [^{18}F]dopamine. The sum of [^{18}F]dopamine, [^{18}F]HVA, and [^{18}F]DOPAC formation is determined by the regional decarboxylation rate. In cerebral tissues other than the striatum, the O-methylated derivative was the principle labeled compound. In arterial plasma of carbidopa-pretreated subjects, the main metabolite after [^{18}F]dopa administration was found to be the O-methylated derivative (8).

Recently, the author and colleagues performed paired PET scans on five healthy volunteers using L-[^{18}F]-6-fluorodopa without and with oral carbidopa (150 mg) pretreatment. As can be seen from Fig. 2, radioactivity uptake in brain was increased by about 30% in both striatal and nondopaminergic regions relative to the arterial radioactivity. The five pairs of PET scans showed similar results. A detailed report is in preparation. An explanation for the findings could be that carbidopa inhibits decarboxylation of the tracer in the endothelial cells of the brain capillaries. On the other hand, a change of metabolite formation in blood by carbidopa might give rise to increased bioavailability of [^{18}F]dopa to the brain. The latter possibility is not supported by the finding of Hoffman and colleagues (9), who reported that carbidopa had no influence on the pattern and concentration of [^{18}F]dopa metabolites. The results of the determination of plasma metabolites in our study are awaited before a firm statement can be made as to which of the two above-mentioned mechanisms is the most likely one.

Further advances in [^{18}F]dopa uptake measurements with PET may arise

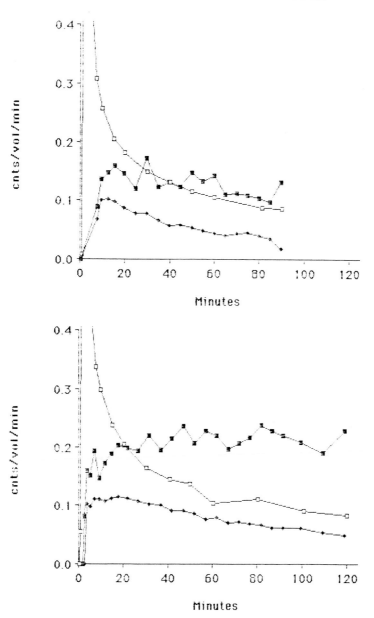

FIG. 2. Graph of L-[18F]6-fluorodopa uptake with time in the putamen, occipital lobe, and arterial plasma in a healthy volunteer scanned twice. **Upper panel:** without carbidopa. **Lower panel:** premedicated with 150 mg oral carbidopa. On both occasions, 75 MBq total radioactivity was injected intravenously. Symbols: open squares denote arterial plasma radioactivity; filled squares indicate mean putamen and filled diamonds indicate mean occipital lobe activity.

from using catechol O-methyltransferase (COMT) inhibitors suitable for human use. Blocking of methylation in the periphery would improve the arterial input curve: the total radioactivity in the plasma might possibly be equivalent to [^{18}F]dopa itself. Blocking of tissue methylation would result in all of the activity being derived from [^{18}F]dopa or a metabolite beyond the decarboxylation step. The kinetic modeling of cerebral [^{18}F]dopa uptake to estimate regional dopamine formation would certainly become easier if such blocking measures could be implemented. The positive effect of a COMT inhibitor on [^{18}F]dopa uptake in rats has been demonstrated by Cumming and colleagues (10).

[^{11}C]nomifensine

Nomifensine (NMF) binds specifically to catecholamine uptake sites on nerve terminals (11,12). In the striatum, specific nomifensine binding is virtually only related to binding to dopaminergic nerve terminals. Unilateral lesions of the nigrostriatal dopaminergic pathway in rats produced a marked (±80%) decrease of specific striatal binding of [^{3}H]nomifensine (12). This decrease was of the same magnitude as the reduction of endogenous striatal dopamine. A unilateral lesion of the locus coeruleus did not change tracer uptake.

Nomifensine labeled with the positron emitting radionuclide carbon-11 ([^{11}C]NMF) has been applied in PET studies (13,14). A similar experiment as reported by Scatton and colleagues in rats using autoradiography and [^{3}H]NMF (12) was performed on a Rhesus monkey using PET and [^{11}C]NMF (14). PET scans were performed before and after administration of MPTP, a neurotoxin specifically damaging or destroying dopaminergic neurons. MPTP was slowly infused as a solution (1.2 mg in total) through a catheter that was positioned into the right internal carotid artery via the femoral artery. Within 2 days, left-sided akinesia developed, occasionally accompanied by marked dystonic postures of the left upper or lower limb. After apomorphine or levodopa, the akinesia disappeared and normal use of the limbs was observed. In addition, during about 45 min rotation to the left occurred.

Striatal [^{11}C]NMF uptake 2 days after the lesion was normal on both sides. However, 9 days after the lesion, the difference between striatal and non-dopaminergic brain tissue activity was reduced between 80 and 90% in the right striatum, but normal on the left side. Apparently, MPTP had been taken up by the nerve terminals in the right hemisphere and resulted in rapid functional but slower structural damage of the dopaminergic nigrostriatal pathway. Six weeks after the lesion, the same [^{11}C]NMF uptake reduction was seen in the right striatum, but after 5 months and 1 year the uptake had recovered to about 50%. Clinically, only mild left-sided hypokinesia was noticeable from several months after the lesion onwards.

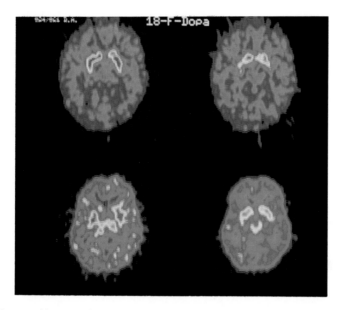

FIG. 3. Summed images of radioactivity distribution in the brain of one healthy volunteer scanned twice: **upper row:** after L-[^{18}F]6-fluorodopa; **lower row:** after [^{11}C]nomifensine. Two cross sections at a higher (**left image**) and lower (**right image**) level cutting through the striatum are displayed. For discussion of the distribution pattern, see the text.

Human studies using [^{11}C]NMF and PET have also been performed. Figure 3 illustrates the distribution of radioactivity in a healthy subject's brain compared to [^{18}F]dopa uptake. Both tracers are seen to concentrate in the striatum, but [^{11}C]NMF is also accumulated in thalamic regions. Since the latter tracer binds to catecholamine uptake sites, it is suggested that striatal [^{11}C]NMF activity is determined by dopaminergic and thalamic [^{11}C]NMF activity by adrenergic uptake sites. An abundance of adrenergic innervation of the rat thalamus has been shown by Lindvall and colleagues (15).

Striatal uptake of [^{11}C]NMF is diminished in patients with Parkinson's disease (Fig. 4). The results presented here were obtained using a racemic mixture of NMF. It is expected that more accurate quantitation can be obtained when only the active labeled isomer is administered. Much further work needs to be carried out before the value of this tracer as indicator for regional catecholaminergic nerve terminal density can be fully assessed.

Postsynaptic Tracers

[^{11}C]methylspiperone

Spiperone is a neuroleptic drug (butyrophenone) and is essentially a dopamine D_2 receptor antagonist. The radiolabeled analogue [^{11}C]methyl-

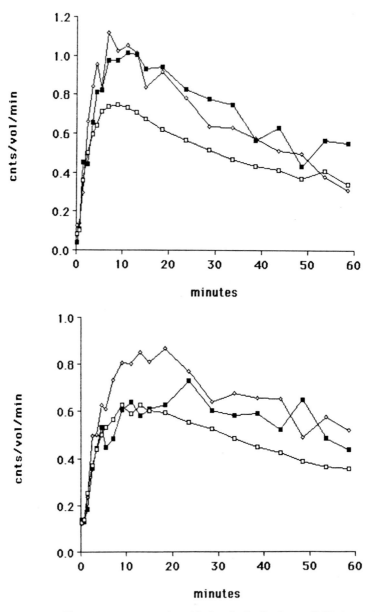

FIG. 4. Graph of [¹¹C]nomifensine uptake with time in the "putamen," "thalamus," and "cerebellum" in a healthy volunteer (**upper panel**) and a patient with Parkinson's disease (**lower panel**). Symbols: open squares indicate occipital lobe radioactivity; filled squares denote mean putamen and open diamonds denote mean thalamic radioactivity.

spiperone ([^{11}C]MSP) therefore binds predominantly to D$_2$ receptors in the striatum, where these receptors are highest in concentration (16). However, binding to serotonin receptors also occurs (17), which particularly dominates binding in cortical regions.

[^{11}C]MSP has been used in humans (18,19) and Eckernäs and colleagues (20) discuss the mathematical modeling associated with quantification of [^{11}C]MSP uptake. Reports about its application in Parkinson's disease have been scarce so far (21,22). Untreated parkinsonian patients showed similar striatal [^{11}C]MSP uptake compared to healthy controls. Levodopa drug treatment seemed to reduce [^{11}C]MSP uptake to some extent (21), but the number of patients studied was small. These findings are in agreement with post-mortem results showing virtually no change of dopamine D$_2$ receptor densities in parkinsonian patients (23). In this chronic disease, the apparently intact postsynaptic dopaminergic system, in the presence of a severe presynaptic lesion, "explains" why dopaminergic drug treatment is effective at all in Parkinson's disease. Patients with other chronic neurodegenerative disease associated with parkinsonian features like Steele–Richardson–Olszewski syndrome do not respond or only slightly on levodopa therapy. In that condition, impaired presynaptic dopaminergic function (7) is accompanied by striatal dopamine D$_2$ receptor decreases (24), probably due to striatal neuronal cell loss.

[^{11}C]raclopride

Raclopride is a neuroleptic drug (a substituted benzamide) and can also be radiolabeled to visualize dopamine receptor binding in human brain with PET (25). This compound is specific for dopamine D$_2$ receptors and quantitative analysis of these receptors can be achieved (26). [^{11}C]Raclopride has not been used extensively in patients with Parkinson's disease yet, but a recent report (27) about two patients showed normal striatal values before and after engraftment of homologous adrenal medulla tissue. The above-mentioned unilaterally lesioned (right internal carotid artery MPTP infusion) Rhesus monkey had also been studied using [^{11}C]raclopride (14). Two days after the lesion, an increased ($\pm 50\%$) specific tracer uptake was found in the lesioned striatum in the presence of a clinically impaired presynaptic dopaminergic function. At 6 weeks after the lesion, increased [^{11}C]raclopride and marked decreased [^{11}C]nomifensine (see above) was found in the lesioned striatum, but normal values on the unlesioned side. After 5 months and 1 year [^{11}C]raclopride uptake was normal again, while the presynaptic function was still impaired. This suggests that *acute* lesions of the nigrostriatal system can provoke a temporary increase of striatal dopamine D$_2$ receptor density. However, a *chronic* lesion of this system seems compatible with normal postsynaptic receptor density, at least in the absence of postsynaptic neuronal cell loss (see the discussion of [^{11}C]MSP).

REFERENCES

1. Huang, S., and Phelps, M.E. (1986): Principles of tracer kinetic modeling in positron emission tomography and autoradiography. In: *Positron Emission Tomography and Autoradiography. Principles and Applications for the Brain and Heart*, edited by M. E. Phelps, J. C. Mazziotta, and H. R. Schelbert, pp. 287–346. Raven Press, New York.
2. Garnett, E. S., Firnau, G., and Nahmias, C. (1983): Dopamine visualised in the basal ganglia of living man. *Nature (Lond.)*, 305:137–138.
3. Firnau, G., Sood, S., Chirakal, R., Nahmias, C., and Garnett, E. S. (1987): Cerebral metabolism of 6-[F-18]Fluoro-L-dopa in the primate. *J. Neurochem.*, 48:1077–1082.
4. Leenders, K. L., Palmer, A. J., Quinn, N., et al. (1986): Brain dopamine metabolism in patients with Parkinson's disease measured with positron emission tomography. *J. Neurol. Neurosurg. Psychiatry*, 49:853–856.
5. Leenders, K. L., Poewe, W. H., Palmer, A. J., Brenton, D. P., and Frackowiak, R. S. J. (1986): Inhibition of L-[^{18}F]fluorodopa uptake into human brain by amino acids demonstrated by positron emission tomography. *Ann. Neurol.*, 20:258–262.
6. Leenders, K. L., Frackowiak, R. J. S., Quinn, N., and Marsden, C. D. (1986): Brain energy metabolism and dopaminergic function in Huntington's disease measured in vivo using positron emission tomography. *Movement Disorders*, 1:69–77.
7. Leenders, K. L., Frackowiak, R. J. S., and Lees, A. J. (1988): Steele–Richardson–Olszewski syndrome. Brain energy metabolism, blood flow and fluorodopa uptake measured by positron emission tomography. *Brain* 111:615–630.
8. Boyes, R. E., Cumming, P., Martin, W. R. W., and McGeer, E. G. (1986): Determination of plasma [^{18}F]-6-fluorodopa during positron emission tomography: elimination and metabolism in carbidopa treated subjects. *Life Sci.*, 39:2243–2252.
9. Hoffman, J. M., Luxen, A., Bahn, M. M., et al. (1987): Carbidopa pretreatment in 6-[^{18}F]-L-Dopa PET studies: is it useful? *J. Cereb. Blood Flow Metab.*, 7(suppl 1):S362.
10. Cumming, P., Boyes, B. E., Martin, W. R. W., Adam, M., Ruth, T., and McGeer, E. G. (1987): Altered metabolism of [^{18}F]-6-fluorodopa in the hooded rat following inhibition of catechol-O-methyltransferase with U-0521. *Biochem. Pharmacol.*, 36:2527–2531.
11. Slater, P., and Crossman, A. R. (1984): Autoradiographic distribution of [3H]-nomifensine in brain. In: *Nomifensine. A Pharmacological and Clinical Profile*, edited by W. Linford-Rees and R. G. Priest, pp. 15–19. The Royal Society of Medicine, London.
12. Scatton, B., Dubois, A., Dubocovitch, M. L., Zahniser, N. R., and Fage, D. (1984): Quantitative autoradiography of 3H-nomifensine binding sites in rat brain. *Life Sci.*, 36:815–822.
13. Aquilonius, S. M., Bergström, K., Eckernäs, S. A., et al. (1987): In vivo evaluation of striatal dopamine reuptake sites using ^{11}C-nomifensine and positron emission tomography. *Acta Neurol. Scand.*, 76:283–287.
14. Leenders, K. L., Aquilonius, S. M., Bergström, K., et al. (1988): Unilateral MPTP lesion in a Rhesus monkey: effects on the striatal dopaminergic system measured in vivo with PET using various novel tracers. *Brain Res.*, 445:61–67.
15. Lindvall, O., Björklund, A., Nobin, A., and Stenevi, U. (1974): The adrenergic innervation of the rat thalamus as revealed by the glyoxylic acid fluorescence method. *J. Comp. Neurol.* 154:317–348.
16. Fowler, J. S., Arnett, C. D., Wolf, A. P., et al. (1986): A direct comparison of the brain uptake and plasma clearance of N-(^{11}C)methylspiroperidol and (^{18}F)N-methylspiroperidol in baboon using PET. *Nucl. Med. Biol.*, 13:281–284.
17. Frost, J. J., Smith, A. C., Kuhar, M. J., Dannals, R. F., and Wagner, H. N., Jr. (1987): In vivo binding of ^{3}H-N-methylspiperone to dopamine and serotonin receptors. *Life Sci.*, 40:987–995.
18. Wagner, H. N., Burns, H. D., Dannals, R. F., et al. (1983): Imaging dopamine receptors in the human brain by positron tomography. *Science*, 221:1264–1266.
19. Wong, D. F., Wagner, H. N., Jr., Dannals, R. F., et al. (1984): Effects of age on dopamine and serotonin receptors measured by positron tomography in the living human brain. *Science*, 226:1393–1396.
20. Eckernäs, S. A., Aquilonius, S. M., Hartvig, P., et al. (1987): Positron emission tomog-

raphy (PET) in the study of dopamine receptors in the primate brain: evaluation of a kinetic model using ^{11}C-N-methyl-spiperone. *Acta Neurol. Scand.*, 75:168–178.
21. Leenders, K. L., Herold, S., Palmer, A. J., et al. (1985): Human cerebral dopamine system measured in vivo using PET. *J. Cereb. Blood Flow Metab.*, 5(suppl):S517–18.
22. Hägglund, J., Aquilonius, S.-M., Eckernäs, S.-Å, et al. (1987): Dopamine receptor properties in Parkinson's disease and Huntington's chorea evaluated by positron emission tomography using ^{11}C-N-methyl-spiperone. *Acta Neurol. Scand.*, 75:87–94.
23. Bokobza, B., Ruberg, M., Scatton, B., Javoy-Agid, F., and Agid, Y. (1984): (3-H)spiperone binding, dopamine and HVA concentrations in Parkinson's disease and supranuclear palsy. *Eur. J. Pharmacol.*, 99:167–175.
24. Baron, J. C., Maziere, B., Loc'h, C., Sgouropoulos, P., Bonnet, A. M., and Agid, Y. (1985): Progressive supranuclear palsy: loss of striatal dopamine receptors demonstrated in vivo by positron tomography. *Lancet*, 2:1163–1164.
25. Farde, L., Ehrin, E., Eriksson, L., et al. (1985): Substituted benzamides as ligands for visualisation of dopamine receptor binding in the human brain by positron emission tomography. *Proc. Natl. Acad. Sci. U.S.A.*, 82:3863–3867.
26. Farde, L., Hall, H., Ehrin, E., and Sedvall, G. (1986): Quantitative analysis of D_2 dopamine receptor binding in the living human brain by PET. *Science*, 231:258–261.
27. Lindvall, O., Backlund, E. O., Farde, L., et al. (1987): Transplantation in Parkinson's disease: two cases of adrenal medullary grafts to the putamen. *Ann. Neurol.*, 22:457–468.

TABLE 1. *Differential diagnosis of buccolinguofacial dyskinesias*

Spontaneous buccolinguofacial dyskinesias in the elderly
Edentulous dyskinesias
Stereotyped movements in schizophrenia
Drug-induced chorea: antiparkinsonian drugs, dopamine antagonistic drugs, central
nervous system stimulants, anticonvulsants, steroids, tricyclic antidepressants, anti-
histaminics, lithium, and flunarizine
Other choreic syndromes: hereditary, metabolic and endocrine choreas, vasculitis,
and basal ganglia stroke

---

of spontaneous oral–facial dyskinesias in the elderly, all other conditions known to cause similar symptoms have to be ruled out (see Table 1).

Edentulous Orofacial Dyskinesia

Edentulous orofacial dyskinesia consists of recurrent jaw openings and involuntary movements of the tongue and lips occurring usually many years after tooth extraction. The most prominent factor in the genesis of dyskinesia appears to be the lack of dentures. Thus, in one study, 16% of edentulous patients without dentures had dyskinesias. However, age would be another important factor because the mean age of these patients was 62 years, but in this study a control group of elderly patients with a mean age of 68 years had no dyskinesias (16). Inadequate dento-oral prosthesis would cause disruption of dental proprioception resulting in dyskinetic searching movements of the oral cavity. Drug therapy with a variety of agents is ineffective and the abnormal movements diminish or completely disappear with proper construction of dentures.

Drug-Induced Chorea

Tardive dyskinesia (TD) is a well-recognized side effect of long-term neuroleptic and antiemetic therapy, and is frequently seen in patients ranging in age from 50 to 70 years. Characteristically, the syndrome consists of repetitive stereotyped movements of tongue twisting and protrusion, lip smacking and puckering, and chewing movements. Usually, a rather rapid onset of the orofacial symptoms occurs with gradual spreading in some cases to limbs and trunk. Although tardive dyskinesia does occur in any age group, increasing age appears to correlate with increased prevalence. Furthermore, TD is generally more severe in elderly patients, and an inverse correlation exists between rates of spontaneous remission and age (17). Tardive dyskinesia of the orolingual masticatory type tends to occur late in the course of neuroleptic therapy, often after the drug dosage is decreased or therapy discontinued. Differential diagnosis is the same as that for buccolinguolfacial dyskinesias in the elderly and is particularly difficult in psychiatric patients who may be receiving numerous other drugs. Pharmacological studies have shown that striatal dopamine is important in the mediation of these involuntary movements, and it is currently speculated that, since neuroleptics block dopamine receptors, tardive dyskinesia results from a supersensitivity of postsynaptic dopamine receptors in the brain. Neuroleptics would produce such a state of dopamine hypersensitivity perhaps by inducing an increase in the number of striatal dopamine receptors.

Choreic dyskinesias can be induced in the elderly by a variety of *other drugs*. Most common are those induced by levodopa and other *antiparkinsonian drugs*. Levodopa-induced dyskinesias may be influenced by the age of the patient, since they tend to develop more frequently and are more severe in young adults with Parkinson's disease and in cases of juvenile parkinsonism.

Dopamine agonists can also induce choreiform movements, especially in patients that are taking levodopa or have previously received it. The anticholinergics can induce buccolingualfacial dyskinesias when given for the treatment of tremor in Parkinson's disease or for other types of tremor. Anticonvulsants, tricyclic antidepressants, central nervous system stimulants, oral contraceptives, antihistaminics, flunarizine, and lithium have been reported to induce dyskinesias that, in some cases, are of the buccal–lingual–facial type (18).

Other Secondary Choreas

Generalized chorea in the elderly, often attributed to degenerative disease, has also been recognized to be a result of a cerebrovascular disease (19), such as caudate infarction, multiple lacunar infarcts in the basal ganglia, and hypertensive putaminal hemorrhage. In this situation, the onset is abrupt and the involuntary jerky movements affect all extremities and the face, accompanied by slurred speech. Neuroimaging techniques such as computed tomography and magnetic resonance help diagnose these cases during life. Neuropathologically, there is evidence of multiple lacunar infarcts bilaterally in the caudates, putamina, and subthalamic nuclei with selective sparing of the globus pallidus. Metabolic and endocrine choreas include those encountered with hyperthyroidism, hyperparathyroidism, acquired hepatocerebral degeneration, and polycythemia vera. Polyarteritis nodosa and lupus erythematosus can also cause chorea, at times only in one-half of the body (hemichorea).

DYSTONIAS

The term dystonia is used to describe a type of involuntary movement that is twisting, repetitive, and continuous. Dystonic spasms are the only or

GASTROINTESTINAL FUNCTION

Various disturbances of the gastrointestinal function occur in Parkinson's disease. *Sialorrhea* is a common late manifestation of the disease, although it is much less obvious (both in frequency and severity) in treated patients. Most probably, sialorrhea arises from poverty of automatic swallowing, and should therefore be regarded as being due to hypokinesia rather than as a purely autonomic manifestation. The rate of saliva production is unimpaired. This symptom responds dramatically to levodopa and its derivatives and is relatively nonresponsive to anticholinergics. In fact, the more mucous consistency of the saliva produced by antimuscarinics may further impair swallowing.

A more advanced manifestation of the same problem causes clinically significant swallowing difficulties, particularly evident for solid foods. Frequently associated chewing problems coexist, with a lower amplitude of chewing movements.

The difficulties in swallowing saliva and solid foods, if not sufficiently responsive to levodopa derivatives, may be relieved by drugs liquefying the saliva. A chance observation by one of our patients who had this problem and responded well to bromhexine has led us to an ongoing prospective study with this drug.

Probably the most common gastrointestinal manifestation of Parkinson's disease is *constipation*. This phenomenon occurs almost universally and although data are not available on the frequency of constipation of age-matched populations, we have data on the frequency among responses which is considerably lower. Patients with Parkinson's disease in many cases report that constipation predated the first motor manifestations; both started concomitantly in a few. In the remainder, where constipation has started after Parkinson's disease was diagnosed, the question of relationship to drugs can be addressed. Our impression is that several antiparkinsonian drugs are incriminated by patients as exacerbating pre-existing constipation, but they rather infrequently *cause* constipation.

The constipation in Parkinson's disease will usually respond to various dietary and drug manipulations, including mild laxatives, but several patients depend on enemas. An occasional patient may develop intestinal pseudo-obstruction, later on leading to paralytic or adynamic *ileus* (Fig. 1). Several patients known to us have undergone exploratory laparotomy and sigmoidostomy for the treatment of their ileus. Several years ago, it was suggested that habitual constipation may respond to naloxone (6). In view of this report, we have given naloxone, 1 to 15 mg i.v. to two patients with severe constipation complicating Parkinson's disease on four different occasions. There was no response to any of these injections.

The most severe patient we had has been treated in various ways but we have found the only practical solution to be the use of cholinomimetic drugs.

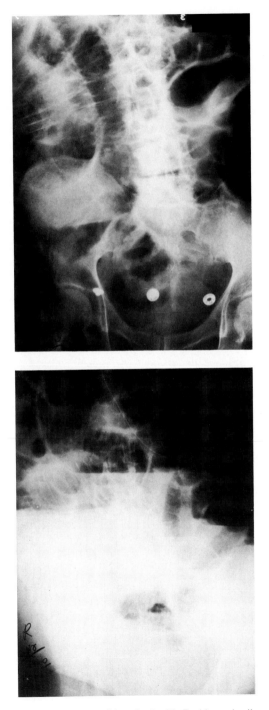

FIG. 1. Paralytic ileus in a 76-year-old patient with Parkinson's disease. This skiagram demonstrates widened ileal loops as well as fluid levels.

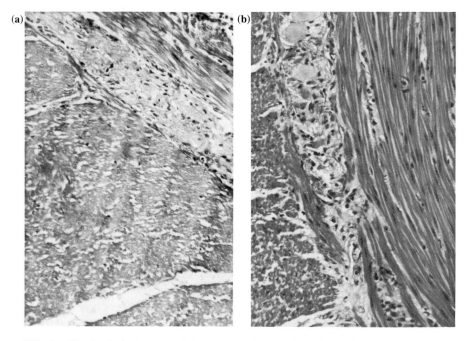

FIG. 2. Histological changes of the autonomic ganglia in the gastrointestinal tract in Parkinson's disease. The preparations in (**a**) are from the same person depicted in Fig. 1, and in (**b**) are from an age-matched control. The myenteric plexus in the muscular coat of the sigmoid colon shows loss of ganglion cells, as well as paucity of fibers in (**a**), as opposed to the control (**b**). Remaining neurons demonstrate picnotic changes. Hematoxylin and eosin, original magnification ×200 (courtesy of Dr. B. Ilie, Dept. of Pathology, Ichilov Hospital, Tel Aviv, Israel).

The patient had no response to oral prostigmine or betanechol. Parenteral betanechol stimulated intestinal motility, audible and even visible through the abdominal wall. However, this had not resulted in fecal evacuation. It therefore became clear that the intestinal pseudo-obstruction was the result of impaired motility in the most distal part of the intestinal tract. We have therefore tried giving the patient betanechol by enema, with surprisingly good results. This patient required the administration of 20–50 mg betanechol by enema (dissolved in a small amount of saline) repeatedly for several years until his death. Postmortem examination revealed (Fig. 2) diminution in the number of fibers and loss of ganglion cells within the muscularis mucosa with picnotic changes in the remaining neurons, particularly in the sigmoid colon and cecum (Dr. B. Ilie). Whether these changes represent an extreme form of a common process or whether they are due to a separate coexistent disorder remains to be investigated.

Weight loss frequently accompanies Parkinson's disease, although the loss is relatively mild (7). Several factors may be thought to contribute to this phenomenon, including the swallowing impairment noted above as well as the anorexia or nausea from dopaminergic therapy. The negative nitrogen balance resulting from hypokinesia and inactivity may also contribute. Interestingly, in a recent study (8), we have found that patients with Parkinson's disease treated with lisuride *gain* weight. This observation is consistent with animal data (9).

CARDIOVASCULAR SYSTEM

There is a clinical impression that patients with Parkinson's disease are less likely than the general population to develop *cardiovascular diseases*, e.g., hypertension and coronary artery disease. Whether this impression is correct should be concluded from more detailed studies, e.g., case-control studies.

Cardiac arrhythmias are rare in patients with Parkinson's disease, but may occur as side effects of levodopa therapy. The use of peripheral decarboxylase inhibitors probably reduces the frequency of such episodes.

Livedo reticularis, or *cutis marmorata*, frequently occurs among patients treated with amantadine and is particularly common in women. The mechanism underlying these phenomena is unclear but may be related to venular dilatation. Although this phenomenon is innocuous, it is important to recognize since it may otherwise lead to unnecessary investigations.

Edema, usually dependent, is another common manifestation. It almost always is absent or less conspicuous when the patient wakes up in the morning and develops during the day. It is only observable in advanced stages of the disease and probably occurs in patients who are hypokinetic and sedentary from the loss of the propelling force on venous flow by muscular massage. It is likely that amantadine may increase the edema, particularly if high doses are being used. On the other hand, ergot alkaloids like lisuride have a positive effect on venomotor tone and thus may decrease venous stasis and edema formation.

The most incapacitating cardiovascular symptom is undoubtedly *orthostatic hypotension*. The hypotension in Parkinson's disease is particularly common following meals (10), although the patients may not be aware of the association with food intake. The occurrence of orthostatic hypotension and postprandial hypotension may suggest that the patient may not be suffering from paralysis agitans but from progressive autonomic failure. However, in Parkinson's disease, other cardinal symptoms of the Shy–Drager syndrome are absent, e.g., pupillary response abnormalities, iris atrophy, and pharmacologic evidence for supersensitivity to direct adrenergic agonists. This may suggest that the problem is central rather than peripheral. In fact, recent data demonstrate normal blood pressure responses to tilt and we have shown that these patients have normal responses to the cold pressor test (Fig. 3).

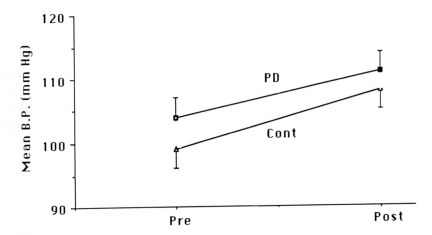

FIG. 3. Cold pressor test in patients with Parkinson's disease (n = 18) and age-matched controls (n = 14). Blood pressure was measured prior to and 15 s after immersion in ice-cold water for 2 min. Mean blood pressure was calculated as diastolic + one-third of the pulse pressure. Data are given as mean ± SD. The differences between the two groups were small and not statistically significant (Rabey, Mulla, and Korczyn, to be published).

An important factor in the evaluation of orthostatic hypotension in patients with Parkinson's disease is the possible contribution of drugs. Several antiparkinsonian agents may cause or exacerbate orthostatic hypotension including levodopa. Levodopa may act through a mechanism similar to that of the antihypertensive drug α-methyldopa, i.e., centrally, although the peripheral conversion to dopamine may also contribute to the hypotension. This component will be eliminated by the use of decarboxylase inhibitors.

Direct-acting dopamine agonists like bromocriptine or lisuride are particularly potent in precipitating hypotension by causing peripheral vasodilation. Activation of dopamine receptors located on sympathetic terminals powerfully inhibits stimulation-induced norepinephrine release. This action is abolished by treatment with the D_2 receptor antagonist domperidone.

PUPILLARY CHANGES

Few reports are available mentioning pupillary abnormalities in Parkinson's disease, and these are all drug-related. However, even if not posing a clinical problem, investigation of pupillary changes may be important since the pupillary size and its responses can be measured accurately and repeatedly using noninvasive techniques. Moreover, the effects of physiological stimuli and of locally applied pharmacologic agents can be studied. The importance of such observations may lie in the fact that using the pupil as

TABLE 1. *Pupillary cycle time (PCT) in Parkinson's disease*

	n	Age (years)	PCT	PCT >1000 ms	
Normal controls	14	68 ± 14	880 ± 54	0/14	(0%)
Stage 1	3	72 ± 2	990 ± 49	0/3	(0%)
Stage 2	16	66 ± 8	1277 ± 266*	13/16	(81%)
Stage 3	7	63 ± 12	1579 ± 325*	7/7	(100%)
All Parkinson's patients	26	66 ± 9	1335 ± 322*	20/26	(77%)

Data are given in years (for age) and in milliseconds (for PCT). The staging of Parkinson's disease is according to the criteria of Hoehn and Yahr (16). Asterisks indicate statistically significant differences from age-matched controls by Student's t test or by χ^2 test, as appropriate.

a model, pathophysiologic mechanisms may be discovered to be relevant to our understanding of other autonomic manifestations.

The size of the pupil is commonly believed to be reduced in parkinsonism, but again reference is to be made to the common miosis in old age (11). In fact, if correction is made for this factor, pupil size appears to be normal in Parkinsonian patients (12).

A relatively new method to evaluate autonomic disorders is the edge-light pupillary cycle time (ELPCT) (13). This method employs the light reflex, the physiology of which is well understood, to the study of the conduction in autonomic nerves. The ELPCT is known to be impaired in optic nerve disease (14) and in patients with autonomic neuropathy (15). We have measured the ELPCT in a small group of patients with Parkinson's disease and have found it to be abnormal in most, with a progressive slowing in more advanced stages of the disease (Table 1). The pathogenesis of this phenomenon is yet unknown. Although abnormal delays in visual-evoked responses have been reported in Parkinson's disease (17), the prolongation is small and unlikely to be responsible for the long delays observed by us. It is possible to count for these abnormalities by considering changes in the nucleus of Edinger–Westphal (18). An alternative explanation is of defective *sympathetic* tone. We have recently shown that the ELPCT is prolonged in patients with Horner's syndrome (19), and the magnitude of the prolongation in patients with Parkinson's disease is suggestive of a sympathetic dysfunction.

CONCLUSIONS

Reviewing the literature as well as our own results have led us to conclude that patients with Parkinson's disease manifest impaired autonomic nervous system activity. The pattern of impairment, with prominent gastrointestinal manifestations, is quite different from the abnormalities observed in progressive autonomic failure. Our understanding of the pathogenesis and pathophysiology of the autonomic dysfunction is still quite unsatisfactory.

An important facet of the autonomic dysfunction relates to drug-induced changes (20). It is yet an open question as to whether the effects of the medication are "normal," i.e., whether the same alterations would be produced in non-parkinsonian subjects when these drugs are given, or whether specific changes predispose patients with Parkinson's disease to develop these side effects. Be this as it may, recognition of these side effects would allow selection of appropriate drugs for the treatment of individual patients with Parkinson's disease.

REFERENCES

1. Appenzeller, O., Gross, J. E., and Albuquerque, N. M. (1971): Autonomic deficits in Parkinson's syndrome. *Arch. Neurol.*, 24:30–57.
2. Rajput, A. H., and Rozdilsky, B. (1976): Dysautonomia in parkinsonism: a clinicopathological study. *J. Neurol. Neurosurg. Psychiatry*, 39:1092–1100.
3. Korczyn, A. D. (1987): Autonomic manifestations in Parkinson's disease. In: *Morbo di Parkinson e Malattie Extrapiramidali*, edited by G. Nappi and T. Caraceni, Pavia, Edizioni Mediche Italiane, pp. 201–205.
4. Den Hartog Jager, W. A., and Bethlem, J. (1960): The distribution of the Lewy bodies in the central and autonomic nervous system in idiopathic paralysis agitans. *J. Neurol Neurosurg. Psychiatry*, 23:283–290.
5. Den Hartog Jager, W. A. (1970): Histochemistry of adrenal bodies in Parkinson's disease. *Arch. Neurol.*, 23:528–533.
6. Kreek, J. J., Schaefer, R. A., Hahn, E. F., and Fishman, J. (1983): Naloxone, a specific opioid antagonist reverses chronic idiopathic constipation. *Lancet*, 1:261–262.
7. Vardi, J., Oberman, Z., Rabey, I., Streifler, M., Ayalon, D., and Herzberg, M. Weight loss in patients treated long-term with levodopa. *J. Neurol. Sci.*, 30:33–40.
8. Rabey, J. M., Treves, T., Streifler, M., and Korczyn, A. D. (1986): Comparison of efficacy of lisuride hydrogen maleate with increased doses of levodopa in parkinsonian patients. *Adv. Neurol.*, 45:569–572.
9. Horowski, R., and Wachtel, H. (1978): Direct dopaminergic action of lisuride hydrogen maleate, an ergot derivative, in mice. *Eur. J. Pharmacol.*, 36:373–383.
10. Micieli, G., Martignoni, E., Cavallini, A., Sandrini, G., and Nappi, G. Postprandial and orthostatic hypotension in Parkinson's disease. *Neurology*, 37:386–393.
11. Korczyn, A. D., Laor, N., and Nemet, P. (1976): Sympathetic pupillary tone in old age. *Arch. Ophthalmol.*, 94:1905–1906.
12. Korczyn, A. D., Rubenstein, A. E., and Yahr, M. D. (1985): The pupil in Parkinson's disease. Proceedings of the 8th International Symposium on Parkinson's Disease, New York, 1985, p. P43.
13. Miller, S. D., and Thompson, H. S. (1978): Edge-light pupil cycle time. *Br. J. Ophthalmol*, 62:495–500.
14. Miller, S. D., and Thompson, H. S. (1978): Pupil cycle time in optic neuritis. *Am. J. Ophthalmol.*, 85:635–642.
15. Martyn, C. N., and Ewing, D. J. (1986): Pupil cycle time: a simple way of measuring an autonomic reflex. *J. Neurol. Neurosurg. Psychiatry*, 49:771–774.
16. Hoehn, M. M., and Yahr, M. D. (1967): Parkinsonism: onset, progression and mortality. *Neurology*, 17:427–442.
17. Bodis-Wollner, I., and Yahr, M. (1978): Measurements of visual evoked potentials in Parkinson's disease. *Brain*, 101:661–671.

18. Hunter, S. (1985): The rostral mesencephalon in Parkinson's disease and Alzheimer's disease. *Acta Neuropathol.*, 68:53–58.
19. Blumen, S. C., Feiler-Ofry, V., and Korczyn, A. D. (1986): The pupil cycle time in Horner's syndrome. *J. Clin. Neuro-ophthalmol.*, 6:232–234.
20. Korczyn, A. D., and Rubenstein, A. E. (1982): Autonomic nervous system complications of therapy. In: *Neurological Complications of Therapy*, edited by A. Silverstein, New York, Futura, pp. 405–418.

Parkinsonism and Aging, edited by
Donald B. Calne et al., Raven Press, Ltd.,
New York © 1989.

Regional Cerebral Blood Flow Reductions in Patients with Parkinson's Disease: Correlations with Normal Aging, Cognitive Functions, and Dopaminergic Mechanisms

Eldad Melamed and Bracha Mildworf

*Laboratories of Cerebrovascular Research and Clinical Neurochemistry,
Department of Neurology, Hadassah University Hospital, Jerusalem, and the
Department of Neurology, Beilinson Medical Center and Tel Aviv University
Sackler School of Medicine, Petah Tiqva, Israel*

The predominating pathological substrate in Parkinson's disease is degeneration of the neuromelanin-containing dopaminergic neurons in the substantia nigra pars compacta, loss of the ascending nigrostriatal axonal projections and their terminal ramifications, with reductions of dopamine concentrations in the caudate and putamen nuclei (1,2). There is evidence that the nigromesolimbic and nigromesocortical dopaminergic neurons are also involved in the degeneration process (3). The causes for the nigrostriatal neuronal loss are unknown, and viral, immune, hereditary, and toxic mechanisms may hypothetically play a role (4).

Although Parkinson's disease may occur in younger subjects, it is generally regarded as a disease affecting mainly the older population. Normal aging itself is associated with progressive loss of dopaminergic neurons. It is therefore possible that in Parkinson's disease there is premature and accelerated aging and degeneration (abiotrophy) of the nigrostriatal neurons. Furthermore, there is a high prevalence of cognitive impairment in Parkinson's disease that may also be due to enhanced aging processes in the central nervous system of afflicted patients (5–9).

In the brain, neuronal function is maintained by the adequacy of the regional cerebral blood flow (rCBF). Among other things, the rCBF is controlled, regulated, and coupled to local tissue metabolic rates (10,11). Therefore, rCBF measurements can serve as a useful probe to obtain information not only on the state of cerebral hemodynamics but also on the metabolic functional aspects of neuronal activity. Thus, previous studies have shown that normal aging is associated with progressive decreases in the rCBF (12). Furthermore, the age-dependent rCBF decline is not limited to elderly subjects but is already present in the younger age groups (12). The mechanisms responsible for this phenomenon are unknown. Since the rCBF reductions linked to advancing age have an early onset, it is unlikely that they are due to changes in the caliber of cerebral microvessels (e.g., by atherosclerosis) or to significant losses of metabolically active neuronal tissue that occur in the older population. It is possible that the rCBF decreases are caused by one or more of the multiple neurochemical alterations that take place in the brain during the normal, "physiological" process of aging. Several studies have shown that the rCBF is also reduced in Parkinson's disease but the underlying causes are undetermined (13–18). Nerve endings of dopaminergic neurons and perhaps also circulatory dopamine may be part of a complex neurochemical machinery that operates to regulate the rCBF (19,20). It was suggested that dopaminergic stimulation of brain vasculature produces vasodilatation and rCBF increases (21–23). One possibility, therefore, is that the rCBF reductions in Parkinson's disease are due to relative vasoconstriction induced by absence of dopamine molecules at target cerebral microvessels. Other experimental and clinical studies demonstrated that destruction of the nigrostriatal projections may cause decreases in the local cerebral metabolic rates of glucose and oxygen (24–27). Consequently, the deficient nigrostriatal, nigromesolimbic, and nigromesocortical dopaminergic transmission in Parkinson's disease may evoke rCBF reductions also secondarily, via suppression of cerebral tissue metabolism.

If, indeed, the rCBF decreases in patients with Parkinson's disease are due to diminished dopamine levels in their brains, the gradual decline in the concentrations of this neurotransmitter during normal aging may also be responsible for the age-dependent decreases in rCBF in the normal population. In addition, rCBF alterations in parkinsonians may theoretically be involved in the development of some of the clinical manifestations of this disorder. For instance, they could be contributory to the emergence of cognitive dysfunction and of the response fluctuations associated with long-term levodopa therapy. We therefore measured the rCBF in a large series of patients with Parkinson's disease under various conditions and in normal controls to determine (a) whether rCBF reductions in patients exceed or are similar to the flow alterations linked to normal aging, (b) whether dopaminergic mechanisms are responsible for the observed rCBF changes, and (c) whether there is a correlation between the presence and severity of cognitive impairment and the extent and pattern of rCBF decreases.

MATERIALS AND METHODS

Subjects

The rCBF was measured in 119 patients with idiopathic Parkinson's disease with age range of 36 to 80 years. We excluded patients whose parkinsonism was due to postencephalitic or multi-infarct states and to drugs and those with extrapyramidal features as part of multisystem central nervous system disorders. The parkinsonian clinical manifestations were predominantly unilateral in 38 patients (right-sided in 17 and left-sided in 21) and bilateral in 81 patients. Disease stage according to Hoehn and Yahr scale (28) at the time of study was 1 in 33, 2 in 40, 3 in 25, and 4 in 20 subjects. Duration of illness was less than 4 years in 52 patients, 5 to 8 years in 24, 9 to 12 years in 13, and more than 13 years in 8 patients. There were 91 patients who were on levodopa therapy while 28 were not on this medication at the time of the study. In 26 patients, the rCBF was measured once before initiation of the treatment with levodopa and a second study was carried out 8 weeks later when all patients had a beneficial response to an optimal daily maintenance dose. In 14 patients on chronic levodopa therapy, rCBF was measured first 1 week after discontinuation of treatment (if tolerated) and again at 4 weeks after renewal of levodopa administration when previous efficacy was reachieved. In 10 patients who developed predictable dose-related response oscillations after chronic levodopa therapy, rCBF and plasma levodopa levels (using HPLC–EC) were measured once during an "off" stage and again at an "on" phase of clinical benefit induced by a single oral dose of levodopa.

In 24 patients, rCBF was first measured before and again at 2.5 to 5 months after initiation of treatment with bromocriptine (parlodel). In 41 patients, rCBF measurement was repeated 1 to 2 years after the first study. A detailed neuropsychological test battery was given to 48 patients undergoing the rCBF study to determine the presence and severity of cognitive impairment. These included the Minimental test as well as a variety of procedures to examine memory, language, constructional skills, visuomotor coordination, visuospatial perception, spatial organization, etc.

The rCBF was measured for comparison in 103 age-matched, healthy, ambulatory, neurologically and mentally intact, normotensive control subjects.

rCBF Measurements

The noninvasive xenon-133 inhalation technique was used to measure the rCBF (29,30). The study was conducted in the resting state in a semidarkened room with patients in a supine position with eyes closed and ears plugged to minimize sensory inputs. The radioisotope tracer was applied through a tight-fitting face mask for 1 min via a nonrebreathing system. The washout of xenon-133 from the brain was monitored by 16 collimated NaI scintillation detectors applied externally, in a standard position over homologous regions of the right and left cerebral hemispheres (eight probes over each) and connected on-line to a computer system. Air, drawn directly from the face mask, was continuously monitored by an additional NaI detector for xenon concentrations in the expired air. The end-expiratory xenon concentrations are analogous to those in the arterial blood. These data were used for correction of the head clearance curves for the recirculation of the inhaled radioisotope. The rCBF was computed for each regional clearance curve as the initial slope index (ISI) derived according to Risberg et al. (31) from the initial slope of the curve between the second and third minutes. The blood–brain partition coefficient was arbitrarily chosen as 1 and the ISI data are presented in ml/100 g tissue/min.

RESULTS AND CONCLUSIONS

For the whole group of patients with Parkinson's disease, the mean brain CBF (calculated from 16 bihemispheric rCBF values in each individual subject) was reduced by an average of $11.4 \pm 1.6\%$ from expected normal, age-matched rCBF (calculated for each patient's age from the regression line through 103 mean flow values obtained in the normal subjects and plotted vs. age). There was no significant effect of age on the extent of rCBF decreases in parkinsonians. The mean brain CBF reductions from age-matched, normal CBF were $12.4 \pm 2.1\%$ in patients younger than 50 years of age, $10.9 \pm 1.5\%$ in the 50 to 59 years age group, $12.7 \pm 2.5\%$ in the 60 to 69 years age group, and $6.2 \pm 1.8\%$ in those older than 70 years. This shows that the rCBF reductions in parkinsonians exceed the "normal" age-dependent flow decline. It also suggests that age *per se* is not a primary cause for the observed rCBF decreases since the phenomenon was already present in the younger (below 50 years of age) patients and was even less pronounced in the older (above 70 years) age group in this series. This is supported by an additional observation. If age plays an important role in reducing the rCBF, it should be even lower when patients grow older. However, in the 41 subjects in whom the rCBF measurement was repeated at 1 to 2 years (mean of 1.7 ± 0.1 years) after the initial study, the rCBF and the extent of its reduction from age-matched control values remained unaltered. Since this is a rather short period in the natural evolution of Parkinson's disease, we intend to carry out additional longitudinal measurements in these patients. If similar findings are obtained, it would strengthen the impression that the rCBF reductions in parkinsonians may already be maximal when first studied regardless of age of patient.

The rCBF reductions were generally similar in the two cerebral hemispheres and in the various (frontal, temporal, parietal, and occipital) brain regions monitored. Furthermore, the degree of rCBF decline was unaffected by unilaterality of the clinical extrapyramidal manifestations. Thus, the right and left mean hemispheric rCBF (calculated as an average of eight rCBF values obtained in each hemisphere) was similar in patients with predominantly right or left unilateral signs. This suggests that the rCBF decline in parkinsonians is a global phenomenon affecting both cerebral hemispheres. The rCBF normally increases (mainly focally) during voluntary movements (32,33). Although we measured the rCBF during the resting state, it could be argued that the bradykinesia may contribute to the observed flow reductions. However, the similar bihemispheric rCBF decreases in patients with predominantly unilateral signs argues against such possibility.

A major question is whether the rCBF decreases in Parkinson's disease are due to deficient dopaminergic neurotransmission in the brains of afflicted patients. The following data do not support such a mechanism.

Striatal dopamine concentrations are lower contralateral to the body side with more marked symptomatology (2). If rCBF decreases were due to the nigrostriatal degeneration, they should have been more pronounced in the contralateral hemisphere. However, the rCBF reductions were similar in both hemispheres in patients with hemiparkinsonism (see above).

There is a linear correlation between the severity of the disease and central dopamine depletion (2). If rCBF decreases are due to lesser dopaminergic function, they should be more marked when the illness is more severe. However, there was no correlation between the extent of rCBF decreases and the severity (stage) of the disease according to the Hoehn and Yahr scale (28). The mean brain CBF reductions from normal, age-matched values were $11.8 \pm 2.6\%$ in patients with stage 1, $9.5 \pm 2.0\%$ in stage 2, $10.0 \pm 2.1\%$ in stage 3, and $10.6 \pm 4.1\%$ in stage 4.

The nigrostriatal dopaminergic lesion is a progressive phenomenon. Therefore, if the rCBF decreases are due to reduced central dopaminergic transmission, they should be more pronounced the longer the duration of the illness. However, there was no correlation between the severity of rCBF reductions and the duration of Parkinson's disease. If at all, reductions were more marked in patients with disease durations of less than 4 years (by a mean of $11.8 \pm 2.0\%$) and 5 to 8 years (by $12.4 \pm 2.7\%$) than in those with longer durations of 9 to 12 years (by $6.4 \pm 2.2\%$) or 13 to 16 years (by $7.7 \pm 2.5\%$). Also, a repeated study in 41 patients (see above) at a mean of 1.7 ± 0.1 years after first measurement and when severity of disease deteriorated mildly from a mean stage of 1.9 to that of 2.3 did not show further decreases in the rCBF.

Treatment with levodopa increases brain dopamine concentrations, corrects the deficient nigrostriatal, nigromesolimbic, and nigromesocortical transmissions, and has a beneficial effect on the signs and symptoms in parkinsonians (2,34–36). Thus, if the rCBF decreases in Parkinson's disease are due to brain dopamine depletions, they should be reversed or, at least, partially corrected after levodopa administration. We tested this possibility using various approaches, but the results were all negative: (a) The rCBF was similar in patients who were on levodopa (n = 91) and in those who were not on this medication at the time of study (n = 28). (b) In treated patients, there was no correlation between the rCBF or the extent of its reductions and the total daily dose of levodopa. (c) The rCBF remained unchanged in 26 *de novo* patients before initiation of levodopa therapy and 8 weeks later although all responded favorably to the treatment. (d) The rCBF remained unaltered in 14 parkinsonians at 7 days after discontinuation of the drug (levodopa "holiday") and again at 4 weeks after renewal of treatment when previous beneficial response was regained. (e) In 10 patients who developed severe dose-related response fluctuations after chronic levodopa therapy (36), the rCBF during the "off" phase was similar to that in the "on" stage induced by a single oral dose of levodopa, although plasma drug levels increased threefold (suggesting also central dopamine elevations).

Treatment with dopaminergic agonists is beneficial in Parkinson's disease mainly through direct stimulation of postsynaptic dopamine receptors and restoration of the deficient nigrostriatal neurotransmission (37). Thus, if rCBF reductions in parkinsonians are linked to suppressed dopamingergic function, administration of such agents might correct the basic flow alterations. However, the rCBF did not increase in a group of 24 patients at 2.5 to 5 months after administration of low doses (10–15 mg) of parlodel. Even if patients were divided into two groups, i.e., those in whom parlodel had a beneficial antiparkinsonian effect (n = 15) and those who showed no response to the drug (n = 9), the posttreatment rCBF was similar in both populations. In fact, during treatment with parlodel, there was a slight tendency for further rCBF reductions. Patients were divided into two groups, according to pretreatment basic rCBF levels, i.e., those in whom rCBF reductions from expected age-matched, normal control values were severe and greater than 15% and those in whom decreases were milder (less than 15%) or absent. It was observed that administration of parlodel did not affect flow in the first group but significantly reduced the rCBF in the second. This finding suggests that parlodel does not change the rCBF in parkinsonians when it is already maximally reduced but decreases it further when it is only partly diminished. The mechanism responsible for this phenomenon is not yet clear. It is unlikely that it is due to dopaminergic stimulation by parlodel since levodopa therapy does not cause a similar reduction. It might be due to a direct effect of parlodel on cerebral microvessels or to its possible interactions with other central neurotransmitter systems.

All of the above data indicate that the rCBF reductions are not due to deficient dopaminergic functions in the parkinsonian brain. There is a high prevalence of dementia in Parkinson's disease. The rCBF is reduced in other dementing disorders such as Alzheimer's disease (38–42). The cause for the cognitive impairment in parkinsonians is not fully established but may be linked, as in Alzheimer's disease (43), to degeneration of cortical cholinergic neurons originating in the nucleus basalis (44–46). There is even a correlation between the severity of cognitive dysfunction and loss of innominatocortical cholinergic neurons in patients with Parkinson's disease (44). Cholinergic neurons innervate cerebral microvessels and cholinergic stimulation produces vasodilation and rCBF increases (47–50). It is theoretically possible that loss of cortical cholinergic neurons causes the rCBF decreases in Parkinson's disease. Another possibility is that the dementia *per se*, through reduced metabolic demand in the cortex (51), secondarily induces the observed flow reductions. In such cases, there should be a close correlation between presence and severity of cognitive impairment and the magnitude of rCBF decreases in patients with Parkinson's disease. In 48 patients subjected to a detailed neuropsychological battery, most cognitive functions were found to be impaired as compared with those in age-matched, normal subjects. However, we found no correlation between the severity of rCBF reductions and the extent of cognitive impairment in this group of parkinsonians. This finding suggests that the rCBF decreases are not due to the dementing process and that both phenomena do not share a common pathogenetic substrate. Since the rCBF reductions in Parkinson's disease do not seem to be caused by either aging, deficient dopaminergic transmission, or cognitive impairment, these might be the result of other, yet unidentified, physiological and/or neurochemical brain alterations in this disorder. Further detailed studies should examine the nature of such mechanisms.

Acknowledgment: This work was supported, in part, by the Karen and Eric Segal Foundation, by the Jacob and Hilda Blaustein Foundation Inc., and by the Benjamin Boshes Endowment Fund for Research of the Neurological Disorder of Aging and Parkinson's Disease.

REFERENCES

1. Greenfield, J. G., and Bosanquet, F. D. (1953): *J. Neurol. Neurosurg. Psychiatry*, 16:213–219.
2. Bernheimer, D., Birkmayer, W., Hornykiewicz, O., et al. (1973): *J. Neurol. Sci.*, 20:415–455.
3. Javoy-Agid, F., and Agid, Y. (1980): *Neurology*, 30:1326–1330.
4. Calne, D., and Langston, J. W. (1983): *Lancet*, 2:1451–1459.
5. Sroka, H., Elizan, T. S., Yahr, M. D., et al. (1981): *Arch. Neurol.*, 38:339–342.
6. Hakim, A. M., and Mathieson, G. (1979): *Neurology*, 29:1209–1214.
7. Pollock, M., and Hornabrook, R. W. (1966): *Brain*, 89:429–448.
8. Leiberman, A., Dziatolowski, M., Kupersmith, M., et al. (1974): *Ann. Neurol.*, 6:355–359.
9. Boller, F., Mizutani, T., Roessman, U., et al. (1980): *Ann. Neurol.*, 7:329–335.
10. Lassen, N. A. (1959): *Physiol. Rev.*, 39:183–238.

11. Raichle, M. E., Grubb, R. L., Gado, M. H., et al. (1976): *Arch. Neurol.*, 33:523–526.
12. Melamed, E., Lavy, S., Bentin, S., and Cooper, G. (1975): *Stroke*, 11:31–35.
13. Lavy, S., Melamed, E., Cooper, G., et al. (1979): *Arch. Neurol.*, 36:344–348.
14. Melamed, E., Lavy, S., Cooper, G., and Bentin, S. (1978): *J. Neurol. Sci.*, 38:341–347.
15. Bes, A., Guell, A., Fabre, N., et al. (1983): *J. Cereb. Blood Flow Metab.*, 30:33–37.
16. Bottcher, J., and Henriksen, L. (1982): *Acta Neurol. Scand.*, suppl. 90:284–285.
17. Leenders, K. L., Wolfson, L., Gibbs, J. M., et al. (1985): *Brain*, 108:171–191.
18. Perlmutter, J. S., and Raichle, M. E. (1985): *Neurology*, 35:1127–1134.
19. Edvinsson, L., Hardebo, J. E., McCulloch, J., and Owman, C. H. (1978): *Acta Physiol. Scand.*, 104:349–354.
20. Ingvar, M., Lindvall, O., and Stenevi, U. (1983): *Brain Res.*, 262:259–269.
21. Lavyne, M. H., Wurtman, R. J., and Moskowitz, M. A. (1975): *Life Sci.*, 16:475–486.
22. Teasdale, G., and McCulloch, J. (1977): *Acta Neurol. Scand.*, 56(suppl. 64):98–99.
23. Edvinsson, L., Hardebo, J. E., Harper, A. M., et al. (1977): *Acta Neurol. Scand.*, 56(suppl. 64):350–351.
24. Schwartz, W. J., Sharp, F. R., Gunn, R. H., and Evarts, E. V. (1976): *Nature (Lond.)*, 261:155–157.
25. Harik, S. I., LaManna, J. C., Snyder, S., et al. (1982): *Neurology*, 32:282–289.
26. Lenzi, G. L., Jones, T., Reid, J., and Moss, S. (1979): *J. Neurol. Neurosurg. Psychiatry*, 42:59–62.
27. Kuhl, D. E., Metter, E. J., and Riege, W. H. (1984): *Ann. Neurol.*, 15:419–424.
28. Hoehn, M. M., and Yahr, M. D. (1967): *Neurology*, 17:427–442.
29. Obrist, W. D., Thompson, H. K., King, C. H., and Wang, H. S. (1967): *Circ. Res.*, 20:124–135.
30. Obrist, W. D., Thompson, H. K., Wang, H. S., and Wilkinson, W. E. (1975): *Stroke*, 6:245–256.
31. Risberg, J., Ali, Z., Wilson, E. M., et al. (1975): *Stroke*, 6:142–148.
32. Roland, P. E., Larsen, B., Lassen, N. A., and Skinhoj, E. (1980): *J. Neurophysiol.*, 43:118–136.
33. Roland, P. E., Meyer, E., Shibuzaki, T., et al. (1982): *J. Neurophysiol.*, 48:467–480.
34. Hefti, F., Melamed, E., and Wurtman, R. J. (1981): *J. Pharmacol. Exp. Ther.*, 217:189–197.
35. Globus, M., and Melamed, E. (1985): *Neurology*, 35(suppl. 1):159–160.
36. Marsden, C. D., Parkes, J. D., and Quinn, N. (1983): In: *Movement Disorders*, edited by C. D. Marsden and S. Fahn, London, Butterworth, pp. 96–122.
37. Lieberman, A., Kupersmith, M., Estey, E., and Goldstein, M. (1976): *N. Engl. J. Med.*, 195:1400–1404.
38. Obrist, W. D., Chivian, E., Cronquist, S., and Ingvar, D. H. (1970): *Neurology*, 20:315–322.
39. Lavy, S., Melamed, E., Bentin, S., et al. (1978): *Ann. Neurol.*, 4:445–450.
40. Simard, D., Olesen, J., Paulson, O. B., et al. (1971): *Brain*, 94:273–288.
41. Melamed, E., Lavy, S., Siew, F., et al. (1978): *J. Neurol. Neurosurg. Psychiatry*, 41:894–899.
42. Yamaguchi, F., Meyer, J. S., Yamamoto, M., et al. (1981): *Arch. Neurol.*, 37:410–418.
43. Whitehouse, P. J., Price, D. L., Struble, R. G., et al. (1982): *Science*, 215:1234–1237.
44. Ruberge, M., Ploska, A., Agid, F. J., and Agid, Y. (1982): *Brain Res.*, 232:129–139.
45. Whitehouse, P. J., Hedreen, J. C., White, C. L., and Price, D. L. (1983): *Ann. Neurol.*, 13:243–248.
46. Candy, J. M., Perry, R. H., Perry, E. K., et al. (1983): *J. Neurol. Sci.*, 59:177–189.
47. Scremin, O. U., Rovere, A. A., Raynold, A. C., and Giardini, A. (1973): *Stroke*, 4:132–239.
48. Edvinsson, L., Falck, B., and Ourman, C. H. (1977): *J. Pharmacol. Exp. Ther.*, 204:117–126.
49. Eckenstein, F., and Baughman, R. W. (1984): *Nature (Lond.)*, 309:153–155.
50. Estrada, C., Hamel, E., and Krause, D. N. (1983): *Brain Res.*, 266:261–270.
51. Cutler, N. R., Haxby, J. V., Duara, R., et al. (1985): *J. Neurol.*, 18:298–309.

Parkinsonism and Aging, edited by
Donald B. Calne et al., Raven Press, Ltd.,
New York © 1989.

Comparison of Normal Senile Gait with Parkinsonian Gait

P. J. Delwaide and Ph. Delmotte

University Department of Neurology, Hôpital de la Citadelle, 4000 Liege, Belgium

Similarities between morphological and biochemical changes in the central nervous system during normal aging and Parkinson's disease have encouraged the view that Parkinson's disease may represent premature or accelerated aging. That hypothesis applies particularly to gait modifications. However, that assumption is difficult to verify as the characteristics of both situations are poorly or very partially described. An agreement is only reached on trivial and rather nonspecific aspects such as slowness and reduced stride length.

In order to make a parallel between parkinsonian and senile gait, it thus appears necessary to specify more clearly the senile gait. The following represents both clinical and electrophysiological studies we conducted.

THE SENILE GAIT: A HETEROGENOUS ENTITY

First of all, it is necessary to define what senile gait is. In aged people, various gait disturbances are observed. Some of them reflect orthopedic, vascular, etc. problems. Others are due to well-identified neurological problems: stroke, polyneuritis, Parkinson's disease, etc. In a remaining group, although gait is clearly modified and sometimes unstable, no evident explanation is available at first sight. We propose to restrict the meaning of senile gait to this last group.

Prior studies have been concerned with senile gait. Imms and Eldhom (1) measured three parameters in a group of 71 subjects aged 60 to 99 years. Table 1 summarizes their results, which are compared to those measured in adult subjects and in parkinsonian patients. These researchers found that mean walking velocities for even the more active older adults were slower than any previous research had reported. It averaged 0.735 ± 0.285 m/s. Stride length was reduced at 0.930 ± 0.274 m whereas stepping frequency

229

TABLE 1. *Results from studies on gait*

	Young adults[a]	Aged adults[b]	Parkinsonian patients[c]
Walking speed (m/s)	0.96–1.35	0.735 ± 0.285	0.56 ± 0.21
Stride length (m)	1.2–1.5	0.930 ± 0.274	0.75 ± 0.29
Stepping frequency (half strides/s)	1.6–1.83	1.579 ± 0.278	1.50 ± 0.21

[a] From ref. 8.
[b] From ref. 1.
[c] From ref. 6.

was 1.579 ± 0.278 half strides/s. The authors found a linear correlation between walking speed and stride length and for that reason they considered senile gait as a homogenous process, where departures from adult values evolved in parallel but not necessarily in terms of age. This view has not been challenged until now. However, the conclusions are difficult to subscribe to since clinical experience indicates that among subjects presenting with senile gait there is an apparent diversity. We made the hypothesis that, aside from the three aforementioned parameters, which are linearly correlated, some others could evolve differently. For that reason, we undertook a new study of senile gait.

   We decided to include patients of both sexes, older than 60 years, free of any identifiable neurological disease, and not demented. They were selected during a hospitalization in a general hospital where they have been admitted for diseases with no direct incidence on gait (for example, hypertension, coronary insufficiency, gastric ulcer, and pulmonary infection). We excluded patients with lower limb problems such as arthrosis, arteritis, marked edema, etc. They all have been submitted to a neurological examination: all had preserved ankle jerks and flexor plantar responses. Patients with overt parkinsonian, cerebellar, or vestibular signs have been rejected. On the basis of these criteria, 181 subjects have been included in the study. The group was composed of 138 females and 43 males; the sex ratio is in agreement with the proportion of both sexes in the aged population of the city. The mean age was 80.17 ± 7.09 years, with values ranging from 60 to 99 years.

   As parameters, we took those used previously by Spielberg (2), Imms and Edholm (1), and Nayak et al. (3), i.e., stride length, walking speed, and stepping frequency. The subjects have been asked to walk at their preferred speed over a distance of 10 m. The number of steps has been measured as well as the time needed. With these measures, it was possible to know the mean stride length (expressed in m) and the walking speed (expressed in m/s). Stepping frequency has been obtained from stride length and speed and is expressed in half strides/s). Every subject has been tested at least

TABLE 2. *Study results*

Walking speed	0.66 ± 0.28 m/s	(reduced)
Stride length	0.784 ± 0.192 m	(reduced)
Stepping frequency	1.64 ± 0.25 half strides/s	(reduced)

two or three times on separate days. If the results in one subject differed more than 10%, the subject has not been considered for mean values. Additional parameters have been measured; vibration sensitivity and degree of flexum are the only two that will be discussed here but the basis of support and oscillations have also been assessed. Vibration sensitivity has been reflected by the number of seconds a patient perceives the stimulus given by a tuning fork (128 Hz) applied on the internal malleolus. The degree of flexion has been scored with quotation ranging from 1 to 5. The angle between hips and trunk was measured with a goniometer after the subjects had been requested to stand as erect as possible. One corresponds to an angle of 180°, 2 when the flexion is comprised between 0 and 10°, 3 between 10 and 20°, 4 between 20 and 30°, and 5 for flexion higher than 30°. In addition, each subject has been questioned about his subjective complaints regarding his gait and, in particular, has been asked if he has experienced falls in the last 3 months before the examination.

The results first indicate that, compared to young adults, the stride length and walking speed are reduced (see Table 2). Our values are a little bit lower than those reported by Imms and Edholm (1). This difference can be attributed to patient selection, Imms and Edholm having chosen subjects living at home with a greater autonomy. Stepping frequency in our series is 1.64 ± 0.25 half stride/s. The results confirm that gait parameters are modified in old age. The results have a normal distribution as confirmed by S and Henri's curves, suggesting that population is homogenous. To see if the various parameters are linked, the correlation coefficient has been calculated between stride length and speed. These two are linearly correlated with average value of 0.9487 (Fig. 1). However, there is no correlation between the results and patient's age.

The values of vibration sensitivity expressed in seconds are not normally distributed. They indicate two peaks, one at 16 s and the other at 4 s. In terms of stride length, no correlation is found for linear, exponential, logarithmic, or hyperbolic functions. For a parabolic function, the r coefficient is more satisfactory (Fig. 2).

The degree of flexion is linked to stride length by a logarithmic function. It is thus clear that at least two parameters–vibration sensitivity and degree of flexion—do not evolve in parallel with stride length and walking speed. This observation, supported by mathematical analysis (4), leads one to con-

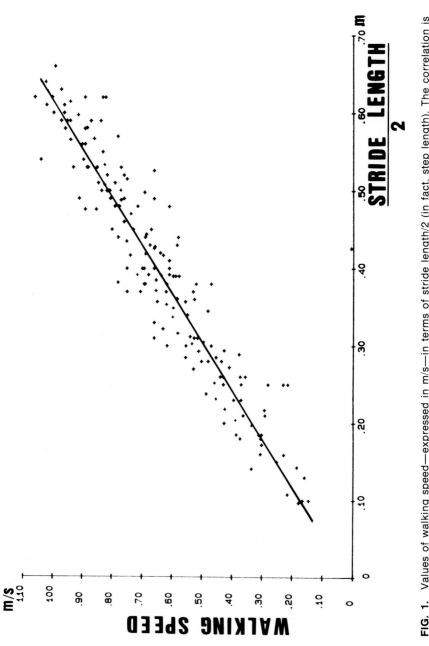
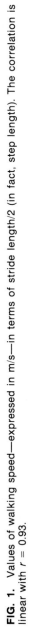

FIG. 1. Values of walking speed—expressed in m/s—in terms of stride length/2 (in fact, step length). The correlation is linear with $r = 0.93$.

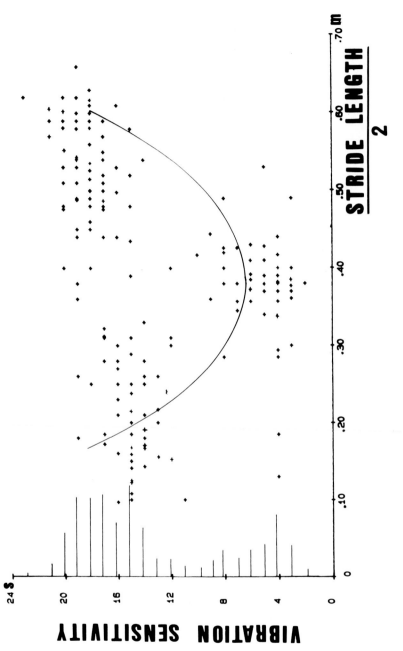

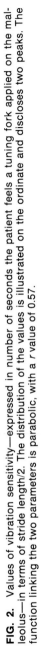

FIG. 2. Values of vibration sensitivity—expressed in number of seconds the patient feels a tuning fork applied on the malleolus—in terms of stride length/2. The distribution of the values is illustrated on the ordinate and discloses two peaks. The function linking the two parameters is parabolic, with a *r* value of 0.57.

TABLE 3. *Analysis of results*

	Pattern A	Pattern B	Pattern C
Walking speed (m/s)	≥0.7	<0.70, >0.58	≤0.58
Stride length (m)	≥0.9	<0.9, >0.68	≤0.68
Vibration sensitivity	Conserved (16 s)	Altered (4 s)	Conserved (14 s)
Posture	Erect	Erect	Flexed
Basis of support	Not enlarged	Enlarged	Not enlarged
	No falls	Frequent falls	Few falls

sider, as far as gait in old people is concerned, three distinct populations or three distinct patterns of gait (Table 3).

The first group—named A—is the closest to adult subjects. Nevertheless, the values of the parameters are clearly different from those measured in a younger population (Table 1). Subjects can be characterized by a stride length equal to or higher than 0.90 m and a walking speed equal to or faster than 0.70 m/s. The posture is erect and the vibration sensitivity is unaltered. It can be added that the basis of support is not enlarged and that subjects of that group do not complain of spontaneous falls.

The second group—named B—is characterized by a stride length of between 0.68 and 0.90 m and a walking speed of between 0.58 and 0.70 m/s. The posture is erect but vibration sensitivity is reduced, to less than 8 s; the basis of support is enlarged. In that group, falls are a frequent complaint.

The third group—named C—presents with a stride length greater to 0.68 m and a walking speed slower than 0.58 m/s. The posture is definitely flexed; vibration sensitivity is felt to be more than 8–10 s; the basis of support is not enlarged. Falls are rare in that group.

Having defined the characteristics of these three groups, we have established in a next step the proportion of each one in a nonselected old population. We have examined 300 subjects aged more than 65 years. Pattern A is clearly the most commonly observed since it applies to more than 50%. Pattern B concerns roughly 15%. Pattern C characterizes another 15% of subjects, the remaining 20% having a well-defined gait disorder: sequelae of stroke, parkinsonism, polyneuropathy (chiefly diabetes), arthritis, etc.

THE PARKINSONIAN GAIT

If parkinsonian gait is well described in neurological textbooks, it is rather unusual to observe at present a patient belonging to stage III and more of Hoehn and Yahr (5) who is not on dopa therapy. In stages I and II, the gait is moderately impaired. We have measured the same gait parameters as above in a limited group of parkinsonian patients at stages I and II, not yet treated by dopa, with a mean age of 63 years. We have also studied them in a special subgroup of patients with long-duration parkinsonism treated by dopa. In this group, the patients had special complaints about their gait. Although our results are interesting, especially in the second group, it is not evident that they are the most representative of the classical parkinsonian gait. To find reliable values, it seems wise to go back before the L-dopa therapy era. Fortunately, a study of Knutson (6) provides values of the various parameters we have studied (Table 1) in a group of parkinsonians, especially at stage III, who have not been treated with L-dopa. In addition to the parameters reported in the table, it can be remembered that in Parkinson's disease the trunk is flexed and that vibration sensitivity is not reduced. It is thus clear that the parameters of parkinsonian gait are very reminiscent of one subgroup of senile gait, the C pattern. They are distinct from those of the A and C patterns. It can be concluded that parkinsonian gait is not similar to senile gait taken as a whole but close to a special subgroup—the C pattern, which corresponds to 15% of aged people.

ELECTROPHYSIOLOGICAL STUDIES

Electrophysiological studies have been conducted in order to characterize better the different gait patterns and to ameliorate the comparisons between senile and parkinsonian gait. We have made use of a very simple method to avoid frightening old patients not accustomed to medical investigations. We have recorded EMG activity with cutaneous electrodes from the tibialis anterior and soleus during usual walking. We review here the preliminary results collected in young adults, old subjects belonging to the C pattern, and patients with a long-standing Parkinson's disease. In the young adults, there are EMG bursts, alternating without overlap in the two muscles. Activity predominates in the extensor muscle. In old patients, there is an almost continuous EMG discharge in the tibialis anterior while EMG bursts in the soleus are small and intermittent. There is evident cocontraction in muscles with antagonistic functions. The gait of parkinsonian patients is similar to that of old patients of the C pattern: continuous activity in the tibialis, very frequent cocontractions, and a reduced activity in the soleus. The recordings of EMG activity are able to interpret the shuffling character of the gait: propulsion due to leg posterior compartment muscles is reduced and, to avoid having the foot tip hook the ground, the tibialis anterior is continuously active. In fact, progression is obtained by pelvic rotation rather than by distal muscle contraction. Simple direct recordings of EMG activity favor resemblances between C pattern and parkinsonian gait (Fig. 3).

However, it could be unwise to assimilate the two types of gait and to consider that they depend on similar mechanisms. In fact, differences can be observed on clinical grounds. If festination and freezing are common in

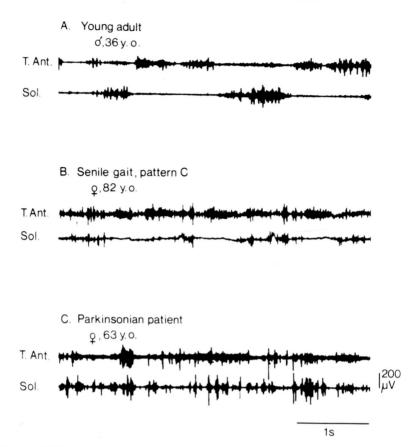

FIG. 3. EMG recordings from cutaneous electrodes fixed on tibialis anterior and soleus during usual deambulation. Three illustrative examples taken from **(A)** a young adult, **(B)** an old subject characteristic of the C pattern of gait, and **(C)** a parkinsonian patient with clinical gait problems. There are similarities between the records in **B** and **C**.

Parkinson's disease, similar abnormalities have never been observed in the old patients we have studied, irrespective of the gait patterns they presented with. Moreover, some spinal mechanisms may be modified in Parkinson's disease and not in normal aging even if subjects belong to group C. We have already reported (7) that, in parkinsonian patients, nonpainful stimulation of the tibial nerve at the ankle elicits frequently synchronous bursts of EMG activity both in the tibialis anterior and soleus. This cocontraction is a general rule in patients with festination or with difficulties in initiating walking but it is also observed in parkinsonian patients without these specific problems. According to our preliminary results, a similar cocontraction is not seen in nonparkinsonian subjects even if they belong to the C gait pattern. In that case, the evoked responses are basically out of phase with some possible overlap.

These observations point to the fact that the differences between senile and parkinsonian gait are not only quantitative but could also be qualitative.

CONCLUSIONS

If similarities exist between parkinsonian gait and gait seen in aged people, resemblances apply only to a special subtype of senile gait that is seen in a minority of old people, not exceeding 15% of them. However, the parallel should be cautious because it seems that parkinsonian gait may be enriched by special features such as festination and freezing that are never observed in normal aging. In addition, among parkinsonian patients, spinal mechanisms may be disturbed and reveal specific troubles, indicating that the channeling of afferent information onto motoneurons is modified. Such a problem is not observed in nonparkinsonian old subjects.

REFERENCES

1. Imms, F. J., and Edholm, O. G. (1981): *Age Ageing,* 10:147–156.
2. Spielberg, P. I. (1940): In: *Investigations on the Biodynamics of Walking Running and Jumping,* Part II, edited by N. A. Bernstein, Moscow, Central Scientific Institute of Physical Culture.
3. Nayak, U. S., Gabell, A., Simons, M. A., and Isaacs, B. (1982): *J. Am. Geriatr. Soc.,* 30:516–520.
4. Delwaide, P. J., Delmotte, P. (submitted for publication).
5. Hoehn, M. M., and Yahr, M. D. (1967): *Neurology,* 17:427–442.
6. Knutsson, E. (1972): *Brain,* 95:475–486.
7. Delwaide, P. J. (1985): *Clinical Neurophysiology in Parkinsonism,* edited by P. J. Delwaide and A. Agnoli, Chap. 3, Amsterdam, Elsevier, pp. 19–30.
8. Imman, F. J., Ralston, H. J., and Todd, F. (1981): *Human Walking,* Baltimore, Williams & Wilkins.

Parkinsonism and Aging, edited by
Donald B. Calne et al., Raven Press, Ltd.,
New York © 1989.

Influence of Treatment on the Natural History of Parkinson's Disease

Marco Trabucchi, *Ildebrando Appollonio, Fiorenzo Battaini,
†Stefano Govoni, and *Lodovico Frattola

*Department of Toxicology, University of Rome, Rome; *Neurological Clinic V,
University of Milan—S. Gerardo Hospital, Monza, Milan; and
†Institute of Pharmacological Sciences, University of Milan, Milan, Italy*

Parkinson's disease (PD) is the first documented example of a neurological disease consistently correlated with a deficiency in a specific neurotransmitter, i.e., dopamine. In fact, following the observations of various research groups indicating that dopamine represents a large proportion of brain catecholamines and is concentrated in basal ganglia (1,2), Hornykiewicz discovered, by studying human brains obtained at postmortem examination, that parkinsonian patients had low brain levels of monoamines, in particular of dopamine (3).

This observation provided the rationale for the introduction of levodopa therapy (4), which represented the first attempt to cure a brain disease by exogenously administering a neurotransmitter precursor. This therapeutic approach raised the hope that levodopa might not only improve the symptoms of PD but also arrest its progression.

This, unfortunately, turned out not to be the case, giving rise to tremendous research efforts aimed at a better characterization of the disease and to the design of a more efficient therapy. Although the primary pathology in PD is the degeneration of dopaminergic cells projecting to the striatum, losses of noradrenergic or serotoninergic neurons are also observed. In addition, since the original description of dopamine deficiency in PD, the neurochemical picture of the brain and of the disease itself has grown in complexity. In the late 1960s–early 1970s, some key points in neurochemistry were confuted and modified, leading to the discovery of many peptide transmitters (5) and to the concept of cotransmission.

Receptors have become measurable entities (6), displaying the unforeseen ability to adapt to transmitter availability changes and families of functionally and pharmacologically distinguishable receptors for a given transmitter have grown.

This is the new context in which pathophysiological changes of PD and levodopa therapy should be examined. Dopamine synaptic activity is complexly regulated by various peptides such as enkephalin (7,8), neurotensin (9), cholecystokinin (CCK) (10), substance P (11), and somatostatin (12). Moreover, subsets of dopamine terminals appear to contain CCK as cotransmitter (13).

Some of these peptides are also affected in PD (14) although it is not known if the defect is primary or consequent to the loss of dopamine. In addition, experimental evidence suggests that treatments affecting dopamine function also modify the status of these accompanying transmitters (15–18). It should be stressed that these regulatory systems as well as the mechanisms regulating dopamine uptake and synthesis may differ in the various dopaminergic areas. An emblematic example is the cocaine binding site controlling dopamine uptake, which is substantially different in the nucleus accumbens in comparison with the striatum (19). As a consequence, these two brain areas may present different, and sometimes opposite, changes in dopamine function in response to experimental manipulation (20,21).

At the postsynaptic level, at least two dopamine receptors (22–24) having a distinct pharmacological profile have been described. Moreover, the machinery providing the transmembrane transduction of the message and the cellular response appears to be highly sophisticated, involving the concurrent action of various proteins (the receptor itself, GTP binding proteins, adenylate cyclase, protein kinases, and protein kinase substrates) (25–29), which may also be modified by the pathophysiological process or by therapeutic intervention.

Due to the predominant appearance of PD in advanced age, another aspect that may interfere in the course of the disease is aging. The neurochemical setting of the brain presents marked age-dependent changes from development to the late stages of life. In general, the results in the literature indicate that synthesis, release, and recognition sites of several neurotransmitters display an age-related decline (30,31). Even if the available data do not allow the identification of a single neuronal population controlling the aging of the brain, significant progress has been made in the attempt to identify and interpret the most relevant age-related changes in brain neurochemistry. Along this line, an age-related decline of dopaminergic transmission is one of the most consistent findings in the literature.

The synaptic deficit of dopaminergic circuits involves the synthesis and the uptake of dopamine (32–34) as well as a complex pattern of changes at the level of postsynaptic dopamine receptors and their associated transducing mechanisms (35–39). PD is superimposed on these age-dependent alterations. It is not known whether the disease represents an "accelerated" aging quantitatively affecting more dopamine neurons or a qualitatively different process. Conversely, it is not known whether aging changes in brain neurochemistry of the parkinsonian patients may affect and participate in the evolution of the disease.

These notes indicate that the unanswered and debated questions of PD therapy (type and sequence of drugs, dosage, and when to start treatment) are intimately linked to the lack of a complete biological characterization of the disease, stressing the importance of both basic neurochemical investigations and careful analysis of the history of the disease before and after treatment. In particular, early or late levodopa treatment remains a controversial argument (40,41): various authors studying different parameters have reached opposite theoretical conclusions on timing for levodopa therapy. The results reported in the present paper are intended to represent a contribution along this line.

PATIENTS AND METHODS

The present study considers subjects examined between 1978 and 1986: they were divided into two groups on the basis of duration of disease before the beginning of levodopa therapy. During the 8 years of study, 47 subjects (28 males and 19 females) were admitted to group A (symptoms for less than 2 years before levodopa was added) and 56 subjects (34 males and 21 females) were admitted to group B (symptoms for more than 2 years and less than 5 years before levodopa treatment was started). All patients had idiopathic Parkinson's disease; the few early misdiagnosed subjects were detected during the time course and excluded from the study. Following Markham (42), we thought it was virtually impossible to form an unbiased group of patients with disease duration of more than 5 years who had never received levodopa.

Exclusion criteria were (a) nonresponders to therapy in the first year of treatment; (b) subjects in the V stage of the Hoehn and Yahr scale at the beginning of the treatment; (c) subjects with a Mini Mental State score below 24 on admission, indicating significant cognitive impairment; and (d) subjects with loss of self-sufficiency at the beginning of the treatment.

All subjects underwent a neurological evaluation and an interview almost twice a year. The following variables were assessed: (a) motor impairment, determined according to Hoehn and Yahr criteria (43); motor decline was defined as the progression of the disease from the starting stage to the following one; (b) response variations to levodopa, comprehensive of on–off and wearing-off phenomena, early morning akinesia, and of complex, resistant fluctuations; they were recorded after clinical observation by two different neurologists; (c) dyskinesias, detected according to the AIMs scale; (d) cognitive impairment, tested using the Mini Mental State by Folstein (44); and (e) activity of daily living (ADL), recorded according to the index worked out by Katz (45); patients were classified as independent if they could independently perform all ADLs.

According to the indicated criteria, it was possible to obtain sample groups sufficiently numerous to perform adequate statistical analysis and sufficiently homogeneous in their baseline profile to be comparable without unrecognized biases. Even if these groups are not representative of the entire situation usually encountered in general practice, they allow us to evaluate the effects of different predopa disease duration on subsequent clinical course of the disease.

During the observation period, a major effort was made to keep the daily dosage of levodopa constant and at the minimal therapeutic level to obtain relief of symptoms. Most patients' dosages were adjusted up or down every few months. Most patients received other antiparkinsonian drugs: anticholinergic drugs, dopamine agonists, such as bromocriptine or lisuride, and monoamine oxidase (MAO) B inhibitors in recent years. These antiparkinsonian drugs were almost equally distributed in the two groups; anticholinergics were withdrawn on starting levodopa treatment.

The appearance of impairment in one of the parameters under study was considered as an end point and the interval between the beginning of therapy and the occurrence of each end point was determined.

For both groups, we computed a cumulative survival curve from these intervals, according to the Kaplan and Meier method (46). The equality of the distributions of the end points for the two groups was tested with the Mantel–Cox test statistic.

RESULTS AND DISCUSSION

Table 1 shows descriptive characteristics of the two groups; it is notable that there are not significant differences with respect to mean age at onset

TABLE 1. *Descriptive statistics of the groups*

	Group A	Group B
Sample size	47	56
Males/females	28/19	35/21
Mean age at onset (years)	55.6 ± 3.3	54.5 ± 3.8
Mean age at beginning dopa treatment (years)	56.5 ± 3.3	57.9 ± 4.0
Mean duration predopa (years)	0.9 ± 0.5	3.4 ± 0.7*
Mean daily dose of L-dopa (mg)		
At the beginning	367	583
After 1 year	412	628
After 4 years	633	864
After 8 years	871	903

All patients took levodopa in combination with a decarboxylase inhibitor.
* $p < 0.05$.

of symptoms and mean age at the beginning of dopa treatment. Analysis of variance showed that duration of the disease before levodopa therapy—the characteristic defining the groups—was significantly different, as expected.

Motor Decline

Motor decline is represented in Fig. 1; the two groups did not differ in any of the year intervals of the study, i.e., the progression of the disease had the same speed regardless of the years of pre-dopa therapy. These data are in partial agreement with the findings by Markham (42,47) and suggest that duration of disease is the determinant factor governing motor decline in PD patients. Markham found a significant difference between groups with different length of pre-dopa illness, but this difference was present since the beginning of the follow-up and then curves increased in a parallel way. Our definition of motor decline is different and allows us to distinguish eventual differences in the temporal range of effectiveness of levodopa therapy in the

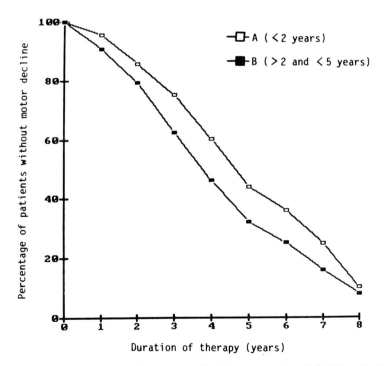

FIG. 1. Two separate curves for the groups with different duration of Parkinson's disease prior to levodopa showing the percentage of patients without motor decline in relation to duration of therapy (years). There are no significant differences in any of the year intervals considered between the two groups.

two groups, which is, however, not detectable. de Jong et al. (48), on the contrary, presented data on motor decline, dividing patients into two groups based on less or more than 5 years of duration of symptoms before levodopa. They did not comment on the data, which, however, clearly show a significant difference in mean Hohen and Yahr stage at the beginning of the treatment that was lost at the end of the follow-up, as if levodopa effectiveness was significantly longer in the group that began treatment later. From our data, levodopa seems able to relieve symptoms for the same span of time in the two groups; so in our opinion, other parameters must be taken into account before deciding on early or later treatment.

Response Variations to Levodopa

A great variety of response variations are known although the classification has yet to be firmly established. In untreated disease, they take the form of freezing and paradoxical akinesis (41,51); after the introduction of levodopa, other types appear, i.e., early morning akinesia and other "off" periods, on–off phenomena, wearing-off, and more complex and resistant fluctuations (52–55). Some symptoms such as freezing, more related to the underlying disease, have not been considered further (47,54). The two principal response fluctuations are the wearing-off, characterized by a progressive shortening of the levodopa effect, and the on–off phenomenon where sudden unpredictable shifts between "on" and "off" period may be seen. They increase in frequency and severity with progression of the disease and duration of therapy and these adverse reactions may predominate and become intolerable (56). Several hypotheses try to explain these paradoxical side effects during long-term treatment, involving peripheral and central pharmacokinetic factors as well as pharmacodynamic mechanisms with the development of supersensitivity in both pre- and postsynaptic components (51,57–59). However, the pathogenesis remains uncertain because of the close relationship between disease duration and levodopa treatment duration. On the whole, all of these hypotheses are based on two opposite theories: (a) PD is a progressive disease and levodopa cannot stop it; so illness length may explain the deterioration in efficacy of levodopa (49,53); and (b) management problems are caused by the prolonged administration of levodopa itself (50,60,61).

Our data support the latter hypothesis (Fig. 2): in fact, we found a progressive decrease of the percentage of patients without response variations that correlated with duration of therapy; at the end of the study, 80% of the subjects had response variations, in accordance with other studies (51). Moreover, there was a significant difference between the two groups from the third to the fifth year of therapy, with group B showing less response variations. So disease duration cannot be considered to be involved in response variations.

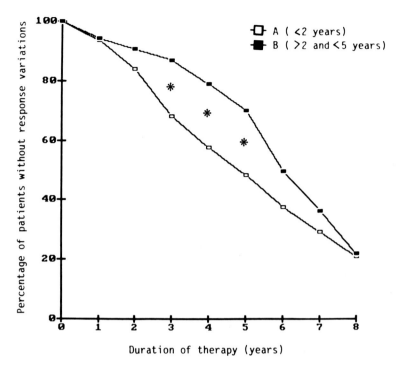

FIG. 2. Two separate curves for the groups with different duration of Parkinson's disease prior to levodopa showing the percentage of patients without response variations to levodopa in relation to duration of therapy (years). There is a significant difference from the third to the fifth year, with group B showing less percentage of patients with response variations.

These data agree and reinforce a previous study (48) where a trend of lower percentage of response variation in patients who began levodopa substitution later was seen. Age at onset of the disease, its duration and severity, and predominant symptoms were not related in this study to the development of fluctuations. Our cumulative curve also shows that the percentage of subjects with response variations is relatively low during the first 3 years of treatment; there is a decrease from the fourth to the sixth year of treatment and then a trend toward a relative stabilization seems to be detectable.

The setting out of the present study does not allow us to take into account and analyze the hypothesized different pathogenetic aspects of the wearing-off and the on–off phenomenon; however, recent studies also suggest that their pathophysiological mechanisms may be different: the former seems to arise from the progressive loss of dopaminergic neurons as a consequence of natural disease progression, thus resulting in a diminished ability to buffer variations in cerebral levodopa availability (57,62).

The on–off phenomenon, on the other hand, appears to require additional postsynaptic changes at the receptor level possibly occurring in response to the chronic nonphysiological fluctuations in synaptic dopamine due to long-term phasic administration of dopaminomimetic therapy (57,62); other studies, however, showed that D_2 receptor density remains constant in treated PD (63).

Hyperkinesias

Dyskinesias can be divided with respect to the interval between the administration of levodopa and their appearance (end-of-dose dyskinesias, peak-dose dyskinesias, and diphasic dyskinesias); even if underlying mechanisms may be different, our patients were not subgrouped due to our aim of studying side effects as a whole. According to Rajput (64) and Markham (47), dystonic reactions were summed to dyskinesias: they were seen in the morning as early morning dystonia (65) and during end-of-dose deterioration and accounted for almost 15–20% of all dyskinesias, without a significant difference between the two groups. Various studies showed that the percentage of subjects with hyperkinesias was related to duration of therapy (61,64,66), even though other studies found no correlation (47,49,50). Our data (Fig. 3) confirmed the occurrence of an increasing prevalence of hyperkinesias during time course; moreover, the percentage of patients with hyperkinesias was not significantly different between the two groups; it may be argued that the increase is independent from disease duration before levodopa, as suggested by some authors (66). Duration of treatment is the major cause of hyperkinesias. Decrease is advanced to the second year from the beginning of levodopa treatment (64,67,68). Dystonias tended to appear later during the follow-up than choreoathetoid movements and accounted for the strong decline of the corresponding survival curve in the advanced years.

It has also been suggested that the mean age at onset of the disease may play a role in the appearance of hyperkinesias, independently from disease duration and mean daily dose of levodopa; in fact, the percentage of subjects developing hyperkinesias seems to be significantly higher in patients whose Parkinson's disease appeared before the age of 50 years (50,66). Our patients, whose mean age at onset was 55.6 ± 3.3 years (SD) for group A and 54.5 ± 3.8 years for group B, and with a very low number of subjects suffering from juvenile PD, could not allow us to discuss this interesting aspect; however, other studies did not confirm the effect of age at onset on the occurrence of response variations (48).

Disability

Figure 4 shows the cumulative curve for the appearance of disability. It is similar to the previous one, but at the third and fourth year intervals,

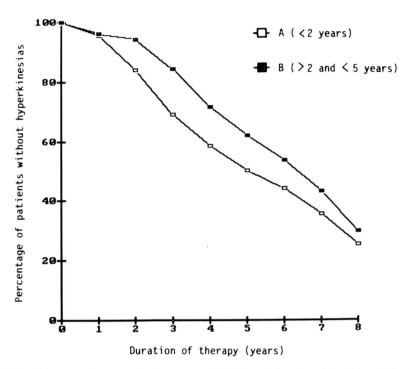

FIG. 3. Two separate curves for the groups with different duration of Parkinson's disease prior to levodopa showing the percentage of patients without hyperkinesias in relation to duration of therapy (years). Groups A and B do not differ in any of the year intervals considered.

group A shows a significantly lower percentage of patients with disability than group B. During the subsequent period, this difference in disability score between the two groups was not apparent. These data agree with previous studies where groups differing in duration of disease differed in disability even when the duration of therapy was held constant (42,47,49). However, in these studies, the differences observed in disability were preserved during the entire follow-up period, until the sixth year of levodopa therapy, while in our study this difference vanished after 4 years. Other studies found that disability scores were correlated with duration of the therapy, while duration of the disease and age of onset did not correlate (50).

So it may be argued that in the first years, after the beginning of levodopa therapy, disability mainly depends on the illness length and consequently on the progression of the disease, while in the following period other factors gain importance; probably, the appearance of important side effects due to levodopa—which predominate in group A—is responsible for the increasing degree of disability in group A, which reaches the same levels of group B.

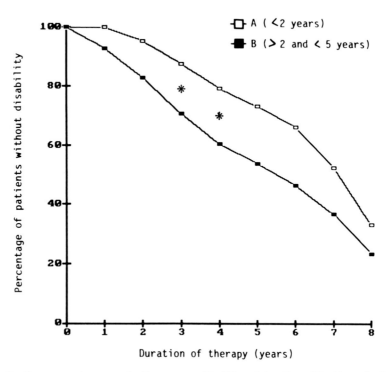

FIG. 4. Two separate curves for the groups with different duration of Parkinson's disease prior to levodopa showing the percentage of patients without disability in activity of daily living in relation to duration of therapy (years). There is a significant difference at the third and fourth year intervals, with group A showing lower percentage of patients with disability than group B.

Therefore, critical determinants for disability are both duration of disease and duration of therapy.

Cognitive Impairment

Various studies during the 1970s underlined the presence in PD both of specific cognitive impairments—such as disorders in visuospatial and motor planning functions or selective memory disturbances (69,70)—and of global intellectual impairment, more common than in age-related controls (70–73). The former deficits seem to signal the appearance of the latter (74). Recent studies differentiated between bradyphrenia and dementia, questioning if they are independent (75) or correlated (76–78). Some authors associated bradyphrenia with the involvement of norepinephrine metabolism (78,79); others suggested it was the specific mental equivalent of bradykinesia (80) and related it to dysfunction in basal ganglia (78,81–83) or to the involvement of the mesolimbic–cortical pathway (75,84–86). Both basal ganglia (81,82,87) and mesolimbic–cortical (86,88) pathways have dopaminergic projections to the frontal lobe, where dopamine deficiency has been found (89).

It is still not known whether dementia is an integral part of the disease (90–92) or whether it is due to concomitant Alzheimer's disease (93,94) without correlation with decreased regional cerebral blood flow (95), although it seems to be associated with different patterns of electrophysiological recordings (96,97). Fluctuations in motor function are associated with only mild changes in cognitive performance during the "off" phases (above all, memory and perseveration) (98–100). The neuropathology of global cognitive impairment showed a correlation with severe neuronal cholinergic loss (101,102) in the nucleus basalis of Meynert (91,103–105) and in the substantia innominata (84,106) with/without the coexistence of Alzheimer-type lesions in the cerebral cortex and hippocampus (92,102,107). Recent studies, however, suggest that estimates of true dementia have been inflated by misdiagnosis: the real percentage should be 15–20% (108–110).

In the present study, the cumulative curve for cognitive impairment shows that in group A the prevalence of cognitive impairment increased from 2.5% after 1 year to 33% after 8 years; in group B, it increased from 2 to 35% (Fig. 5). The two curves are flattened and there is only a trend to a progressive increase during years that can probably be explained by the in-

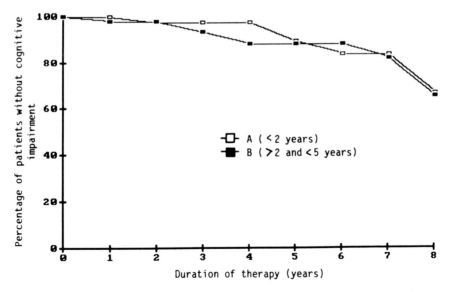

FIG. 5. Two separate curves for the groups with different duration of Parkinson's disease prior to levodopa showing the percentage of patients without cognitive impairment in relation to duration of therapy (years). There are no significant differences between groups A and B.

creasing age of the subjects (64,66). This lack of relation between cognitive impairment and length of illness has been repetitively detected (64,66,72). Data are not in contrast with previous findings (42) underlying major cognitive impairment in the group with longer duration of symptoms before levodopa, because in these studies the difference in cognitive impairment appeared from the beginning of the follow-up and was maintained during its course, with the curves rising in parallel. The cognitively impaired patients were excluded from the present study; thus, the possible, initial difference between the two groups was eliminated.

CONCLUSIONS

Timing of levodopa therapy in PD is still a main topic of discussion (40,41). We can summarize our results as follows: Cognitive impairment in PD seems to be independent both from illness length and number of years of levodopa. Response variations are dependent only on duration of the treatment; 3–4 years of therapy represent a critical period for the appearance of these symptoms. Hyperkinesias are also dependent only on duration of the treatment, although their appearance is more precocious in comparison with response variations. Motor decline is related to illness length and independent of treatment. Disability is related both to illness length (particularly in the first years) and with duration of levodopa treatment. These data may be interpreted as represented in Fig. 6.

In the present study, we chose not to consider life expectancy for various reasons: at first, mortality is not a direct consequence of PD, so that it would

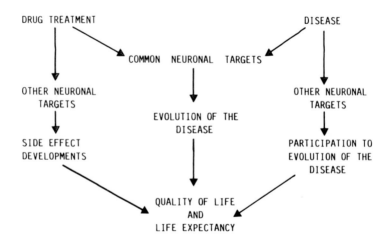

FIG. 6. Outline of the relationship between drug treatment and disease and of its impact on the quality of life and life expectancy.

be necessary to distinguish between parkinsonian-related and non-parkinsonian-related causes of death (56,67), but there is no general agreement on which causes of death can be related to the first or to the second category. Moreover, causes of death, as listed in death certificates, are known to be inaccurate (111). Several reports suggest that levodopa therapy substantially improves the life expectancy in PD in comparison with the predopa period (43,61,112,113); other studies also indicate that early levodopa treatment offers a more favorable prognosis, with less mortality on a long-term than later treatment (47,111,114). Recent observations, however, pointed out the need for more critical analysis on these optimistic interpretations, indicating that the favorable outcome in patients treated with levodopa can be attributed to a bias resulting from selection of healthier patients for treatment (67,115). Lastly, the present study was not broad and long enough to allow statistical manipulation of data from this point of view.

Markham and Diamond asserted that, despite the profoundly divergent theoretical assumptions, "those physicians with considerable familiarity in treating PD show surprisingly little disagreement on when to start levodopa treatment in individual cases" (42). We agree with this statement and we believe that, if possible, levodopa treatment should be delayed over the first 2 years after the appearance of clinical symptoms so as to reserve the beneficial effects of the drug for the late stages and avoid as long as possible its disabling side effects (48,56,64,116,117). However, if we consider the natural history of the disease, 2 years after symptom onset can still be considered as an early phase for starting levodopa treatment.

REFERENCES

1. Bartler, A., and Rosengren E. (1959): *Experientia*, 15:10–11.
2. Carlsson, A. (1959): *Pharmacol. Rev.*, 11:490–495.
3. Hornykiewicz, O. (1966): In: *Biochemistry and Pharmacology of the Basal Ganglia*, edited by E. Costa, L. J. Coté, and M. D. Yahr, New York, Raven Press, pp. 171–185.
4. Birkmayer, W., and Hornykiewicz, O., eds. (1966): *Advances in Parkinsonism; Biochemistry, Physiology, Treatment*, 5th International Symposium on Parkinson's disease, Vienna, Basel, Roche.
5. Hoekfelt, T., Johansson, O., Ljungdahl, A., Lundberg, J. M., and Schultzberg, M. (1980): *Nature (Lond.)*, 284:515–521.
6. Snyder, S. H. (1984): *Science*, 224:22–31.
7. Govoni, S., Missale, C., Arminio, M., and Trabucchi, M. (1984): In: *New Research Strategies in Biological Psychiatry*, edited by D. Kemali, P. V. Horozon, and G. Toffano, London, J. Libbey, pp. 54–57.
8. Diamond, B. I., and Borrison, E. (1978): *Neurology*, 28:1085–1088.
9. Nemeroff, C. B., and Cain, S. T. (1985): *Trends Pharmacol. Sci.*, 6:201–205.
10. Fuxe, K., Andersson, K., Locatelli, V., et al. (1980): *Eur. J. Pharmacol.*, 67:329–331.
11. Cheramy, A., Nieguillon, A., Michelot, R., and Glowinski, J. (1977): *Neurosci. Lett.*, 4:105–109.
12. Beal, M. F., and Martin, J. B. (1984): *Neurosci. Lett.*, 44:271–276.
13. Hokfelt, T., Rehefeld, J. F., and Skirboll, L. (1980): *Nature (Lond.)*, 285:476–478.
14. Beal, M. F., and Martin, J. B. (1986): *Ann. Neurol.*, 20:547–565.

15. Tang, F., Costa, E., and Schwartz, J. (1983): *Proc. Natl. Acad. Sci. U.S.A.*, 80:3841–3844.
16. Hong, J. S., Yang, H. Y. T., Costa, E. (1978): *Neuropharmacology*, 17:83–85.
17. Pasinetti, G., Govoni, S., Di Giovine, S., Spano, P. F., and Trabucchi, M. (1984): *Brain Res.*, 293:364–367.
18. Govoni, S., Hong, J. S., Yang, H. Y. T., and Costa, E. (1980): *J. Pharmacol. Exp. Ther.*, 215:413–417.
19. Missale, C., Castelletti, L., Govoni, S., Spano, P. F., Trabucchi, M., and Hanbauer, I. (1985): *J. Neurochem.*, 45:51–56.
20. Govoni, S., Lucchi, L., Missale, C., Memo, L., Spano, P. F., and Trabucchi, M. (1986): *Brain Res.*, 381:138–142.
21. Govoni, S., Memo, M., Spano, P. F., and Trabucchi, M. (1979): *Toxicology*, 12:343–349.
22. Seeman, P. (1980): *Pharmacol. Rev.*, 32:229–313.
23. Spano, P. F., Carboni, E., Garan, L., Memo, L., Govoni, S., and Trabucchi, M. (1982): In: *Receptors as Supramolecular Entities*, edited by G. Biggio et al., Oxford, Pergamon Press, pp. 131–138.
24. Staff, J. C., and Kebabian, J. W. (1981): *Nature (Lond.)*, 294:366–368.
25. Litosch, L. (1987): *Life Sci.*, 41:251–258.
26. Schiamm, M., and Selinger, Z. (1984): *Science*, 275:1350–1356.
27. Worley, P. F., Barban, J. M., and Snyder, S. H. (1987) *Ann. Neurol.*, 21:217–229.
28. Nestler, E. J., Waalas, S. I., and Greengard, P. (1984): *Science*, 225:1357–1364.
29. Hugamir, R. L., and Greengard, P. (1987): *Trends Pharmacol. Sci.*, 8;472–477.
30. Govoni, S., and Battaini, F., eds. (1987): *Modification of Cell to Cell Signals, During Normal and Pathological Aging*, NATO Asi Series on Cell Biology, Vol. 9, Heidelberg, Springer-Verlag, p. 297.
31. Pradham, S. N. (1980): *Life Sci.*, 26:1643–1656.
32. Finch, C. E. (1973): *Brain Res.*, 52:261–276.
33. Jonec, V., and Finch, C. E. (1975): *Brain Res.*, 91:197–215.
34. Missale, C., Govoni, S., Pasinetti, G., et al. (1987): *J. Gerontol.*, 41:134–136.
35. Govoni, S., Leddo, P., Spano, P. F., and Trabucchi, M. (1977): *Brain Res.*, 138:565–570.
36. Memo, L., Lucchi, L., Spano, P. F., and Trabucchi, M. (1980): *Brain Res.*, 202:488–492.
37. Govoni, S., Rivz, R. A., Battaini, F., Spano, P. F., and Trabucchi, M. (1986): In: *Neuroendocrine System and Aging*, edited by P. Vezzadini et al., Eurage Series Vol. 8, Paris, pp. 147–152.
38. Henry, J. M., and Roth, G. S. (1986): *J. Gerontol.*, 41:129–135.
39. Severson, J. A., Marcusson, J., Winblad, B., and Finch, C. E. (1982): *J. Neurochem.*, 39:1623–1631.
40. Hachinski, V. (1986): *Arch. Neurol.*, 43:407.
41. Duvoisin, R. C. (1987): *Ann. Neurol.*, 22:2–3.
42. Markham, C. H., and Diamond, S. G. (1986): *Arch. Neurol.*, 43:405–407.
43. Hoehn, M. M., and Yahr, M. D. (1967): *Neurology*, 17:427–442.
44. Folstein, H. F., Folstein, S. S., and McHugh, P. R. (1975): *J. Psychiatr. Res.*, 12:189–198.
45. Katz, S., and Ford, A. B. (1963): *J.A.M.A.*, 185:914–919.
46. Kaplan, E. R., and Meier, P. (1958): *J. Am. Stat. Assoc.*, 53:451–481.
47. Markham, C. H., and Diamond, S. G. (1986): *Ann. Neurol.*, 19:365–372.
48. de Jong, G. J., Meerwaldt, J. D., and Schmitz, P. I. M. (1987): *Ann. Neurol.*, 22:4–7.
49. Markham, C. H., and Diamond, S. G. (1981): *Neurology*, 31:125–131.
50. Lesser, P. R., Fahn, S., Snider, S. R., Cote, L. J., Isgreen, W. P., and Barrett, R. E. (1979): *Neurology*, 29:1253–1260.
51. de Jong, G. J., and Meerwaldt, J. D. (1984): *Neurology*, 34:1507–1509.
52. Marsden, C. D., and Parked, J. D. (1976): *Lancet*, 1:292–296.
53. Marsden, C. D., and Parkes, J. D. (1977): *Lancet*, 1:345–349.
54. Marsden, C. D., Parkes, J. D., and Quinn, N. (1982): In: *Movements Disorders*, edited by C. D. Marsden and S. Fahn, London, Butterworths, pp. 96–122.
55. Rinne, U. K. (1981): *J. Neural Transm.*, 51:161–174.
56. Melamed, E. (1986): *Arch. Neurol.*, 43:402–404.
57. Fabbrini, G., Juncos, J., Mouradian, M. M., Serrati, C., and Chase, T. N. (1987): *Ann. Neurol.*, 21:370–376.

58. Nutt, J. G., and Woodward, W. R. (1986): *Neurology*, 36:739–744.
59. Nutt, J. G. (1987): *Ann. Neurol.*, 22:535–540.
60. Fahn, S., and Calne, D. B. (1978): *Neurology*, 28:5–7.
61. Sweet, R. D., and McDowell, F. H. (1975): *Ann. Intern. Med.*, 83:456–463.
62. Mouradian, M. M., Juncos, J. L., Fabbrini, G., and Chase, T. N. (1987): *Ann. Neurol.*, 22:475–479.
63. Guttman, M., Seeman, P., Reynolds, G. P., Riederer, P., Jellinger, K., and Tourtelotte, W. W. (1986): *Ann. Neurol.*, 19:487–492.
64. Rajput, A. H., Stern, W., and Laverty, W. H. (1984): *Neurology*, 34:991–996.
65. Melamed, E. (1979): *Arch. Neurol.*, 36:308–310.
66. Caraceni, T. A., Giovannini, P., Girotti, F., Scigliano, G., Soliveri, P., and Geminiani, G. (1987): In: *Atti del II corso di aggiornamento sul morbo di Parkinson e malattie extrapiramidali*, edited by G. Nappi and T. Caraceni, Pavia, EMI, pp. 345–362.
67. Barbeau, A. (1976): *Arch. Neurol.*, 33:333–338.
68. Calne, D. B. (1983): *Can. J. Neurol. Sci.*, 10:11–15.
69. Matthews, C. G., and Haaland, K. Y. (1979): *Neurology*, 29:951–956.
70. Liebermann, A., and Dziatolowkski, M. (1979): *Ann. Neurol.*, 6:355–358.
71. Loranger, A. W., and Goodel, H. (1972): *Brain*, 95:405–412.
72. Rajput, K. H., and Offord, K. (1984): In: *Advances in Neurology*, Vol. 40, edited by R. G. Hassler and J. F. Christ, New York, Raven Press, pp. 229–234.
73. Rajput, A. H., Offord, K. P., Beard, C. M., and Kurland, L. T. (1987): *Neurology*, 37:226–232.
74. Pirozzolo, F. J., and Hausch, E. C. (1982): *Brain Cogn.*, 1:71–83.
75. Scatton, B., Javoiy-Agid, F., and Agid, Y. (1984): *Neurology*, 34:265–266.
76. Piccirilli, M., Piccinin, G. L., and Agostini, L. (1984): *Neurology*, 34:265.
77. Pillon, B., and Dubois, B. (1986): *Neurology*, 36:1179–1185.
78. Mayeux, R., and Stern, Y. (1987): *Neurology*, 37:1130–1134.
79. Cash, R., and Dennis, T. (1987): *Neurology*, 37:42–46.
80. Mortimer, J. A., Pirozzolo, F. J., Hausch, E. C., and Webster, D. D. (1982): *Neurology*, 32:133–137.
81. Taylor, A. E., Saint-Cyr, J. A., Lang, A. E., and Kenny, F. T. (1986): *Brain*, 109:279–282.
82. Taylor, A. E., Saint-Cyr, J. A., and Lang, A. E. (1986): *Brain*, 109:845–883.
83. Rafal, R. D., Posner, M. I., Walker, J. A., and Friedrich, F. J. (1984): *Brain*, 107:1083–1094.
84. Agid, N., Ruberg, M., Dubois, B., and Javoy-Agid, F. (1984): In: *Advances in Neurology*, Vol. 40, edited by R. G. Hassler and J. F. Christ, New York, Raven Press, pp. 211–218.
85. Lees, A. J., and Smith, E. (1983): *Brain*, 106:255–270.
86. Torack, R. M., and Morris, J. C. (1986): *Arch. Neurol.*, 43:1074–1078.
87. Price, K. S., and Farley, I. J. (1978): *Adv. Biochem. Psychopharmacol.*, 19:283–300.
88. Javoid-Agid, F. (1981): *J. Neurochem.*, 36:2101–2105.
89. Scatton, B., Rouquier, R., Javoy-Agid, F., and Agid, Y. (1982): *Neurology*, 32:1039–1040.
90. Rinne, U. K., and Laakso, K. (1985): In: *Normal Aging, Alzheimer Disease and Senile Dementia*, edited by C. G. Gottfries, Brussels, Editions de l'Université, pp. 135–146.
91. Chui, H. C., Mortimer, J. A., Slager, U., Zarow, C., Bondareff, W., and Webster, D. D. (1986): *Arch. Neurol.*, 43:991–995.
92. Jellinger, R. K. (1987): *Arch. Neurol.*, 44:190–191.
93. Hakim, A. M., and Mathieson, G. (1979): *Neurology*, 29:1209–1214.
94. Boller, F., and Mizutani, T. (1980): *Ann. Neurol.*, 7:329–335.
95. Globus, M., Mildworf, B., and Melamed, E. (1985): *Neurology*, 35:1135–1139.
96. Hausch, E. K., Syndulko, K., Cohen, S. N., Goldberg, E. I., Potvin, A. P., and Tourtelotte, W. W. (1982): *Ann. Neurol.*, 11:599–607.
97. Goodin, D. S., and Aminoff, M. J. (1987): *Ann. Neurol.*, 21:90–94.
98. Delis, D. D., Direnfeld, L., Alexander, M. P., and Kaplan, E. (1982): *Neurology*, 32:1049–1052.
99. Brown, R. C., Marsden, C. D., Quinn, N., and Nyke, M. A. (1984): *J. Neurol. Neurosurg. Psychiatry*, 47:454–465.
100. Huber, S. J., Shulman, H. G., Paulson, G. W., and Shuttleworth, E. C. (1987): *Neurology*, 37:1371–1375.

101. Ruberg, M., Ploska, A., and Javoy-Agid, F. (1982): *Brain Res.*, 28:217–22.
102. Gaspar, P., and Grey, F. (1984): *Acta Neuropathol.*, 64:43–52.
103. Candy, J. M., Perry, R. M., Perry, E. K., et al. (1983): *J. Neurol. Sci.*, 59:277–289.
104. Perry, E. K., and Curtis, M. (1985): *J. Neurol. Neurosurg. Psychiatry*, 48:413–421.
105. Xuereb, J. H., Tomlinson, B. E., Perry, R. M., Perry, E. K., Fairbairn, A., and Blessed, G. (1987): In: *Atti del II Corso di Aggiornamento sul Morbo di Parkinson e Malattie Extrapiramidali*, edited by G. Nappi and T. Caraceni, Pavia, EMI, pp. 47–56.
106. Whitehouse, P. J., Hedreen, J. C., White, C. L., III, and Price, D. L. (1983): *Ann. Neurol.*, 13:243–248.
107. Hornykiewicz, O., and Kish, S. J. (1984): *Can. J. Neurol. Sci.*, 11(suppl.):185–190.
108. Brown, R. G., and Marsden, C. D. (1984): *Lancet*, 2:1262–1265.
109. Lees, A. J. (1985): *Lancet*, 1:43–44.
110. Taylor, A., Saint-Cyr, J. A., and Lang, A. E. (1985): *Lancet*, 1:1037.
111. Diamond, S. G., Markham, C. H., Hoehn, M. M., McDowell, F. H., and Muenter, M. D. (1987): *Ann. Neurol.*, 22:8–12.
112. Martilla, R. J., Rinne, U. K., Sietola, T., and Sonninen, V. (1977): *J. Neurol.*, 216:147–153.
113. Hoehn, M. M. (1983): *J. Neural Transm.*, 19(suppl.):253–264.
114. Hoehn, M. M. (1985): *Acta Neurol. Scand.*, 71:97–106.
115. Rajput, A. H., Offord, K. P., Beard, C. M., and Kurland, L. T. (1984): *Ann. Neurol.*, 16:278–282.
116. Battistin, L., Bracco, F., and Saladini, M. In: *Atti del I Corso di Aggiornamento sul Morbo di Parkinson e Malattie Extrapiramidali*, edited by G. Nappi and T. Caraceni, Pavia, EMI, pp. 183–193.
117. Fahn, S., and Bressman, S. B. (1984): *Can. J. Neurol. Sci.*, 11(suppl.):200–206.

Parkinsonism and Aging, edited by
Donald B. Calne et al., Raven Press, Ltd.,
New York © 1989.

New Strategies in the Treatment of Parkinson's Disease

U. K. Rinne

Department of Neurology, University of Turku, Turku, Finland

There is no doubt that today the substitution of striatal dopamine deficiency with levodopa remains the most effective treatment for Parkinson's disease (PD). However, the drug loses its efficacy with time, and many problems are associated with long-term therapy, especially fluctuations in disability (7,13,14). New therapeutic strategies are therefore needed. For this purpose, I have been studying whether dopamine agonist therapy alone, or in early combination with levodopa, might be a better long-term treatment than levodopa alone (8,9,11).

INITIATION OF DOPAMINERGIC TREATMENT

The timing of the initiation of levodopa treatment is still a controversial issue: early or late, and alone or in combination with other drugs? However, it is only now, when information has accumulated on the different responses to long-term levodopa therapy, that enough data are available to provide evidence on how to resolve the open questions, and in this way to be able to provide optimal long-term treatment for the patients. Indeed, in addition to the loss of efficacy and development of daily fluctuations in disability, the patients' survival is a further factor that also critically influences the decision on when to start levodopa therapy in Parkinson's disease.

Levodopa treatment is not believed to retard or prevent the progression of the underlying brain pathology of Parkinson's disease. However, it is well documented that levodopa therapy increases the life expectancy of parkinsonian patients by decreasing the excess mortality (1,5,14). Furthermore, follow-up studies by us (6,12) and by others (2–4) have clearly demonstrated that early initiation of levodopa therapy results in better survival than later initiation. Moreover, analyses of possible risk factors contributing to the development of fluctuations in disability showed that neither the pretreatment duration of the disease nor the disability stage of the disease was associated with the development of fluctuations in disability, thus not arguing against early treatment. Since prolonged high-dose levodopa therapy, however, seems to be a significant risk factor for the development of fluctuations (8), a better long-term treatment than levodopa alone should be adopted. Our recent studies (8–11) suggest that early combination of a dopamine agonist and a low dose of levodopa seems to provide the kind of treatment needed. With this combination treatment, it seems to be possible to initiate the dopaminergic treatment in the early stages of the disease (Hoehn and Yahr stage 1–2), and thus offer for the patients more years with a better quality of life, due to the decreased frequency of disabling fluctuations in disability.

DOPAMINE AGONIST ALONE

The dopamine agonists available for clinical trials, stimulating D_2 and D_1 or D_2 dopamine receptors alone, do seem to have significant antiparkinsonian efficacy alone in the treatment of *de novo* patients with Parkinson's disease. However, the degree of therapeutic response is only moderate, and significantly less than that achieved with levodopa. Furthermore, only a small proportion of the patients have long-term benefit during treatment with a dopamine agonist alone. Thus, after 2 years one-third, after 3 years one-fourth, and after five years only 5 to 13% of the patients had a satisfactory therapeutic response with bromocriptine, pergolide, or lisuride alone (Table 1). Although the improvement in primary parkinsonian disability during treatment with a dopamine agonist alone is not so prominent, the therapeutic response seems to be very good, and better than with levodopa with respect to the development of fluctuations in disability. Indeed, no end-of-dose failure developed and there were only a few cases with dyskinesias or randomly occurring freezing episodes during periods of 3 to 5 years of treatment (9–11).

TABLE 1. *Number of* de novo *parkinsonian patients under long-term treatment with bromocriptine, pergolide, or lisuride*

| | | Duration of treatment (years) | | | | | | | | |
| | | 1 | | 2 | | 3 | | 4 | | 5 | |
Drug	Initially, N	N	(%)	N	(%)	N	(%)	N	(%)	N	(%)
Bromocriptine	76	32	(42)	22	(29)	21	(28)	13	(17)	5	(7)
Pergolide	20	12	(60)	7	(35)	5	(25)	2	(10)	1	(5)
Lisuride	30	16	(53)	10	(33)	6	(20)	5	(17)	4	(13)

EARLY COMBINATION OF A DOPAMINE AGONIST AND LEVODOPA

Bromocriptine and Pergolide

The early addition of levodopa to the regimen of patients who showed insufficient therapeutic response to initial treatment with bromocriptine (9,11) or pergolide (10) alone resulted in a significant increase in therapeutic benefit. In these trials, the long-term tolerance of the combined treatment was significantly better than that with a dopamine agonist alone. Furthermore, during combined treatment, the daily dose of levodopa needed for optimal therapeutic response was significantly lower than when using levodopa alone; yet the improvement in parkinsonian disability was equal to that with high-dose levodopa alone, but with significantly fewer end-of-dose disturbances and dyskinesias.

Lisuride

For further clarification, a randomized, prospective trial was carried out with lisuride alone, or in early combination with levodopa, in comparison to levodopa alone, in the long-term treatment of *de novo* parkinsonian patients (10). Ninety *de novo* patients with Parkinson's disease were randomly allocated to treatment with levodopa alone, lisuride alone, or combined levodopa and lisuride. If the therapeutic response to lisuride alone was insufficient after 3 months of treatment, levodopa was added to the regimen, thus forming a second group with the early combination of lisuride and levodopa.

Initially, during the first 3 months of treatment, lisuride alone produced a significantly lower therapeutic response than levodopa alone. Furthermore, only a small proportion of the patients seems to have obtained really long-term benefit during treatment with lisuride alone. However, in these few patients with a good long-term response to lisuride, the improvement in parkinsonian disability was at the same level as in other treatment groups (Table 2).

With optimal daily doses, the early combination of levodopa and lisuride resulted in an improvement in parkinsonian disability equal to that achieved with significantly higher doses of levodopa alone. The addition of levodopa to the lisuride regimen in patients with initial insufficient therapeutic response resulted in a significant further improvement in the patients, reaching the same level as in the patients treated with levodopa alone (Table 2).

On treatment with lisuride for 3 years, there were no end-of-dose disturbances or peak-dose dyskinesias and only one patient had early-morning dystonia and random freezing episodes (Table 3). Moreover, in both groups with an early combination of lisuride and levodopa, there were significantly

TABLE 2. *Dosage (mg) and improvement in parkinsonian disability (PD) during 3 years of treatment of parkinsonian patients with levodopa, lisuride, or levodopa in combination with lisuride*

Variable	Levodopa (N = 26)	Lisuride (N = 6)	Levodopa + lisuride (N = 28)	Lisuride + levodopa (N = 19)
Dosage (mg)				
Levodopa	700 ± 44	—	459 ± 30*	611 ± 42
Lisuride	—	1.2 ± 0.2	1.1 ± 0.2	0.8 ± 0.1
Improvement of PD (%)	38 ± 3	40 ± 16	47 ± 3	34 ± 3

* $p < 0.001$ as compared to levodopa alone or lisuride alone, Student's t test.

fewer end-of-dose disturbances and dyskinesias than with high-dose levodopa alone (Table 3).

CONCLUSIONS

The increased survival pattern observed with levodopa indicates the early initiation of levodopa treatment (at Hoehn and Yahr stages 1–2).

Although prolonged high-dose levodopa therapy seems to be a significant

TABLE 3. *Occurrence of fluctuations in disability during long-term treatment of parkinsonian patients with levodopa, lisuride, or levodopa in combination with lisuride for 3 years*

Disability	Levodopa (N = 26) N	(%)	Lisuride (N = 6) N	(%)	Levodopa + lisuride (N = 28) N	(%)	Lisuride + levodopa (N = 19) N	(%)
1. End-of-dose failure	11	(42)	0	(0)	2**	(7)	4	(21)
2. Early-morning akinesia	8	(31)	0	(0)	1**	(4)	1*	(5)
3. Nocturnal akinesia	3	(12)	0	(0)	1	(4)	0	(0)
4. Freezing episodes, dose-related	1	(4)	0	(0)	1	(4)	0	(0)
5. Freezing episodes, random	2	(8)	1	(17)	1	(4)	2	(11)
6. Early-morning dystonia	5	(19)	1	(17)	1	(4)	1	(5)
7. Daily dystonia	8	(31)	0	(0)	3	(11)	1*	(5)
8. Peak-dose dyskinesia	16	(62)	0**	(0)	2***	(7)	4*	(21)

* $p < 0.05$, ** $p < 0.01$, *** $p < 0.001$ as compared to levodopa, Mantel–Haenszel test.

risk factor for the development of fluctuations in disability, a better long-term treatment than levodopa alone should be used.

Only a small proportion of parkinsonian patients seems to have long-term benefit and tolerance during treatment with a dopamine agonist alone.

Dopamine agonists alone, therefore, do not seem to be useful antiparkinsonian agents as the primary treatment for the majority of patients, despite the fact that they produce less fluctuations in disability.

Long-term follow-up showed that the early combination of low, submaximal doses of levodopa and a dopamine agonist such as bromocriptine, pergolide, or lisuride seems not only to improve parkinsonian disability, but also to inhibit the development of fluctuations in disability, especially end-of-dose disturbances and dyskinesias.

This kind of combined treatment with a dopamine agonist and levodopa seems to offer a better long-term treatment than high-dose levodopa, presumably by maintaining the normal functioning of the striatal dopamine neurotransmission for a longer period than does levodopa alone.

It is therefore possible with this combination to initiate the dopaminergic treatment in the early stage of the disease and thus offer the patient more years with a better quality of life.

Thus, in the new treatment policy, it appears advisable that the management of parkinsonian patients should begin in the early phase of the disease, with a dopamine agonist combined with low, submaximal doses of levodopa.

Acknowledgment: This work was supported by a grant from the Medical Research Council, Academy of Finland (Project No. 09/037).

REFERENCES

1. Diamond, S. G., and Markham, Ch. H. (1976): Present mortality in Parkinson's disease: the ratio observed to expected deaths with a method to calculate expected deaths. *J. Neural Transm.*, 36:259–269.
2. Diamond, S. G., Markham, Ch. H., Hoehn, M. M., McDowell, F. H., and Muenter, M. D. (1987): Multi-center study of parkinson mortality with early versus later dopa treatment. *Ann. Neurol.*, 22:8–12.
3. Hoehn, M. M. (1985): Result of chronic levodopa therapy and its modification by bromocriptine in Parkinson's disease. *Acta Neurol. Scand.*, 71:97–106.
4. Markham, Ch. H., and Diamond, S. G. (1986): Long-term follow-up of early dopa treatment in Parkinson's disease. *Ann. Neurol.*, 19:365–372.
5. Marttila, R. J., Rinne, U. K., Siirtola, T., and Sonninen, V. (1977): Mortality of patients with Parkinson's disease treated with levodopa. *J. Neurol.*, 216:147–153.
6. Marttila, R. J., Rinne, U. K., and Sonninen, V. (1984): Levodopa in Parkinson's disease: effect on mortality. *Acta Neurol. Scand.*, 69(suppl. 98): 45–46.
7. Rinne, U. K. (1981): Treatment of Parkinson's disease: problems with a progressing disease. *J. Neural Transm.*, 51:161–174.
8. Rinne, U. K. (1983): New ergot derivatives in the treatment of Parkinson's disease. In: *Lisuride and Other Dopamine Agonists*, edited by D. B. Calne, R. Horowski, R. J. McDonald, and W. Wuttke, New York, Raven Press, pp. 431–442.
9. Rinne, U. K. (1985): Combined bromocriptine–levodopa therapy early in Parkinson's disease. *Neurology*, 35:1196–1198.

10. Rinne, U. K. (1986): Dopamine agonists as primary treatment in Parkinson's disease. In: *Advances in Neurology*, edited by M. D. Yahr and K. J. Bergmann, New York, Raven Press, pp. 519–523.
11. Rinne, U. K. (1987): Early combination of bromocriptine and levodopa in the treatment of Parkinson's disease: a 5-year follow-up. *Neurology*, 37:826–828.
12. Rinne, U. K., and Marttila, R. J. (1987): Initiation of levodopa treatment: early versus late. *Neurology*, 37(suppl. 1):271.
13. Rinne, U. K., Sonninen, V., and Siirtola, T. (1976): Long-term treatment of parkinsonism with L-dopa and decarboxylase inhibitor: a clinical and biochemical approach. In: *Advances in Parkinsonism*, edited by W. Birkmayer and O. Hornykiewicz, Basel, Editiones Roche, pp. 555–565.
14. Yahr, M. D. (1976): Evaluation of long-term therapy in Parkinson's disease: mortality and therapeutic efficacy. In: *Advances in Parkinsonism*, edited by W. Birkmayer and O. Hornykiewicz, Basel, Editiones Roche, pp. 435–443.

Parkinsonism and Aging, edited by
Donald B. Calne et al., Raven Press, Ltd.,
New York © 1989.

A Long-Term Comparative Study of Lisuride and Levodopa in Parkinson's Disease

J. M. Rabey, M. Streifler, T. Treves, and A. D. Korczyn

*Department of Neurology, Tel-Aviv Medical Center, Ichilov Hospital,
Sackler School of Medicine, Tel Aviv University, Tel Aviv, Israel*

In Parkinson's disease (PD), levodopa administration compensates initially for the deficiency of dopamine due to degeneration of the nigrostriatal dopaminergic pathway, by increasing dopamine synthesis by the surviving neurons (1). With progression of the disease, the system may be incapable of generating enough dopamine to stimulate the receptors even when levodopa is supplied (2,3). Therefore, it was assumed that drugs that bypass the degenerating nigrostriatal dopaminergic neurons and stimulate the dopamine receptors directly, would be beneficial.

Lisuride hydrogen maleate, N-(D-6 methyl-8-isoergolenyl-N'-N'-diethyl-carbamide), is a semisynthetic ergot alkaloid that was shown to be effective *in vitro* and in animal models of PD (4,5). Positive data were also reported in human trials (6–8) and encouraged us to test the drug in parkinsonian patients who have shown signs of progressive deterioration, comparing the results with those obtained in a group that has received increasing dose of levodopa. The favorable results of a 6 month clinical trial of lisuride were previously reported by our group (9), and have prompted us to continue the treatment for a period of 4 years.

PATIENTS AND METHODS

Patients

Candidates for the study were patients suffering from idiopathic parkinsonism and having been treated in the past with conventional drugs, after obtaining their formal consent. The study was conducted in an open fashion and approved by the local Helsinki committee. All of the patients had responded previously to levodopa, but later the treatment needed to be sub-

TABLE 1. *Characteristics of patients before starting in trial*

	Lisuride N = 24	Levodopa N = 20
Mean age (years)	64.7 (48–76)	66 (52–83)
Mean disease duration (years)	7.54 (5–12)	7 (2–10)
Stage (mean) (Hoehn–Yahr)	2–5	2–4
Dopa before trial (mg), mean	590 (250–750)	531 (250–750)

stantially changed because of increased motor disability with diminishing response to levodopa, marked fluctuation of symptoms, and/or dyskinesias. They had never previously received direct dopaminergic agonists. Patients with significant cardiovascular, renal, or hepatic diseases were excluded, as were patients with serious psychiatric disorders.

Upon admission, 44 ambulatory patients (24 men and 20 women) were clinically evaluated (see the following paragraph). Laboratory screening included hemogram, and tests of liver, renal, and thyroid functions. They were then randomly allocated into two groups.

(a) The lisuride group consisted at the start of 24 patients; 4 withdrew, 3 because there was no improvement after 1 month, and they suffered side effects (acroparesthesias, vertigo, and confusional episodes), and 1 because of severe dizziness with initial dose of lisuride. In the extended observation of 4 years, one patient died of bronchopneumonia after 3 years and four others abandoned the treatment because of severe dizziness (one patient) and persistent confusion (three patients) within the third year.

By the end of the study after 4 years, 15 patients were available for comparison (see Tables 1 and 2). By the beginning of the study, patients in the lisuride group were taking levodopa in a mean dose of 590 mg (range of 250–

TABLE 2. *Effects of lisuride (n = 15)*

Motor Function	Baseline	Final	Significance
Total disability score	38.7 ± 2	28.8 ± 1.8	$p < 0.005$
Bradykinesia	2.8 ± 0.2	2.06 ± 0.2	$p < 0.005$
Rigidity	7.4 ± 1.1	5.1 ± 0.9	$p < 0.005$
Tremor	4.13 ± 0.5	3.86 ± 0.6	N.S.
Gait	2.6 ± 0.3	1.8 ± 0.2	$p < 0.005$
"Off" (min) (n = 11)	212.5 ± 30	143 ± 25	$p < 0.005$
Dyskinesia (n = 10)	11.1 ± 2.2	7.56 ± 2.0	$p < 0.005$

Based on overall symptoms severity ratings (mean ± SEM) obtained from patients before and after completing 4 years of treatment; p = statistical significant; N.S. = not significant. The number in parentheses beside "off" and "dyskinesia" express the number of patients who showed the incapacity.

TABLE 3. *Effects of dopa (n = 13)*

Motor function	Baseline	Final	Significance
Total disability score	35.3 ± 4	28 ± 2.3	$p < 0.005$
Bradykinesia	2.6 ± 0.2	1.9 ± 0.3	$p < 0.005$
Rigidity	8.2 ± 0.9	5.5 ± 0.8	$p < 0.005$
Tremor	3.6 ± 0.8	3.5 ± 0.7	N.S.
Gait	2.3 ± 0.3	1.5 ± 0.3	$p < 0.005$
"Off" (min) ($n = 9$)	217.5 ± 30	180 ± 25	$p < 0.01$
Dyskinesia ($n = 11$)	7.1 ± 0.9	8.1 ± 1.0	N.S.

Based on overall symptoms severity ratings (mean ± SEM) obtained from patients before and after completing 4 years of treatment. p = statistical significance; N.S. = not significant. The number in parentheses beside "off" and "dyskinesia" express the number of patients who showed the incapacity.

750 mg). They also took other adjuvants (alone or combined), which were kept unchanged on a fixed dose during the trial: trihexyphenydil, amantadine, and amitriptyline.

Patients in the lisuride group were kept on a fixed dose of levodopa during the trial (divided into 6–8 daily doses) and were given increased doses of lisuride hydrogen maleate (Dopergin, Schering, Berlin, F.R.G.), starting with 0.1 mg t.i.d. Increments were gradually made over a period of 4 to 6 weeks until a maximal beneficial clinical response was obtained. By this time, lisuride was administered in 4–6 daily ingestions. The maximal daily dose of lisuride was 5 mg.

(b) The levodopa group included 20 patients, all of whom completed the first 6 months trial period. They were taking levodopa in a mean dose of 531 mg (range of 276.5–750 mg) + 53 mg (27.6–75 mg) carbidopa before the medication was increased. They also took other drugs: 10 took trihexyphenydil, 3 took orphenadrine, 9 took amantadine, 4 took amytriptyline, and 1 took maprotiline. Patients in this group were given increased doses of levodopa + carbidopa (Dopicar, Teva, Israel, each tablet containing 250 mg levodopa and 25 mg carbidopa). Of the 20 patients originally treated with increased doses of levodopa, two had died (MI within the second year and bronchopneumonia within the third year). Two were lost to follow-up, and in three, psychiatric disorders obliged us to reduce considerably the levodopa doses. By the end of the study after 4 years, 13 patients were available for comparison (see Tables 1 and 3).

Clinical Evaluation

The patients were graded according to a modification of the Columbia University scale, when the following parameters were examined in each patient: facial expression, seborrhea, sialorrhea, speech, tremor, rigidity, finger dexterity, successive alternating movements, foot tapping, rising from a chair, posture, postural stability, gait, and bradykinesia. Each variable was graded between 0 (normal or no impairment) to 4 (maximal disability). The maximal score (disability) was 100. Dyskinesia was evaluated on a separate scale ranging from 0 (no dyskinesia) to 4 (severe dyskinesias) and the maximal score was 28 (four limbs, trunk, face, and mouth). The amount of "off" episodes was evaluated by the patients and their relatives, and they were requested to score on different days during the "wake" hours the mobility as follows: 0—normal; 1—gait impairment; 2—no gait. A score of 2 was considered "off." The total amount of daily akinetic episodes (expressed in minutes) before and after the 4 year trial was evaluated and compared in each patient. During the build-up period, the patients were seen once weekly or more frequently if necessary. Later on, they were examined and evaluated once in 6 weeks, and later once in 2 months for 4 years. Once in 6 months we repeated the laboratory screening (CBC and SMA 12) on everyone.

RESULTS

After completing 4 years of treatment, patients on lisuride were taking the following doses: 11 patients were on a final dose of 0.4 to 1 mg daily and four patients were taking 1.2 to 2 mg daily. The mean final dose of lisuride was 1.07 mg. Patients on levodopa after 4 years of treatment were taking a mean daily dose of 625 mg (range of 187.5–750 mg, see Table 4). The side effects of lisuride were as follows: eight patients showed confusional states and agitation, which were alleviated with a diminution of the doses in four but obliged interruption of treatment in the other four. Three patients reported dizziness, three patients reported finger paresthesias, and four patients reported increased appetite with weight gain (about 5%). For statistical

TABLE 4. *Lisuride and levodopa doses within the 4 years of follow-up*

Lisuride (n = 15)	Levodopa (n = 13)
Within the first 6 months	
11 patients: 0.6–1.0 mg/day	
3 patients: 1.0–3.0 mg/day	
4 patients: 3.0–5.0 mg/day	
Mean: 1.95 mg/day	Mean: 788.4 mg/day (500–1,000)
Within the fourth year	
11 patients: 0.4–1.0 mg/day	
4 patients: 1.2–2.0 mg/day	
Mean: 1.07 mg/day	Mean: 625 mg/day (187.5–750)

TABLE 5. *Comparison of relative effects of lisuride and levodopa on motor parameters*

Motor function	Lisuride	Levodopa	Signficance
Total disability score	−9.9	−7.3	N.S.
Bradykinesia	−0.74	−0.7	N.S.
Rigidity	−2.3	−2.7	N.S.
Tremor	−0.27	−0.1	N.S.
Gait	−0.8	−0.8	N.S.
"Off" (min)	−69.5 (33%)	−27.5 (15%)	$p < 0.005$
Dyskinesia	−2.53 (23%)	−1.0 (10%)	$p < 0.005$

The effect is expressed as the difference of the mean score for each group at baseline and on completion of the trial.

analysis, we used the two-tailed *t* test, paired or unpaired, as required. There was no difference in age, sex, disease duration, grading (according to Hoehn and Yahr), or for each main motor function tested; and for "off" and dyskinesias, between the two groups, before the start of the trial (see Table 1). The evaluation of the effect of each drug on the parameters of the motor function tested (see Tables 2, 3, and 5), showed a similar positive effect of lisuride and levodopa on the total disability score, bradykinesia, rigidity, gait, and "off." Neither drug altered significantly the tremor during the trial period. Lisuride improved dyskinesia, whereas levodopa did not substantially alter this feature.

Comparison of the two groups (see Table 5) revealed that lisuride was as effective as levodopa in controlling bradykinesia, rigidity, and gait, but was more effective in treating "off" episodes (about 33% relief against 15% in the levodopa group), and dyskinesia (about 23% improvement). The laboratory screening (CBC and SMA 12) remained normal in each patient after 4 years of evaluation.

DISCUSSION

The decreased effectiveness of levodopa in parkinsonian patients, after some years of treatment, has been related mainly to disease progression, because most patients deteriorate in spite of therapy (3). The subsequent failure of levodopa to compensate for the dopamine deficiency may be due to the fact that the remaining neurons are unable to synthesize a sufficient amount of dopamine. The benefit that these patients may derive from direct dopamine agonists, which bypass the degenerating presynaptic neurons and directly stimulate the postsynaptic dopamine receptors, supports this hypothesis.

The high dopaminomimetic activity of lisuride has been confirmed by biochemical studies in reserpinized rats (10,11). In various binding assays, lisuride was the most potent dopamine agonist among the compounds tested and its receptor affinity was clearly higher, as was the case with bromocriptine, apomorphine, and dopamine. Under *in vitro* conditions, lisuride has been shown to displace [^{3}H]spiroperidol binding at lower concentrations than haloperidol or apomorphine (12).

Lisuride is a semisynthetic ergot alkaloid, 10–20 times more potent on a milligram basis than bromocriptine. Its duration of activity is shorter than that of bromocriptine, and appears to be independent of either dopamine synthesis or dopamine stores (5).

In our study, which included patients with advanced parkinsonism, lisuride was as effective as levodopa in controlling bradykinesia, rigidity, and gait. Tremor was substantially unchanged by either medication during the trial period, but lisuride was considerably preferable for the management of "off" episodes and dyskinesias, compared to levodopa (see Table 5). This effect could be due to more prolonged and stable stimulant activation of striatal receptors by lisuride (the plasma half-life of lisuride in parkinsonian patients is 2.2 hr) (13).

In addition to its dopaminergic activity, lisuride also has a very high affinity for different types of serotonin receptors (10). Depending on the neuronal system, preferential stimulation of the pre- or postsynaptic serotonin receptors will result either in functional agonism or antagonism of the system (14). This finding may explain the weight gain observed in some of our patients. A similar observation reported also by other investigators (8) could have a significant clinical importance, since it is well known that many parkinsonian patients lose weight during the progression of the disease (15).

As was shown in our study, one of the most common side effects of lisuride was the production of confusion and/or agitative behavior, which responded to diminishing the dose of the drug. Therefore, by the end of the fourth year, the mean dose of lisuride in the patients group was about 1 mg daily, which means about one-half of the daily dose taken by the patients by the end of the first 6 months of the study (2 mg). It is important to stress the fact that lisuride at low doses was still a potent dopamine agonist after a long-term follow up, suggesting the possible potentiation of its effect after chronic administration as was found in animal studies (16). It is remarkable to point out also that this persistent dopaminergic effect observed with lisuride contrasts with the tachyphylaxis reported in the treatment of PD with bromocriptine (17,18) and pergolide (19).

In conclusion, our results suggest that combined treatment with low doses of lisuride (a selective agonist of D_2 non-adenylate cyclase linked receptors) and levodopa (which activates the D_1 cyclase linked striatal receptors) is more effective than levodopa alone, supporting the idea that the stimulation of different populations of receptors makes it possible to treat patients for a longer time with less fluctuation in the motor response, and less side effects (20).

REFERENCES

1. Agid, Y., Javo, Y. F., and Glowinski, J. (1973): Hyperactivity of remaining neurons after partial destruction of the nigrostriatal dopaminergic system in the rat. *Nature (Lond.)*, 245:150–151.
2. Hornykiewicz, O. (1974): The mechanism of action of levodopa in Parkinson's disease. *Life Sci.*, 15:1249–1259.
3. Marsden, C. D., and Parkes, J. D. (1977): Success and problems of long-term levodopa in Parkinson's disease. *Lancet*, 1:345–349.
4. Goldstein, M., Lew, J., and Engel, A. (1980): The dopaminephilic properties of ergoline derivatives. In: *Ergot Compounds and Brain Function: Neuroendocrine and Neuropsychiatric Aspects*, edited by D. Calne, M. Goldstein, A. N. Lieberman, and M. Thorner, New York, Raven Press, pp. 237–252.
5. Horowski, R., and Wachtel, H. (1976): Direct dopaminergic action of lisuride hydrogen maleate, an ergot derivative, in mice. *Eur. J. Pharmacol.*, 36:373–383.
6. Schachter, M., Sheehy, M. P., Parkes, J. D., and Marsden, C. D. (1980): Lisuride in the treatment of parkinsonism. *Acta Neurol. Scand.*, 62:382–385.
7. Gopinathan, G., Teravainen, H., Dambrosia, J. M., et al. (1981): Lisuride in parkinsonism. *Neurology*, 31:371–376.
8. Lieberman, A. N., Goldstein, M., and Neophytides, A. (1981): Lisuride in Parkinson's disease: efficacy of lisuride compared to levodopa. *Neurology*, 31:961–965.
9. Rabey, J. M., Treves, T. A., Streifler, M., and Korczyn, A. D. (1986): Comparison of efficacy of lisuride hydrogen maleate with increased doses of levodopa in Parkinsonian patients. In: *Advances in Neurology, Vol. 45, Parkinson's Disease*, edited by M. D. Yahr and K. J. Bergman, New York, Raven Press, pp. 569–572.
10. Kehr, W. (1976): Effect of lisuride and other ergot derivatives on monoaminergic mechanisms in rat brain. *Eur. J. Pharmacol.*, 41:261–273.
11. Pieri, L., Keller, H. H., Burkhard, W., and Da Prada, M. (1978): Effects of lisuride and LSD on cerebral monoamine systems and hallucinosis. *Nature (Lond.)*, 272:278–280.
12. Fujita, N., Saito, K., Yonehara, N., and Yoshida, H. (1978): Lisuride inhibits 3H-spiroperidol binding to membranes isolated from striatum. *Neuropharmacology* 17:1089–1091.
13. Burns, R. S., and Calne, D. B. (1983): Disposition of dopaminergic ergot compounds following oral administration. In: *Lisuride and Other Dopamine Agonists: Basic Mechanism and Endocrine and Neurological Effects*, edited by D. B. Calne, R. Horowski, R. J. McDonald, W. Wuttke, New York, Raven Press, pp. 153–160.
14. Da Prada, M., Bonetti, E. P., and Keller, H. H. (1977): Induction of mounting behaviour in female and male rats by lisuride. *Neurosci. Lett.*, 6:349–353.
15. Vardi, J., Oberman, Z., Streifler, M., et al. (1976): Weight loss in elderly parkinsonian patients on long-term L-dopa therapy. *J. Neurol. Sci.*, 30:33–40.
16. Horowski, R., and Wachtel, H. (1979): Pharmacological effects of lisuride in rodents mediated by dopaminergic receptors: mechanism of action and influence of chronic treatment with lisuride. In: *Dopaminergic Ergot Derivatives and Motor Function*, edited by K. Fuxe and D. B. Calne, Oxford, Pergamon Press, pp. 237–251.
17. Grimes, J. D. (1984): Bromocriptine in Parkinson's disease. Results obtained with high and low dose therapy. *Can. J. Neurol. Sci.*, 11:225–228.
18. Rascol, A., Montastruc, N. L., and Rascol, O. (1984): Should dopamine agonists be given early or late in the treatment of Parkinson's disease. *Can. J. Neurol. Sci.*, 11:229–232.
19. Lieberman, A. N., Goldstein, M., and Leibowitz, M. (1984): Long term treatment with pergolide: decreased efficacy with time. *Neurology*, 34:223–226.
20. Calne, D. B. (1983): Current views on Parkinson's disease. *Can. J. Neurol. Sci.*, 10:11–15.

Parkinsonism and Aging, edited by
Donald B. Calne et al., Raven Press, Ltd.,
New York © 1989.

Oral and Parenteral Use of Lisuride in Parkinson's Disease: Clinical Pharmacology and Implications for Therapy

R. Horowski, R. Dorow, P. Löschmann, I. Runge,
H. Wachtel, and *J. A. Obeso

*Clinical and Experimental Research Laboratories, Schering AG, Berlin/
Bergkamen, West Germany and *Department of Neurology,
University of Pamplona, Pamplona, Spain*

Lisuride is a semisynthetic ergot derivative synthesized by Zikan and Semonsky (85) that has an outstanding affinity for dopamine (DA) receptors (54,76).

As the first 8-α-aminoergoline in clinical use, it is devoid of the "classical" ergot effects on the smooth muscles of blood vessels and the uterus, but has been shown to have strong dopaminergic and prolactin-lowering properties and thus has been marketed in European countries as a prolactin-lowering drug similar to bromocriptine for the last few years. Its use in these endocrinological indications has been reviewed separately (30). The high affinity of lisuride not only to dopamine but also to 5-HT$_1$ and 5-HT$_2$ receptors is the basis for the use of lisuride in the prophylaxis of migraine (33,53).

The combination of dopaminergic effects with a functional 5-HT antagonism (due to autoreceptor stimulation in high doses) in rats induces a strong male-type mounting behavior and hypersexuality, which is independent of endogenous gonadal hormones, by lisuride (17,3,29). A similar induction of hypersexuality by high doses of lisuride has not, however, been observed in other species.

Dissimilarities and similarities with D-LSD have been used as a tool for studying mechanisms of hallucination in animals (54,84) but trained rats generalize lisuride as a DA agonist whereas D-LSD is generalized as a 5-HT partial agonist (84). D-LSD-like hallucinations have never been observed in healthy volunteers or patients except those suffering from neurological disease, where all dopaminergic drugs can induce psychotic symptoms (27).

As an ergot-derived dopamine agonist, lisuride is unique because it is

TABLE 1. *Differences between lisuride and bromocriptine*

Lisuride has a 10–100 times higher affinity for D_2 receptors than bromocriptine (76,16)

Lisuride has a stronger intrinsic activity than bromocriptine (e.g., in the induction of stereotyped behavior) (21,26)

Lisuride may have antagonistic or stabilizing effects on D_2 receptors and autoreceptors depending on their state and functional activity (22)

Lisuride is still active in restoring motor activity after complete DA depletion (by reserpine and α-methyl-*p*-tyrosine) while bromocriptine needs exogenous or endogenous DA receptor stimulation for its efficacy (26,11,87,34)

Lisuride can be used on an i.v. or s.c. basis (19)

effective at such low doses that effective concentrations of this drug can be dissolved in water and lisuride, therefore, can also be used in a parenteral, e.g., i.v. or s.c., form (19,64,48). Although both lisuride and bromocriptine lower plasma prolactin levels and can be used to treat hyperprolactinemia independent of its etiology, both drugs differ in other respects (see Table 1). The unique profile of lisuride is the reason why this drug and other 8-α-aminoergoline derivatives have become a standard for new developments. There are several reviews about its pharmacological and clinical effects (7,39,83,44,24).

From the "classical" DA agonist apomorphine, lisuride differs by its higher affinity to the DA receptor, but weaker intrinsic activity (e.g., lower emetic potency), its effects on other systems, e.g., the 5-HT-receptor, its more specific and longer-lasting prolactin-lowering effect, and its oral efficacy (31).

The effects of lisuride on D_1 receptors are less clear; in biochemical studies under *in vitro* conditions, it acts as a D_1 antagonist (i.e., it inhibits the DA-induced cAMP increase), but under other conditions it behaves like an agonist (67,70) and thus may be considered as a "mixed D_1 agonist/antagonist" whose effects depend on state and function of the system tested. Dopamine depletion may be a special situation in both animals and humans, because "empty" receptors may be more sensitive; in these systems (e.g., after reserpine + α-methyl-*p*-tyrosine pretreatment), lisuride restores motor activity in a similar way as apomorphine and L-dopa and is different from bromocriptine, which is ineffective (34).

If one accepts the hypothesis of a positive interaction of D_1 and D_2 receptors in such a situation (for review, see ref. 13), then lisuride must clearly have at least some functional D_1 agonist properties in this system, which resembles the situation in patients with advanced Parkinson's disease. D_1-agonistic effects of lisuride are also supported by the observation that rolipram, a phosphodiesterase inhibitor that prevents cAMP degradation, is able to enhance motor effects of lisuride (78). Whatever the difference, both pharmacological and clinical data support a stronger efficacy of lisuride not only on a dosage basis, but also in "intrinsic" dopaminergic activity, and this way lisuride resembles more apomorphine than bromocriptine. It differs from apomorphine, however, because its effects are influenced by the state of the dopamine systems, as is well known for other ergot derivatives that interact, for example, with noradrenergic receptors, and, like them, its effects may be long lasting and do not seem to correlate directly with drug plasma levels. In rats, apomorphine has a clear and strong dose-dependent inhibitory effect on tyrosine hydroxylase and L-dopa formation (36,10), whereas lisuride has similar properties only after surgical or biochemical denervation (37) but rather weak effects in intact animals that are even reversed at higher dosages (35). This biochemical observation fits well into a hypothesis coming from neurophysiological studies (45,22) that lisuride and its derivatives are high-affinity/low-activity drugs concerning normal receptors but display a high activity in "empty" neurons. Indeed, Gessa (22) has observed opposite dose-dependent effects within the same dosage range depending on the pretreatment of the animals.

Furthermore, his group as well as others have observed that exposure of DA neurons to lisuride—in contrast to apomorphine—results (after the well-known initial inhibitory effects on the firing rate) in a form of "stabilization" of autoreceptors, because subsequent doses of apomorphine and haloperidol fail to induce any of the expected effects (46,82). In nonanesthetized rats, lisuride not only prevented but even reversed apomorphine effects on DA cell activity (46). Mixed agonist–antagonist properties of lisuride might also be an explanation of why changes in DA receptor sensitivity may be less after chronic treatment as compared to treatment with "pure" DA agonists.

However, the changes occurring with repeated oral treatment in rats are quite spectacular: some effects undergo a functional supersensitivity development (e.g., motor activation and sexual stimulation) while others develop tolerance (e.g., hypothermogenic effect in cold environment and inhibitory effects in motility at low doses) and others, still in the same animals, remain unchanged (e.g., prolactin-lowering effect), a phenomenon that we reported earlier (32) as "dissociated functional tolerance/supersensitivity development" (28). In addition to the distinction between effects mediated by D_1 and D_2 receptors whose clinical significance is still unclear, we indeed propose, for all practical purposes, a classification of dopaminergic effects based upon the changes they undergo on chronic treatment, as well as upon the inhibitory effects of domperidone on effects that are caused by DA receptors outside the blood–brain barrier (see Table 2).

All of these effects and their time pattern could be observed in volunteers or patients treated with high oral or parenteral doses of lisuride and we and others have observed them in other dopaminergic drugs as well. With the

TABLE 2. *Dopaminergic effects*

Effect	Pathway and substrate	Inhibition by domperidone	On chronic treatment	
			Tolerance	Supersensitivity
Prolactin-lowering effect, GH-lowering effect in 50% of acromegalics	Tuberoinfundibular system (DA receptors on PRL cells in anterior pituitary)	++	-	-
GH increase, inhibition of TRH-induced TSH increase	Dopaminergic neurons in the hypothalamus	++	++	-
Nausea, emesis	CTZ in medulla oblongata	++	+	-
Reduction of sympathetic tone	Diencephalospinal pathway (?)	++	++	-
Orthostatic hypotension	?	-	++	-
Sedation	?	-	++	-
Headache	?	-	++	-
Antiparkinson effects	Nigroneostriatal system	-	-	(+)
Dyskinesias[a]	"Basal ganglia"	-	-	+
Psychosis[a]	Mesolimbic and mesocortical DA systems	-	-	+

[a] Especially with high-dose therapy in PD.

exception of headache and sedation, they have known dopaminergic systems as a basis, as shown in the table. In clinical pharmacological studies, we and others (8,18,72) have investigated which of these effects can be antagonized by low doses of sulpiride or, more recently, domperidone. This distinction is of importance since this procedure does not disturb the expected antiparkinson effects of the drug to a relevant degree.

It is unclear how the changes over time that these dopaminergic effects undergo, can be explained.

Biochemical investigations performed postmortem so far have failed to demonstrate important changes in dopamine receptor affinity or number—in contrast to some animal models where functional deafferentiation or overstimulation is followed by adaptive biochemical changes. Clearly, the local interaction between different systems is of greater importance; it can be speculated that, for example, a release of growth hormone by whatever dopaminergic stimulus is followed immediately by a compensatory increase in somatostatin synthesis and release that in chronic treatment even prevents all further dopaminergic effects on growth hormone and its releasing peptide (or, with the same result, a decline in GRF production and release can follow chronic dopaminergic treatments). The rapid tolerance with which nausea and emesis develop on chronic dopaminergic therapy, but even when lisuride infusion is slowly increased to higher blood levels, resembles observations from neurophysiology where a threshold to sudden depolarization can be elevated by slowly increasing the exogenous electric current. Peptides as cotransmitters or modulators can play a role, in a similar way as substance P has been shown to reduce postsynaptic effects of the release of high amounts of serotonin in the cervical ganglion; they may interfere with postreceptorial cAMP changes or changes in ion flux caused by dopaminergic drugs. Autoreceptors, of course, can play an important role in maintaining homeostasis of dopaminergic input, even if we have the impression that they have more of an acute role but are of less importance for chronic treatment and, of course, even more so for a state of denervation. It may be relevant, however, that in contrast to nigrostriatal systems, dopaminergic neurons of the mesolimbic and mesocortical systems have been reported to have no autoreceptors on their cell body.

The different neuronal connections and networks may give pharmacologists a chance to influence selectively simple dopaminergic systems by drugs acting not on the dopaminergic receptors but on systems influenced by them. This is well known for the cholinergic systems within the striatum that are under inhibitory dopaminergic control; clinical observations, of course, have shown that at least some symptoms caused by dopamine deficiency in the substantia nigra can be improved if anticholinergics are used to reduce the cholinergic hyperactivity caused by the loss of dopaminergic function. Unfortunately, anticholinergics tend, in elderly patients, to cause confusion and thus are of only limited value. Another example comes from observations by G. L. Gessa (personal communication, 1987), who described a hypothalamic dopaminergic mechanism causing yawning and penile erection in several species. In this system, dopaminergic neurons seem to act on oxytocin systems so that this dopaminergic effect can be blocked not only by haloperidol (which, of course, blocks all other dopaminergic receptors as well) but also by oxytocin antagonists in a specific way. Just another example involves the dopamine receptors of the chemoreceptor trigger zone, which are thought to activate an endorphinergic vomiting center; therefore, apomorphine-induced nausea and emesis could be inhibited in a specific way by naloxone without, probably, any interference with this drug's antiparkinson effects. Of course, the aim can be better achieved by using domperidone, an orally active dopamine antagonist that does not penetrate the blood–brain barrier (see Table 2), and this gives us an example of selective interaction with a limited number of dopaminergic systems.

For dopamine agonists, domperidone may become what the development of peripheral decarboxylase inhibitors like benserazide and carbidopa has been for the extended use of levodopa in parkinsonism, i.e., a pharmacological way of reducing peripheral side effects including dopaminergic influences on gastrointestinal motility and thus drug absorption.

Of even greater importance would be the availability of dopamine antagonists that act on mesolimbic and mesocortical structures in a more selective way than conventional neuroleptics. Indeed, studies with parenteral dopaminergic drugs have shown that, by this technique, good motor results can be achieved even in quite advanced cases but that now dopaminergic psychosis may become the limiting factor in the chronic treatment of these patients. Clozapine could be a first example of such a drug, as proposed recently (66).

Another new pharmacological strategy involves the use of dopamine agonists or mixed agonists/antagonists with more selective effects on denervated, "empty" dopamine receptors. We have been among the first to test this strategy using terguride, a drug that, depending on dopaminergic activity, acts as an agonist or antagonist (79,80) and future developments in this field can be expected.

Another difference can be found in the time course of dopamine effects (see Table 3, here described for the effects of lisuride) and, finally, we may learn something about clinical effects of dopaminergic drugs by observing effects caused by an acute overdose (Table 4).

It is reassuring that, so far, no casualty was reported related to lisuride overdose. From a theoretical point of view but also from our experience in clinical pharmacology, probably all side effects of lisuride can be treated (and often be abolished in a few minutes) by injecting sulpiride (or haloperidol). This inhibitory effect of D_2 antagonists again indicates the crucial role of D_2 receptors in clinical effects of dopaminergic drugs, at least as a common final pathway to D_1 and D_2 receptor activation. Another important

TABLE 3. *Duration of the effects of lisuride after oral administration of 0.2 mg*

≤ 30 min:
  GH increase
  Emetic effect
  Orthostatic hypotension
1–6 hr:
  Antiparkinsonian effect
  Lowering of GH in acromegalics
6–12 hr:
  Prolactin-lowering effect
  After chronic treatment, prolactin remains low for several days
Possible reasons for these differences:
  Rapid adaption of receptors
  Enhanced sensitivity of "empty" receptors
  Accumulation near or at the receptor
  Activation/inhibition of synergistic/antagonistic systems

observation is that we have never learned about psychic disturbances as a symptom of acute overdose; these symptoms did occur only after prolonged exposure to dopaminergic treatment especially in neurological disease.

CLINICAL STUDIES

The results of a few pivotal studies with oral lisuride in Parkinson's disease are summarized in Table 5. Not unexpectedly for a dopamine agonist, lisuride is effective as monotherapy as well as in combination with levodopa in early and advanced forms of this disease. Early in the disease, a similar degree of efficacy can be achieved by the combination in the majority of patients with less acute dopaminergic side effects. This may be related to the different and somehow synergistic mechanisms of both drugs where levodopa is taken up (and, thereby, "buffered") by the neurons while lisuride

TABLE 4. *Symptoms of overdose of dopamine agonists*

Acute overdose:
  Nausea and emesis
  Severe hypotension and sedation
  Dyskinesias and psychosis *not* observed so far
  Duration: some hours up to 2 days
  Treatment: supportive therapy, peripheral dopamine antagonists
Chronic overdose (in parkinsonian patients):
  Dyskinesias
  Sleep disorders
  Visual hallucinations and psychosis
  Duration: several days (up to 2 weeks)
  Treatment: dose reduction; in severe cases, central dopamine antagonists

TABLE 5. Selected studies with oral lisuride in Parkinson's disease

	Authors	Study design	General results
I. Monotherapy	Lieberman et al. (41) Agnoli et al. (1) Rinne (58)	Open, after levodopa withdrawal Single-blind dose-finding study Open vs. bromocriptine	Dose-dependent efficacy at 1–3 mg p.o./day, dose-dependent dopaminergic side effects, no difference to other dopaminergic therapies
II. Combination therapy with L-dopa	Schachter et al. (65) Gopinathan et al. (25) Lieberman et al. (42,43) LeWitt et al. (40) Lees and Stern (38) Caraceni et al. (9) Agnoli et al. (1)	Open vs. bromocriptine Single-blind placebo substituted Double-blind placebo substituted Double-blind vs. bromocriptine Single-blind placebo control Open vs. bromocriptine Single-blind	Significant improvement in all symptoms and/or reduction in levodopa dose by ~ 30%, improvement in hours "off" and dyskinesias in advanced disease; tendency for higher efficacy than bromocriptine
III. Long-term studies	Rinne (59,60) Rabey et al. (55,56) Caraceni et al. (9)	Prospective random combination vs. monotherapy over 3 and 5 years High levodopa monotherapy vs. combination therapy	Good long-term efficacy in combination, levodopa reduction, significantly less fluctuations in mobility than with levodopa monotherapy

acts directly on the postsynaptic receptors. Those patients, however, who benefit enough from dopamine agonist monotherapies seem to have a considerably lower risk to develop long-term problems, i.e., fluctuations in mobility consisting of alternating dyskinesia and akinesia ("on–off"). The occurence of these motor fluctuations can be postponed when lisuride is combined early on with levodopa (see ref. 60). It is not yet clear whether these better long-term prospects of the early combination therapy are related to differential effects of both drugs on D_1 and D_2 receptors, or whether they are due to different kinetics of both drugs at the receptor level (resulting in a more continuous dopaminergic stimulation that is more reminiscent of the physiological tonic activity of the nigroneostriatal dopamine neurons). This hypothesis, i.e., the induction of motor fluctuations by the discontinuous receptor stimulation caused by repeated oral levodopa intake, could be tested, as proposed by S. Ruggieri, A. Agnoli, and F. Stocchi, in a study with continuous s.c. infusion of lisuride as the only therapy in beginning Parkinson's disease.

A "stabilization" of presynaptic receptors as observed in animal studies by Gessa (22) that prevents feedback inhibition of tyrosine hydroxylase could be also discussed; for testing this hypothesis, a combination of levodopa with terguride, a dopamine partial agonist, could be investigated.

Last, but not least, a simple levodopa sparing effect may be concerned if one feels that levodopa or, more likely, some of its metabolites are the cause of the fluctuations as a kind of long-term levodopa syndrome.

Whatever the mechanisms for a preventive or postponing effect of the early lisuride–levodopa combination are, it is clear that, in advanced Parkinson's disease, addition of lisuride to levodopa is superior to increasing the levodopa dose. In this situation, not only the "off" periods are better controlled, but also the occurrence of peak-dose dyskinesias is reduced as shown by an elegant study of Rabey et al. (56,55). Whether here again different receptor kinetics of both drugs play a role, or whether lisuride acts here as a state-dependent dopamine partial agonist, or whether simply again the reduction of levodopa (and thus its metabolites) plays the crucial role is still unclear and may be resolved only by PET studies in patients.

In addition to these and many other reports on the use of lisuride in patients suffering from Parkinson's disease (for review, see refs. 39, 44, and 75), the drug has also been used in a variety of other neurological disorders where it was effective in some cases even when other dopaminergic therapies have failed (39). The same author summarizes the effects of lisuride in Table 6.

PARENTERAL STUDIES WITH DOPAMINERGIC DRUGS IN PARKINSON'S DISEASE

Parenteral use of dopaminergic drugs (as summarized in Table 7) was very helpful for the clinical–pharmacological investigation of dopaminergic ther-

TABLE 6. *Applications for lisuride therapy in parkinsonism*

Reverses all cardinal features of parkinsonism as monotherapy
May improve loss of levodopa efficacy and worsening of parkinsonian stage
May lessen severity of wearing-off and on–off phenomena, abnormal involuntary
    movements, and dystonic features
Available for intravenous as well as oral administration
Possibly less potential for causing long-term problems (such as on–off effect and
    dyskinesia associated with chronic levodopa therapy)
Tolerance may develop to adverse effects; antiparkinsonian efficacy is sustained

---

From ref. 24.

apy and its mechanisms. The underestimated role of the kinetics of drug application became quite clear by these studies, and new therapeutic strategies now arise from these results.

In the first studies with parenteral dopaminergic therapy, apomorphine was used, a drug whose 100% first-pass effect prevents oral application. With quite different ideas about its potential role, Schwab et al. (68) and Struppler (74) found independently a clear antiparkinson effect that was most pronounced on the tremor. These results later were confirmed and extended by a study inaugurated by us, where Strian et al. (73) could observe, using a double-blind design with i.v. apomorphine infusion, a clear antiparkinson effect but also typical side effects including severe orthostatic hypotension and reversible psychosis when therapy was continued with high oral doses.

The failure to achieve stable effective drug concentrations without oscillation and overdose was the reason why this and other attempts with parenteral and oral use of apomorphine or its derivatives (12,14) could not compete with the success of the levodopa therapy. Birkmayer and Hornykiewicz (4) were the first to use parenteral levodopa (due to a shortage in drug supply and with the idea to make the investigations better controllable); much later, Shoulson and co-workers (69) followed by many others used this approach in order to demonstrate the importance of pharmacokinetic factors for the effects and problems (especially fluctuations) associated with long-term levodopa treatment. In these studies, levodopa was infused only for limited periods because very large volumes needed to be infused, which caused local irritations in veins. Recently, water solubility and thus extension of use was improved by the use of levodopa methyl ester by Ruggieri and his colleagues (61). Lisuride was first tested as an i.v. bolus by Dorow et al. (19) and its diagnostic use in endocrine and, subsequently, neurological diseases was proposed (51,52). Other studies with parenteral lisuride were performed by Agnoli and co-workers (1), Birkmayer's group (57), and Frattola et al. (20). Obeso et al. (48,50) were the first to make long-term infusion studies followed by the first introduction of a s.c. infusion pump in neurology by the same group (49), followed by Ruggieri et al. (62,63), Bittkau and Przuntek (5), Critchley et al. (15), and others.

TABLE 7. Parenteral use of dopaminergic therapies

Drug and application	Authors	Remarks
L-dopa i.v. infusion	Birkmayer et al. (4) Shoulson et al. (69)	Short-term therapeutic test Pharmacokinetic study in fluctuating patients, large volume necessary, local toxic effects
L-dopa methyl ester i.v. infusion	Ruggieri et al. (86)	Less volume necessary, only i.v. use possible (bad local tolerance s.c.)
Bromocriptine LAR i.m. injectable depot	Lancranjan et al. (personal communication)	Less side effects than oral; plasma levels quite variable; use only in endocrine disease so far
Apomorphine s.c.	Schwab et al. (68) Struppler (74) Cotzias et al (14)	Therapeutic efficacy (especially tremor, short-lasting effect, side effects)
Apomorphine i.v. infusion	Strian et al. (73)	Effective, but only short-term trials, sometimes severe side effects (including psychosis)
Apomorphine s.c. infusion	Stibe et al. (71)	Up to 6 months; so far only one psychic side effect
PHNO i.v. infusion, transdermal	Parkes et al. (to be published)	Only very preliminary studies
Lisuride i.v. injection	Dorow et al. (19) Parkes et al. (51) Riederer et al. (57)	Diagnostic test, clinical–pharmacological studies, treatment of severe akinesia
Lisuride i.v. infusion	Obeso et al. (48,50) Stocchi et al. (72)	
Lisuride s.c. infusion	Obeso et al. (49)	Good effects on fluctuations
Lisuride s.c. infusion (with nightly intervals)	Stocchi et al. (72)	

TABLE 8. *Continuous dopaminergic stimulation (e.g., by lisuride infusion)*

Enhances effects on motor function in parkinsonian patients with a great reduction of fluctuations

Reduces peripheral side effects (e.g., nausea, emesis, hypotension), which can be further reduced by initial domperidone medication

Therefore, higher drug plasma levels can be achieved (but risk of central side effects, dyskinesia, and psychosis)

Therefore, rapid dosage adjustment must be possible and close monitoring is necessary

Important: patients and relatives must be informed about early warning symptoms of psychosis!

These initial studies have been summarized recently (47) and the main conclusions are in Table 8. These studies were performed mostly in patients with very severe and advanced Parkinson's disease and high doses of lisuride (up to 5 mg) were infused in a continuous way over 24 hr.

The motor improvements even in these patients were often quite striking and thus an indication that fluctuations and loss of sufficient response to oral therapy are not simply a consequence of an irreversible impairment of dopaminergic cells, receptors, transmission, or effector systems as often believed. On the contrary, the rediscovery of the crucial role of the kinetics of dopaminergic drugs and their application may be the basis for new insights and therapies.

It remains to be seen whether continuous dopaminergic stimulation becomes a method to prevent the development of motor fluctuations that is seen after many years of levodopa therapy. Drugs with predictable bioavailability and long duration of effects may ultimately prove superior even to levodopa therapy.

Also, dopaminergic effects clearly undergo a dissociated functional tolerance/supersensitivity development and it became even more obvious that some peripheral side effects, in spite of high plasma levels, soon develop tolerance while the motor effects even increase with time. This, unfortunately, also applies to the psychosis associated with this as well as other forms of dopaminergic therapies (see Table 7) and, indeed, development of this side effect (or, even more, exacerbation of a pre-existing psychosis) has been the main limiting factor for this therapy so far.

Strategies against this problem include the use of a 12-hr infusion schedule, a lower daily dose, an exclusion of patients with a history of psychosis as well as a search for antidotes against these treatment-limiting side effects (66). It now becomes very clear that the mode of administration, i.e., discontinuous versus continuous, may become quite relevant for our understanding of this disease and its development, but possibly also for other neurological and medical disorders.

In conclusion, our work with lisuride may have been of some value for the investigation of dopaminergic effects and stresses the importance of pharmacokinetics and clinical neuropharmacology for improving therapy in neurology. Future developments will involve better application systems or improved bioavailability, while research will also focus on disturbances that precede the dopamine depletion as well as on events beyond the dopamine receptor.

REFERENCES

1. Agnoli, A., Baldassarre, M., Ruggieri, S., Falaschi, P., Urso, R. D., and Rocco, A. (1981): Prolactin response as an index of dopaminergic receptor function in Parkinson's disease. Correlation with clinical findings and therapeutic response. *J. Neural Transm.*, 51:123–134.
2. Ahlenius, S., and Larsson, K. (1980): Stimulating effects of lisuride on masculine sexual behavior of rats. *Eur. J. Pharmacol.*, 64:47–51.
3. Ahlenius, S., and Larsson, K. (1985): Antagonism by lisuride and 8-OH-DPAT of 5-HPT-induced prolongation of the performance of male rat sexual behavior. *Eur. J. Pharmacol.*, 110:379–381.
4. Birkmayer, W., and Hornykiewicz, O. (1961): Der L-3,4-Dihydroxyphenylalanin (=DOPA)-Effekt bei der Parkinson-Akinese. *Wien. Klin. Wochenschr.*, 73:787–789.
5. Bittkau, S., and Przuntek, H. (1986): Psychosis and the lisuride pump. *Lancet*, 2:349.
6. Braham, J., Sarova-Pinhas, I., and Goldhammer, Y. (1970): Apomorphine in parkinsonian tremor. *Br. Med. J.*, 3:768.
7. Calne, D. B., Horowski, R., McDonald, R. J., and Wuttke, W., eds. (1983): *Lisuride and Other Dopamine Agonists*, New York, Raven Press.
8. Cangi, F., Fanciullacci, M., Pietrini, U., Boccuni, M., and Sicuteri, F. (1985): Emergence of pain and extra-pain phenomena from dopaminomimetics in migraine. In: *Updating in Headache*, edited by V. Pfaffenrath, P. O. Lundberg, and O. Sjaastad, Berlin/Heidelberg, Springer-Verlag, pp. 276–280.
9. Caraceni, T., Giovannini, P., Parati, E., Scigliano, G., Grassi, M. P., and Carella, F. (1984): Bromocriptine and lisuride in Parkinson's disease. In: *Advances in Neurology*, Vol. 40, edited by R. G. Hassler and J. F. Christ, New York, Raven Press, 531–535.
10. Carlsson, A., Kehr, W., and Lindqvist, M. (1977): Agonist–antagonist interaction on dopamine receptors in brain, as reflected in the rates of tyrosine and tryptophan hydroxylation. *J. Neural Transm.*, 40:99–113.
11. Carruba, M. O., and Mantegazza, P. (1983): Behavioral pharmacology of ergot derivatives. In: *Lisuride and Other Dopamine Agonists*, edited by D. B. Calne, R. Horowski, R. J. McDonald, and W. Wuttke, New York, Raven Press, pp. 65–77.
12. Castaigne, P., Laplane, D., and Dordain, G. (1971): Clinical experimentation with apomorphine in Parkinson's disease. *Res. Commun. Chem. Pathol. Pharmacol.*, 2:154–158.
13. Clark, D., and White, F. J. (1987): Review: D1 dopamine receptor—the search for a function: a critical evaluation of the D1/D2 dopamine receptor classification and its functional implications. *Synapse*, 1:347–388.
14. Cotzias, G. C., Papavasiliou, P. S., Fehling, C., Kaufmann, G., and Mena, J. (1970): Similarities between neurologic effects of L-DOPA and of apomorphine. *N. Engl. J. Med.*, 282:31–33.
15. Critchley, P., Grandas Perez, F., Quinn, N., Coleman, R., Parkes, D., and Marsden, C. D. (1986): Psychosis and the lisuride pump. *Lancet*, 2:349.
16. Cronin, M. J., Valdenegro, C. A., Perkins, S. N., and MacLeod, R. M. (1981): The 7315a pituitary tumor is refractory to dopaminergic inhibition of prolactin release but contains dopamine receptors. *Endocrinology*, 109:2160–2166.

17. Da Prada, M., Bonetti, E. P., and Keller, H. H. (1977): Induction of mounting behaviour in female and male rats by lisuride. *Neurosci. Lett.*, 6:349–353.
18. Dorow, R., Breitkopf, M., Gräf, K. J., and Horowski, R. (1983): Neuroendocrine effects of lisuride and its 9,10-analog in healthy volunteers. In: *Lisuride and Other Dopamine Agonists*, edited by D. B. Calne, R. Horowski, R. J. McDonald, and W. Wuttke, New York, Raven Press, pp. 161–174.
19. Dorow, R., Gräf, K.-J., Nieuweboer, B., and Horowski, R. (1980): Intravenous lisuride: a new tool for testing responsiveness to dopaminergic agonists and neuroendocrine function. *Acta Endocrinol. (Copenh.)*, 94(suppl. 234):9(Abstract).
20. Frattola, L., Albizzati, M. G., Bassi, S., Ferrarese, C., and Trabucchi, M. (1982): "On–off" phenomena, dyskinesias and dystonias. *Acta Neurol. Scand.*, 66:227–236.
21. Fuxe, K., Fredholm, B. B., Gren, S.-O., Agnati, L. F., Hökfelt, T., and Gustafsson, J.-A. (1978): Ergot drugs and central monoaminergic mechanisms: a histochemical, biochemical and behavioral analysis. *Fed. Proc.*, 37:2181–2191.
22. Gessa, G. L. (1988): Agonist and antagonist actions of lisuride on dopamine neurons: electrophysiological evidence. *J. Neural Transm.*, 27(suppl.):201–210.
23. Giovannini, P., Scigliano, G., Piccolo, I., Soliveri, P., Suchy, I., and Caraceni, T. (1988): Lisuride in Parkinson's disease: 4-year follow-up. *Clin. Neuropharmacol.*, 11:201–211.
24. Gopinathan, G., Horowski, R., and Suchy, I. (1988): Lisuride pharmacology and treatment of Parkinson's disease. In: *Drugs for the Treatment of Parkinson's Disease, Handbook of Experimental Pharmacology*, edited by D. B. Calne, Heidelberg, Springer-Verlag, (in press).
25. Gopinathan, G., Teräväinen, H., Dambrosia, J. M., et al. (1981): Lisuride in Parkinsonism. *Neurology*, 31:371–376.
26. Horowski, R. (1978): Differences in the dopaminergic effects of the ergot derivatives bromocriptine, lisuride and d-LSD as compared with apomorphine. *Eur. J. Pharmacol.*, 51:157–166.
27. Horowski, R. (1986): Psychiatric side-effects of high-dose lisuride therapy in parkinsonism. *Lancet*, 2:510.
28. Horowski, R. (1987): Clinical neuropharmacology of DA agonists in Parkinson's disease. *Neuroscience*, 22(suppl.):S107.
29. Horowski, R., and Dorow, R. (1981): Influence of estradiol and other gonadal steroids on central effects of lisuride and comparable ergot derivatives. In: *Gonadal Steroids and Brain Function*, edited by W. Wuttke and R. Horowski, Berlin, Springer-Verlag, pp. 169–181.
30. Horowski, R., Dorow, R., Scholz, A., DeCecco, L., and Schneider, W. H. F. (1984): Lisuride—a new drug for treatment of hyperprolactinaemic disorders. In: *Advances in Fertility Control and the Treatment of Sterility*, edited by R. Roland, Lancaster, MTP Press Ltd., pp. 37–49.
31. Horowski, R., and Wachtel, H. (1976): Direct dopaminergic action of lisuride hydrogen maleate, an ergot derivative in mice. *Eur. J. Pharmacol.*, 36:373–383.
32. Horowski, R., and Wachtel, H. (1979): Pharmacological effects of lisuride in rodents mediated by dopaminergic receptors: mechanism of action and influence of chronic treatment with lisuride. In: *Dopaminergic Ergot Derivatives and Motor Function*, edited by K. Fuxe and D. B. Calne, Oxford/New York, Pergamon Press, pp. 237–251.
33. Horowski, R., Wachtel, H., and Dorow, R. (1986): Dopamine as a deuteragonist in migraine: implications for clinical pharmacology of dopamine agonists. In: *The Neurobiology of Dopamine Systems*, edited by W. Winlow and R. Markstein, Manchester, Manchester University Press, pp. 415–426.
34. Jackson, D. M., and Jenkins, O. F. (1985): Hypothesis bromocriptine lacks intrinsic dopamine receptor stimulating properties. *J. Neural Transm.*, 62:219–230.
35. Kehr, W. (1977): Effect of lisuride and other ergot derivatives on mono-aminergic mechanisms in rat brain. *Eur. J. Pharmacol.*, 41:261–273.
36. Kehr, W., Carlsson, A., and Lindqvist, M. (1977): Catecholamine synthesis in rat brain after axotomy: interaction between apomorphine and haloperidol. *Arch. Pharmacol.*, 297:111–117.
37. Kehr, W., and Speckenbach, W. (1978): Effect of lisuride and LSD on monoamine synthesis after axotomy or reserpine treatment in rat brain. *Naunyn-Schmiedeberg's Arch. Pharmacol.*, 301:163–169.

38. Lees, A. J., and Stern, G. M. (1981): Pergolide and lisuride for levodopa-induced oscillations. *Lancet*, 2:577.
39. LeWitt, P. A. (1986): Clinical and pharmacological aspects of the antiparkinsonian ergolene lisuride. In: *Recent Developments in Parkinson's Disease*, edited by S. Fahn et al., New York, Raven Press, pp. 347–354.
40. LeWitt, P. A., Gopinathan, G., Ward, C. D., et al. Lisuride versus bromocriptine treatment in Parkinson disease: a double-blind study. *Neurology*, 32:69–72.
41. Lieberman, A., Goldstein, M., Neophytides, A., et al. (1981): Lisuride in Parkinson disease: efficacy of lisuride compared to levodopa. *Neurology*, 31:961–965.
42. Lieberman, A. N., Goldstein, M., Gopinathan, G., et al. (1983): Lisuride in Parkinson's disease and related disorders. In: *Lisuride and Other Dopamine Agonists*, edited by D. B. Calne, R. Horowski, R. J. McDonald, and W. Wuttke, New York, Raven Press, pp. 419–429.
43. Lieberman, A. N., Gopinathan, G., Neophytides, A., Leibowitz, M., Walker, R., and Hiesiger, E. (1983): Bromocriptine and lisuride in Parkinson disease. *Ann. Neurol.*, 13:44–47.
44. McDonald, R. J., and Horowski, R. (1983): Lisuride in the treatment of parkinsonism. *Eur. Neurol.*, 22:240–255.
45. Mereu, G., Hu, X. T., Wang, R. Y., Westfall, T. C., and Gessa, G. L. (1987): Failure of subchronic lisuride to modify A10 dopamine autoreceptors' sensitivity. *Brain Res.*, 408:210–214.
46. Mereu, G., Muntoni, F., Collu, M., Boi, V., and Gessa, G. L. (1986): Delayed blockade of dopamine autoreceptors by lisuride. In: *Modulation of Central and Peripheral Transmitter Function*, edited by G. Biggio, F. P. Spano, G. Toffano, and G. L. Gessa, Padova, Liviana Press, pp. 597–601.
47. Obeso, J. A., Horowski, R., and Marsden, C. D. (1988): Continuous dopaminergic stimulation in Parkinson's disease. *J. Neural Transm.*, 27(suppl.):249–251.
48. Obeso, J. A., Luquin, M. R., and Martinez Lage, J. M. (1983): Lisuride infusion for Parkinson's disease. *Ann. Neurol.*, 14:134.
49. Obeso, J. A., Luquin, M. R., and Martinez-Lage, J. M. (1986): Lisuride infusion pump: a device for the treatment of motor fluctuations in Parkinson's disease. *Lancet*, 1:467–470.
50. Obeso, J. A., Luquin, M. R., and Martinez-Lage, J. M. (1986): Intravenous lisuride corrects oscillations of motor performance in Parkinson's disease. *Ann. Neurol.*, 19:31–35.
51. Parkes, J. D., Schachter, M., Marsden, C. D., Smith, B., and Wilson, A. (1981): Lisuride in parkinsonism. *Ann. Neurol.*, 9:48–52.
52. Parkes, J. D., Schachter, M., Quinn, N., Lang, A., and Horowski, R. (1981): Bromocriptine, lisuride and pergolide in the treatment of Parkinson's disease. 12th World Congress of Neurology, Kyoto/Japan, September 1981, p. 1020(Abstract).
53. Peroutka, S. J., Lebovitz, R. M., and Snyder, S. H. (1981): Two distinct central serotonin receptors with different physiological functions. *Science*, 212:827–829.
54. Pieri, L., Keller, H. H., Burkard, W., and Da Prada, M. (1978): Effects of lisuride and LSD on cerebral monoamine systems and hallucinosis. *Nature (Lond.)*, 272:278–280.
55. Rabey, J. M., Streifler, M., Treves, T., and Korczyn, A. D. (1987): Long-term lisuride in Parkinson's disease. *Ital. J. Neurol. Sci.*, 5(suppl. 7):55.
56. Rabey, J. M., Treves, T., Streifler, M., and Korczyn, A. D. (1986): Comparison of efficacy of lisuride hydrogen maleate with increased doses of levodopa in parkinsonian patients. In: *Advances in Neurology*, Vol. 45, edited by M. D. Yahr and K. J. Bergmann, New York, Raven Press, pp. 569–572.
57. Riederer, P., Reynolds, G. P., Danielczyk, W., Jellinger, K., and Seemann, D. (1983): Desensitization of striatal spiperone-binding sites by dopaminergic agonists in Parkinson's disease. In: *Lisuride and Other Dopamine Agonists*, edited by D. B. Calne, R. Horowski, R. J. McDonald, and W. Wuttke, New York, Raven Press, pp. 375–381.
58. Rinne, U. K. (1983): New ergot derivatives in the treatment of Parkinson's disease. In: *Lisuride and Other Dopamine Agonists*, edited by D. B. Calne, R. Horowski, R. J. McDonald, and W. Wuttke, New York, Raven Press, pp. 431–442.
59. Rinne, U. K. (1986): The importance of an early combination of a dopamine agonist and levodopa in the treatment of Parkinson's disease. In: *Lisuride: A New Dopamine Agonist*

and Parkinson's Disease, edited by J. van Manen and U. K. Rinne, Amsterdam, Excerpta Medica, 64–71.

60. Rinne, U. K. (1988): New strategies in the treatment of Parkinson's disease. In: *Parkinsonism and Aging*, edited by B. C. Calne, R. Horowski, and M. Trabucchi, New York, Raven Press, pp. 255–260.

61. Ruggieri, S., Jenner, P., Carta, A., Agnoli, A., Marsden, C. D., and Stocchi, F. (1988): L-dopa methylester in the treatment of Parkinson's disease. 9th Int. Symp. Parkinson's Disease, p. 79 (Abstract).

62. Ruggieri, S., Stocchi, F., and Agnoli, A. (1986): Lisuride infusion pump for Parkinson's disease. *Lancet*, 2:348–349.

63. Ruggieri, S., Stocchi, F., Antonini, A., Bellantuono, P., Carta, A., and Agnoli, A. (1987): Lisuride infusion in chronically treated fluctuating Parkinson's disease: effects of continuous dopaminergic stimulation. *New Trends Clin. Neuropharmacol.*, 1:55–60.

64. Schachter, M., Bédard, P., Debono, A. G., et al. The role of D-1 and D-2 receptors. *Nature (Lond.)*, 286:157–159.

65. Schachter, M., Sheehy, M. P., Parkes, J. P., and Marsden, C. D. (1980): Lisuride in the treatment of parkinsonism. *Acta Neurol. Scand.*, 62:382–385.

66. Scholz, E., and Dichgans, J. (1985): Treatment of drug-induced exogenous psychosis in parkinsonism with clozapine and fluperlapine. *Eur. Arch. Psychiatry Neurol. Sci.*, 235:60–64.

67. Schorderet, M. (1978): Dopamine-mimetic activity of cyclic AMP in isolated retinae of the rabbit. *Gerontology*, 24(suppl. 1):86–93.

68. Schwab, R. S., Amadori, L. V., and Lettoni, J. Y. (1951): Apomorphine in Parkinson's disease. *Am. Neurol. Assoc.*, 76:251.

69. Shoulson, I., Glaubiger, G. A., and Chase, T. N. (1975): On–off response: clinical and biochemical correlations during oral and intravenous levodopa administration in parkinsonian patients. *Neurology*, 25:1144–1148.

70. Spano, P. F., Saiani, L., Memo, M., and Trabucchi, M. (1980): Interaction of dopaminergic ergot derivatives with cyclic nucleotide system. In: *Ergot Compounds and Brain Function: Neuroendocrine and Neuropsychiatric Aspects*, edited by M. Goldstein et al., New York, Raven Press, pp. 95–102.

71. Stibe, C. M. H., Lees, A. J., Kempster, P. A., and Stern, G. M. (1988): Subcutaneous apomorphine in parkinsonian on–off oscillations. *Lancet*, 1:403–406.

72. Stocchi, F., Ruggieri, S., Brughitta, G., and Agnoli, A. (1986): Problems in daily motor performances in Parkinson's disease: the continuous dopaminergic stimulation. *J. Neural Transm.*, 22(suppl.):209–218.

73. Strian, F., Micheler, E., and Benkert, O. (1972): Tremor inhibition in Parkinson syndrome after apomorphine administration under L-dopa and decarboxylase-inhibitor basic therapy. *Pharmacopsychiatry*, 5:198–205.

74. Struppler, A. (1953): Die therapeutische Beeinflussbarkeit des Tremors. *Med. Wochenschr.*, 73:157–160.

75. Suchy, I., and Horowski, R. (1984): Use of ergot derivative lisuride in Parkinson's disease. In: *Advances in Neurology*, Vol. 40, edited by R. G. Hassler and J. F. Christ, New York, Raven Press, pp. 515–521.

76. Suchy, I., Schneider, H. H., Riederer, P., and Horowski, R. (1983): Considerations on the clinical relevance of differences in receptor affinity of various dopaminergic ergot alkaloids. *Psychopharmacol. Bull.*, 19:743–746.

77. Wachtel, H. (1983): Central dopaminergic and antidopaminergic effects of ergot derivatives structurally related to lisuride. In: *Lisuride and Other Dopamine Agonists*, edited by D. B. Calne, R. Horowski, R. J. McDonald, and W. Wuttke, New York, Raven Press, pp. 109–125.

78. Wachtel, H. (1983): Neurotropic effects of the optical isomers of the selective adenosine cyclic 3′,5′-monophosphate phosphodiesterase inhibitor rolipram in rats in-vivo. *J. Pharm. Pharmacol.*, 35:440–444.

79. Wachtel, H., and Dorow, R. (1983): Dual action on central dopamine function of trans-dihydrolisuride, a 9,10-dihydrogenated analogue of the ergot dopamine agonist lisuride. *Life Sci.*, 32:421–432.

80. Wachtel, H., Dorow, R., and Sauer, G. (1984): Novel 8α-ergolines with inhibitory and stimulatory effects on prolactin secretion in rats. *Life Sci.*, 35:1859–1867.

81. Wachtel, H., Kehr, W., and Schlangen, M. (1986): Involvement of dopamine auto- and postsynaptic receptors in locomotor effects of lisuride in rats after systemic or intracerebral administration. In: *Lisuride: A New Dopamine Agonist and Parkinson's Disease*, edited by J. van Manen and U. K. Rinne, Amsterdam, Excerpta Medica, pp. 11–23.
82. Walters, J. R., Baring, M. D., and Lakoski, J. M. (1979): Effects of ergolines on dopaminergic and serotonergic single unit activity. In: *Dopaminerigic Ergot Derivatives and Motor Function*, edited by K. Fuxe and D. B. Calne, Oxford, Pergamon Press, pp. 207–221.
83. White, F. J. (1986): Comparative effects of LSD and lisuride: clues to specific hallucinogenic drug actions. *Pharmacol. Biochem. Behav.*, 24:365–379.
84. White, F. J., and Appel, J. B. (1982): Lysergic acid diethylamide (LSD) and lisuride: differentiation of their neuropharmacological actions. *Science*, 216:535–537.
85. Zikan, V., and Semonsky, M. (1968): Mutterkorn-Alkaloide: 31. Mitt.: Ein Beitrag zur Herstellung von N-(D-6-Methyl-8-isoergolenyl)-N',N'-diäthylharnstoff. *Pharmazie*, 23:147–148.

Parkinsonism and Aging, edited by
Donald B. Calne et al., Raven Press, Ltd.,
New York © 1989.

Latest Therapeutic Strategies in Complicated Parkinson's Disease

A. Agnoli, A. Carta, F. Stocchi, G. Brughitta,
L. Giorgi, and S. Ruggieri

*I Clinic of Neurology, Department of Neurological Sciences,
"La Sapienza" University, Viale dell' Universita' 30, 00185, Rome, Italy*

Since 1975, the continuous intravenous infusion of L-dopa has shown a remarkable efficacy in controlling oscillations of the motor response in patients with idiopathic Parkinson's disease (PD) (1). Unfortunately, it was also clear that although very effective, L-dopa infusion could not be used in long-term treatment because of the low solubility and high acidity of the drug (2–4). Only a few years later, the high solubility of a potent dopamine agonist drug, lisuride (5), and the availability of computerized micropumps already used in diabetics allowed continuous subcutaneous administration in complicated PD patients. Therefore, it was technically possible to perform, for the first time in 1985, a continuous dopaminergic stimulation by means of a new drug delivery system (6–8).

Interestingly, shortly after the first encouraging clinical results of the subcutaneous delivery of dopaminergic agonist compounds (lisuride and afterwards apomorphine), two new formulations of L-dopa were produced: the slow-release preparations and the methyl ester oral solution. The relevance of these different L-dopa formulations will be the matter of further discussion. Let us first analyze the clinical efficacy results of 3 years of lisuride subcutaneous administration.

LISURIDE SUBCUTANEOUS TREATMENT

Over the last 3 years, we have been treating a number of parkinsonian patients who presented severe fluctuations of motor response secondary to chronic treatment with L-dopa with continuous subcutaneous infusion. To date, we have treated 24 patients (13 males, 11 females) who had been chronically taking oral L-dopa in daily doses of 500 to 1250 mg together with a peripheral dopa decarboxylase inhibitor (DDI) (for not less than 4 years and for a maximum of 15 years).

All patients presented "wearing off" phenomena with dyskinesias and dystonias due to L-dopa. Patients older than 65 years and/or having a history of psychiatric disturbances were excluded from this trial.

We usually prefer a 12-hr infusion regimen with subcutaneous lisuride, allowing a drug-free night (from 8.00 A.M. to 8.00 P.M.) (7). Nonetheless, 4 out of the 24 patients were treated at the onset of the trial with a 24 h regimen because of the severity of their symptoms. We observed, though, a higher incidence of systemic and psychiatric side effects in these patients. This evidence suggested the use of the 24-hr regimen only in the more severely affected patients.

The infusional technique was as follows: lisuride 2 mg was diluted in 2 ml of sterile water. The initial infusion rate was defined on the basis of previously performed lisuride intravenous infusions in the same patient, and then it was optimized during the first days of the following subcutaneous stage. In those patients who did not completely show a satisfactory response, a small amount of oral L-dopa was added (100–875 mg/day). All patients orally took 60 mg/day of domperidone to prevent systemic side effects.

Nine patients dropped out of the study: three because of psychiatric disturbances (two of them were on the 24-hr infusion regimen), one for a concurrent myocardial ischemia, one because of vomiting, one for untreatable diarrhea, and the remaining three withdrew for personal "uneasy feelings" against computerized and unusual therapy (Table 1). At present, 15 out of these 24 patients are still on, and experiencing beneficial effects from the subcutaneous treatment. It is possible to separate these subjects into two groups: 7 of them are on lisuride single treatment (0.065 mg/hr; 0.80 mg/12 hr), while the remaining 8 are assuming a combined therapy with relatively small amounts of oral L-dopa. In fact, these patients need an average of 384 mg/day of L-dopa in association with 0.08 mg/hr (0.96 mg/12 hr) of subcutaneous lisuride infusion, while their average L-dopa intake during standard oral therapy was 812.3 mg/day.

TABLE 1. *Subcutaneous lisuride drop-out patients*

Patient	Months of treatment	Drop-out reasons
F.M.	7	Acoustic hallucinations
P.G.	10	Mental confusion
C.G.	1	Visual hallucinations
C.A.	6	Myocardial ischemia
Z.D.	1	Vomiting
D.E.	5	Diarrhea
T.F.	6	Not related to therapy
L.L.	3	Not related to therapy
L.P.	9	Not related to therapy

TABLE 2. *Comparison between patients still on subcutaneous lisuride and patients dropped out from the study*

No. of patients	Still on treatment 15	Dropped out 9
Age (years)	52.00 (9.32)	54.00 (6.88)
Years of disease	12.92 (6.75)	10.25 (2.93)
Years of therapy	9.42 (3.20)	8.75 (2.18)
Years of LTS	3.25 (1.06)	3.75 (1.14)
Previous L-dopa (mg/day)	827.5 (227.3)	775.0 (225.1)
Lisuride (mg/hr)	0.080 (0.023)	0.077 (0.023)
Associated L-dopa (mg/day)	305.0 (125.1) (10 patients)	368.6 (245.2) (8 patients)

However, each group of patients experienced a consistent reduction of the hours spent in the "off" condition, in comparison with conventional oral therapy: 0.7 hr versus 4.8 hr for the associated therapy group; 0.5 hr vs. 3.8 hr in the single therapy group.

Considering the overall clinical data, no substantial differences are evident between the responses of the two groups of patients to lisuride. Therefore, it seems that there are no predictive elements at present to distinguish in advance those patients who will respond to lisuride single treatment from those who will need additional stimulation with L-dopa.

Unfortunately, it was also impossible to detect significant differences between patients responding to therapy and those patients dropping out (Table 2). We noted, though, that all drop-outs took place at an early stage of treatment (not beyond the 12th month) (Table 3).

Another important remark is the fact that the clinically effective lisuride dosage remained practically unchanged for several months in almost all patients studied, without additional tablets of L-dopa. Conversely, the improvement of dyskinesias in such patients appears to be poor, probably due to the already compromised function of the dopamine receptor system, provoked by the long-term oral L-dopa treatment.

Stibe et al. reported satisfactory clinical results in fluctuating parkinson-

TABLE 3. *Follow-up of patients in subcutaneous lisuride treatment*

Number of patients	5	6	5	2	2	1
(drop-outs)	(2)	(4)	(2)			
Lisuride (μg/hr)	68.00	71.67	74.00	90.00	87.5	65.0
(SD)	(15.25)	(11.25)	(11.40)	(42.43)	(31.8)	
Off (hr)	0.42	0.60	0.57	0.61	0.49	0.50
(SD)	(0.44)	(0.60)	(0.60)			
Months of treatment	1	6	12	16	25	31

ians with a combined therapy of oral L-dopa plus a 12 hr subcutaneous administration of apomorphine (9). Interestingly, they reported a lower incidence of psychiatric side effects in comparison with lisuride-treated patients.

We administered apomorphine intravenously in three different PD patients. In one patient who had responded well to lisuride infusion (0.08 mg/hr), 2 mg/hr of apomorphine insured a good clinical state without "off" periods. On the contrary, the other two patients had a limited benefit with apomorphine, showing "off" periods even at 3 and 4 mg/hr: the first one was a partial responder to 0.15 mg/hr of lisuride and the other did not respond at all even to 0.2 mg/hr of lisuride.

Such results suggest an almost equivalent action of the two drugs in terms of pure clinical response. Our subcutaneous apomorphine experiment is still in progress and at present our data are too poor to be compared with Stibe's results.

L-DOPA METHYL ESTER AND LONG-ACTING PREPARATIONS

As previously stated, L-dopa preparations other than the standard formulation were administered in recent years to fluctuating PD patients. Different experiences did not report entirely satisfactory results using the slow-release L-dopa preparations (10,11). In our study, performed on 10 PD patients, we obtained a consistent reduction of the hours spent in the "off" condition, associating standard L-dopa to the slow-release compound (Madopar HBS): this result always implied an increase in total daily intake of L-dopa (Table 4).

A longer latency to achieve "on" clinical conditions, a higher amount of dosages required, and the frequent necessity to associate standard L-dopa tablets seem the most relevant negative aspects of this slow-release preparation, although in some selected individual cases the clinical results were brilliant indeed (12).

At present, the administration of a highly soluble L-dopa prodrug, the methyl ester (13), in an easily drop by drop dosable formulation seems more interesting. Different clinical studies had previously demonstrated the good

TABLE 4. *Time spent in off by 10 PD patients before and after Madopar HBS treatment*

	Baseline	6 weeks
"Off" (min)	267	141[a]
Madopar standard (mg/day)	631	240
Madopar HBS (mg/day)		1050

[a] $p < 0.001$ vs. baseline.

TABLE 5. "Off" reduction after oral methyl ester (eight patients)

	Baseline	7 days	14 days	21–30 days
"Off" (min)	206	162	197	162
Drug	L-dopa	Methyl ester	Methyl ester	Methyl ester
Dose	837 mg/day	837 mg/day	837 mg/day	1004 mg/day

antiparkinsonian activity of repeated L-dopa methyl ester intravenous infusions (14,15).

In a preliminary study performed on six PD patients, we found that peak values of L-dopa plasma levels were achieved in a shorter time after single administration of an oral methyl ester solution (200 mg) rather than with an equivalent L-dopa tablet (26.7 vs. 37.5 min); on the contrary, the two different formulations virtually insured the same duration of clinical benefit (145.8 min with methyl ester vs. 150 min after conventional L-dopa) (14).

Finally, we treated eight fluctuating PD patients with methyl ester drops for 30 days. We performed a milligram per milligram replacement of their previous dosage of standard L-dopa (600–1600 mg daily). While the duration of individual "on" periods remained practically unchanged, the latency time to achieve clinical benefit ("on" phase) was significantly shorter after the methyl ester assumption. The most probable explanation for this evidence seems to be the more rapid gastrointestinal absorption of the methyl ester (16). In fact, most patients overcame their postprandial and midafternoon "off" periods, thus consistently increasing their total daily periods of clinical well-being.

A further reduction of the hours spent in the "off" condition by the patients was obtained by using the methyl ester vs. L-dopa replacement schedule on the basis of equimolar ratios (Table 5).

Acknowledgments: We gratefully acknowledge Schering AG, Berlin, F.R.G., for providing intravenous and subcutaneous lisuride and apomorphine, Roche, Milan, for Madopar HBS, and Chiesi Farmaceutici, Parma, for methyl ester oral and intravenous solution.

REFERENCES

1. Shoulson, I., Glaubiger, G. A., and Chase, T. N. (1975): On–off response. Clinical and biochemical correlations during oral and intravenous L-dopa administration in parkinsonian patients. *Neurology*, 25:1144–1148.
2. Fahn, S. (1983): Fluctuations of disability in Parkinson's disease: pathophysiology. In: *Movement Disorders*, edited by C. D. Marsden and S. Fahn, London, Boston, Butterworth, pp. 123–145.
3. Quinn, N. P., Marsden, C. D., and Parkes, J. D. (1983): Complicated response fluctuations in Parkinson's disease: response to intravenous infusion of L-dopa. *Lancet*, 2:412–415.

4. Marion, M. H., Stocchi, F., Quinn, N. P., Jenner, P., and Marsden, C. D. (1986): Repeated L-dopa infusions in fluctuating Parkinson's disease: clinical and pharmacokinetic data. *Clin. Neuropharmacol.*, 9:165–181.

5. Obeso, J. A., Luquin, M. R., and Martinez-Lage, J. M. (1983): Lisuride infusion for Parkinson's disease. *Ann. Neurol.*, 14:134.

6. Obeso, J. A., Luquin, M. R., and Martinez-Lage, J. M. (1986): Lisuride infusion pump: a device for the treatment of motor fluctuations in Parkinson's disease. *Lancet*, 1:467–470.

7. Ruggieri, S., Stocchi, F., and Agnoli, A. (1986): Lisuride infusion pump for Parkinson's disease. *Lancet*, 2:860.

8. Stocchi, F., Ruggieri, S., Brughitta, G., and Agnoli, A. (1986): Problems in daily motor performances in Parkinson's disease: the continuous dopaminergic stimulation. *J. Neural Transm.*, 22(suppl.):223–229.

9. Stibe, C. M. H., Lees, A. J., Kempster, P. A., and Stern, G. M. (1988): Subcutaneous apomorphine in parkinsonian on–off oscillations. *Lancet*, 1:403–406.

10. Marion, M. H., Stocchi, F., Quinn, N. P., Jenner, P., and Marsden, C. D. (1986): Single-dose study of slow release preparation of levodopa and benserazide (Madopar HBS) in Parkinson's disease. In *Advances in Neurology*, Vol. 45, edited by M. D. Yahr and K. J. Bergmann, New York, Raven Press, pp. 493–496.

11. Goetz, C. G., Tanner, C. M., Klawans, H. L., Shannon, K. M., and Carroll, V. S. (1987): Parkinson's disease and motor fluctuations: long-acting carbidopa/levodopa (CR-4-Sinemet). *Neurology*, 37:875–878.

12. Juncos, J. L., Fabbrini, G., Mouradian, M. M., and Chase, T. N. (1987): Controlled release levodopa–carbidopa (CR-5) in the management of parkinsonian motor fluctuations. *Arch. Neurol.*, 44:1010–1012.

13. Cooper, D. R., Marrel, C., Testa, B., et al. (1984): L-dopa methyl ester: a candidate for chronic systemic delivery of L-dopa in Parkinson's disease. *Clin. Neuropharmacol.*, 7:89–98.

14. Agnoli, A., Stocchi, F., Carta, A., Antonini, A., Bragoni, M., and Ruggieri, S. (1988): Continuous dopaminergic stimulation in the management of complicated Parkinson's disease. *Mt. Sinai J. Med.*, 55:62–66.

15. Juncos, J. L., Mouradian, M. M., Fabbrini, G., Serrati, C., and Chase, T. N. (1987): Levodopa methyl ester treatment of Parkinson's disease. *Neurology*, 37:1242–1245.

16. Nutt, J. G., Woodward, W. R., Hammerstad, J. P., Carter, J. H., and Anderson, J. L. (1984): The on–off phenomenon in Parkinson's disease. Relation to L-dopa absorption and transport. *N. Engl. J. Med.*, 310:483–488.

Subject Index

DATE DUE